Diagnostic
and Structured
Interviewing

A Handbook
for Psychologists

Richard Rogers, Ph.D., ABPP

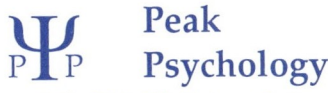

**Peak
Psychology**
*Suite 5G & 5H, Business Centre
North Mill, Bridgefoot, Belper,
Derbyshire DE56 1YD.
Tel: 01773 880222   Fax: 01773 880703*

Diagnostic and Structured Interviewing

A Handbook for Psychologists

Richard Rogers, Ph.D., ABPP

PAR Psychological Assessment Resources, Inc.
P.O. Box 998/Odessa, Florida 33556/Toll-Free 1-800-331-TEST

Library of Congress Cataloging-in-Publication Data

Rogers, Richard, 1950-

    Diagnostic and structured interviewing: a handbook for psychologists / Richard Rogers.

        p.   cm.

    Includes bibliographical references and index.

    ISBN 0-911907-20-3

    1. Interviewing in psychiatry. 2. Mental illness—Diagnosis.

I. Title.

    [DNLM: 1. Interview, Psychological—methods. 2. Mental Disorders—diagnosis. WM 141 R728d 1995]

RC480.7.R64 1995

616.89'075—dc20

DNLM/DLC

for Library of Congress
                                        94-42415
                                          CIP

9 8 7 6 5 4 3 2 1   Reorder #RO-2891   Printed in the United States of America

Acknowledgments

I would like to thank the students from my diagnostic interview course who kindly endured an early draft of this book, offering their critical comments and genuine support. I would like to thank especially Karen Ustad, Vianey Rheinhart, and Randy Salekin for their kindness and commitment to endless library searches and xerox fatigue syndrome. I would also like to acknowledge the unwavering support of family and friends which allowed me to undertake this important challenge.

Contents

Part III: Focused Structured Interviews

Part IV: Summary Chapters

Appendices

Indices

1

The Nature of Diagnostic and Structured Interviewing

Assessment methods in clinical psychology have traditionally rested on unstructured interviews, behavioral assessment, and psychometric measures. Within these three assessment categories exists a panoply of evaluative tools. Evaluation within psychology is largely the product of assessment traditions and philosophies that are defined by training programs and refined by professional settings. Without being iconoclastic, I would argue that diagnostic and structured interviewing deserves its own prominent place in psychological assessment.

I often encounter resistance to structured interviewing, particularly among more experienced clinicians. When voiced, their objections are frequently encapsulated in the question, "What's wrong with traditional interviews?" I believe that this is the wrong question; it promotes the either/or fallacy in which acceptance of structured interviewing is tantamount to a disavowal of unstructured interviews. The question is best reframed as, "Under what circumstances will diagnostic and structured interviewing assist me in meeting my objectives?" To answer the latter question, I will review the essential features of structured interviewing and discuss its advantages and disadvantages.

The essence of structured interviewing is its standardization of the interview process. With unstructured interviews, psychologists typically formulate clinical inquiries that are tailored to the particular patient and record in their own individualistic style the patient's responses and the psychologist's clinical observations. In frank contrast, structured interviewing standardizes (a) the clinical inquiries and subsequent probes, (b) the sequencing of clinical inquiries, and (c) the systematic ratings of patient responses. The resulting uniformity allows for direct comparisons across psychologists, clinical settings, and diagnostic groups. With structured interviewing we can easily ascertain the reliability of our efforts and its generalizability to specific populations and settings. We can also address questions of predictive validity by systematically studying such matters as the course of mental disorders and treatment outcome.

This chapter provides an overview of structured interviewing and its role in the assessment of diagnosis, psychopathology, and other indices of impairment. Both this chapter and the book as a whole emphasize the accurate diagnosis and differential diagnosis of mental disorders. This emphasis is not intended to detract from the importance of psychopathology, indices of impairment, or attention to response styles. Rather, it reflects the current status of structured interviewing in which the preponderance of research is focused on diagnostic methods.

This chapter is composed of four sections. First, I will address the question "Why structured interviewing?" and delineate the advantages and disadvantages of this assessment method. In order to understand how structured interviewing relates to diagnosis, I will then focus our attention on the validity of disorders and how mental health professionals have established what constitutes a disorder. Next, I will provide a conceptual framework for understanding and evaluating important dimensions of structured interviewing. Finally, I will offer a brief rationale for the organization of the remaining chapters.

Advantages and Disadvantages of Structured Interviews

Clinical interviews play a preeminent role in diagnostic evaluations and are instrumental to all psychological assessments. The chief advantages of structured interviewing over traditional methods encompass the following:

1. *Reliability.* The idiosyncratic nature of traditional interviews precludes the possibility of establishing the interrater reliability among psychologists as well as the stability of reported symptoms in the form of test-retest reliability. As previously noted, structured interviewing provides a systematic method for determining reliability.

2. *Level of measurement.* Traditional interviews do not allow psychologists to evaluate clinical characteristics and symptomatology in anything but nominal terms (i.e., presence or absence). In contrast, structured interviewing incorporates systematic ratings that provide for ordinal ratings of psychopathology (see Rogers & Ewing, 1992). In other words, psychologists who employ structured interviewing are often able to make reliable gradations with respect to severity and impairment.

3. *Reduction of information and criterion variance.* In a seminal article, Ward, Beck, Mendelson, Mock, and Erbaugh (1962) described the fundamental reasons for diagnostic disagreement in terms of information and criterion variance (see Table 1.1). When psychologists ask different questions and impose disparate meaning on patient responses, then the accuracy of diagnosis is necessarily constrained. For example, Gauron and Dickinson (1966) found that experienced clinicians are very diversified in how they organize and utilize clinical data. More recently, Blashfield (1992) found that clinicians employing unstructured methods often do not systematically apply diagnostic criteria; the result of this criterion variance was misdiagnoses in approximately 60% of the cases studied. To address these problems with heterogeneity, structured interviewing minimizes the information variance through standardization of clinical inquiries and reduces criterion variance through systematic ratings of clinically relevant information.

Table 1.1
Why Do Clinicians Disagree? A Distillation of Ward et al. (1962)

Source of disagreement	Proportion of cases
Information variance Variations among clinicians in what questions are asked, which observations are made, and how the resulting information is organized	32.5%
Criterion variance Variations among clinicians in applying standards for what is clinically relevant (e.g., when does dysphoric mood qualify as depression?), and when diagnostic criteria are met	62.5%
Patient variance Variations within the same patient that result in substantial differences in clinical presentation and subsequent diagnosis	5.0%

Note. For further discussion, see Murphy, Woodruff, and Herjanic (1974); Rogers (1986) and Ward, Beck, Mendelson, Mock, and Erbaugh (1962). Spitzer, Endicott, and Robins (1975a) elaborated on Ward et al.'s model, perhaps unnecessarily, by subdividing patient variance as "subject variance" (e.g., different disorders at different times) and "occasion variance" (e.g., different stages of the same disorder at different times).

In addition to reducing information variance, the use of structured interviewing also standardizes the sequencing of clinical inquiries. Although empirically untested,[1] the order and progression of questions may influence patients' self-report and further confound information variance. Again, structured interviewing systematizes the sequencing of clinical inquiries and reduces the potential variation due to the discontinuity of questioning.

4. *Comprehensiveness.* Traditional interviews are often focused on presenting problems and concomitant symptomatology (Rogers, 1986, Chapter 9). The process of successive hypothesis generation and testing may miss critical symptoms and/or diagnoses. As observed by Harkness (1992), clinicians tend to stop the diagnostic investigation after the first mental disorder is established. We should not be surprised to find that traditional interviews often miss diagnoses (Wyndowe, 1987), particularly among disorders which occur infrequently (Ford, Hillard, Giesler, Lassen, & Thomas, 1989).

The use of structured interviewing also prevents psychologists from allowing implicit assumptions, such as "the patient is well-functioning," from truncating the assessment process. A disturbing study by Jones, Badger, Ficken, Leeper, and Anderson (1988) suggests that such

---

[1]Findings from Rogers, Bagby, and Dickens (1992) suggest that major modifications in the order of clinical inquiries may affect patient endorsement.

assumptions on the part of health-care professionals may result in under-diagnosis and omission of many mental disorders from classification and treatment.

Several disadvantages may result from overreliance on structured interviewing. These include a routinization of the assessment process and neglect of diagnosis not covered by the structured protocols.

1. *Routinization of the assessment process.* As noted by Ruegg, Ekstrom, Dwight, and Golden (1990) in a study of mental status examinations, clinicians may become "protocol-bound" and miss other important clinical data. In other words, structured interviewing should never be a substitute for establishing rapport, engaging in an unstructured interview, or paying attention to important clinical features which are not otherwise covered. If the assessment process becomes overly routinized, patients may become alienated from the diagnostic procedures. Rosenthal (1989) stressed the importance of rapport-building and the education of patients regarding the value of more structured procedures. Studies suggest, however, that structured interviews appear comparable to their unstructured counterparts for establishing rapport (Saghir, 1971) and do not otherwise impede rapport (Helzer, 1981).

2. *Missed diagnoses.* Even the more comprehensive diagnostic interviews, such as the Schedule of Affective Disorders and Schizophrenia (SADS; Spitzer & Endicott, 1978a) and Structured Clinical Interview for *DSM-III-R* (SCID; Spitzer, Williams, & Gibbon, 1987b), are not exhaustive in their coverage of mental disorders. Some diagnoses are neglected entirely, while others are given only cursory attention. As with all assessment measures, psychologists must know the limitations as well as the strengths of structured interviewing.

The Validity of Mental Disorders

The validity of diagnostic interviewing is inextricably tied to the validity of diagnosis itself. A simple convergence between diagnostic criteria and structured diagnostic interviews is hardly more than a tautological exercise. Indeed, how do we know that mental disorders, which we attempt to assess through structured interviewing, are nothing more than pejorative judgments enshrining social mores and reflecting arbitrary distinctions?

Syndeham Criteria and Diagnostic Validity

Syndeham in 1753 is credited with the definition of disease in operational terms (see Murphy, Woodruff, Herjanic, & Fischer, 1974). He stated that a disorder was composed of three necessary elements: inclusion criteria (What are the core characteristics of a disorder?), exclusion criteria (How does the disorder differ from related disorders?—i.e., differential diagnosis), and outcome criteria (What is the likely course of the disorder?). The first two criteria define the differentiating characteristics of the disorder, while the third predicts a singular, if not unique, outcome. Modern theorists have added little to this definition. Prominent investigators (e.g., Feighner et al., 1972; Murphy, Woodruff, Herjanic, & Fischer, 1974; Robins & Guze, 1970) suggested that the validity of a disorder could be enhanced through external correlates such as laboratory and familial studies. Although etiological models are unpopular with *Diagnostic and Statistical Manual of Mental Disorders* (3rd ed., rev.) (*DSM-III-R;* American Psychiatric Association [APA], 1987) and, more recently, *Diagnostic and Statistical Manual of Mental Disorders* (4th ed.) (*DSM-IV;* APA, 1994), Harkness (1992) and Perry (1990) have underscored their importance in the establishment of mental disorders. Interestingly, both etiology and the course of the disorder serve to furnish a longitudinal dimension to diagnosis (i.e., outcome criteria).

Within the Syndeham framework, I will discuss broadly the facets of inclusion, exclusion, and outcome criteria. The goal of this discussion is to deepen your understanding of the complexity of diagnostic validity as well as the sustained undercurrents that shape our mental disorders.

Inclusion Criteria

Diagnosticians frequently debate the core characteristics that define mental disorders. Historically, schizophrenia has served as the flashpoint for acrimonious debates between the Kraeplin conceptualization of schizophrenia as an irreversible illness resulting in a generalized state of "psychic weakness," and the Bleuler model with its cardinal features: loosening of associations, blunted affect, autism, and ambivalence (see Kendell, 1985). Conflict over the core characteristics of schizophrenia have not abated over time, as observed with the emergence of Schneider's symptoms of first rank (e.g., auditory hallucinations, thought insertion, thought withdrawal, thought broadcasting, bizarre sensations, delusional perceptions, and delusions of control). As further evidence of this conceptual divergence, the transition from the *Diagnostic and Statistical Manual of Mental Disorders* (2nd ed.) (*DSM-II;* APA, 1968) to the *Diagnostic and Statistical Manual of Mental Disorders* (3rd ed.) (*DSM-III;* APA, 1980) decreased the diagnosis of schizophrenia by approximately 50% (Carson, 1991). More recently, attempts have been made to compare diagnostic systems for schizophrenia including the New Haven, RDC, Feighner, Schneiderian, and *DSM-III* criteria (see Kendell, 1985; Stephens, Astrup, & Carpenter, 1982) with concordance rates ranging from 44 to 86 (*M* concordance = 61.7% for these five systems) with modest kappa coefficients (*M* = .27). The diagnostic picture is further clouded when we include cross-cultural dimensions of schizophrenia (Murphy, 1986).

A further example of the pervasive problems in establishing core characteristics of mental disorders is found with antisocial personality disorder (APD; see Rogers & Dion, 1991; Rogers, Dion, & Lynett, 1992). Early formulations (American Psychiatric Association, 1968) emphasized character defects that led to irresponsibility, impaired social relationships, and an incapacity to conform to societal expectations. In marked contrast, *DSM-III* instituted a polythetic model of APD based on overt behavioral disturbances and dyssocial behavior. More recently, *DSM-III-R* has refocused attention on violent delinquent behavior.[2] Nor has the dust settled; *DSM-IV* has introduced further changes in what constitutes

---

[2]Interestingly, this focus on violent childhood behavior may have been stimulated by the need to differentiate inclusion criteria for two other diagnostic categories, conduct disorder and oppositional defiant disorder (see Loeber, Lahey, & Thomas, 1991).

the core characteristics of APD (American Psychiatric Association, 1994; see also Hare, Hart, & Harpur, 1991; Widiger, Frances, Pincus, Davis, & First, 1991). Surprisingly, the major theoretical and empirical work diverges substantially from the *DSM* variations and involves the operationalization of Cleckley's criteria and other formulations (see Hare, 1991).

The first requirement of inclusion criteria should be their reliable measurement. Unfortunately, most validation research has neglected the interrater reliability of the individual inclusion criteria and has been satisfied with aggregate reliability estimates for the disorders themselves. One notable exception is research on personality disorders conducted by Pfohl, Coryell, Zimmerman, and Stangl (1986). Across all personality disorders, they found low kappa coefficients (< .40) for 36 of the inclusion criteria; for five of the inclusion criteria, these coefficients were negligible (< .10). Obviously, similar analyses are needed in the refinement of the *DSM-IV* and have apparently been implemented on a selective basis (Nathan, 1994).

Cloninger, Guze, and Clayton (1985) elaborated on the nature of inclusion criteria in the diagnosis of mental disorders. They argued that the inclusion criteria should represent an intercorrelated group of symptoms which remain constant across time (stability) and within diagnosis (homogeneity). In understanding how diagnoses are rendered, Medin and his colleagues (Medin, Altom, Edelson, & Freko, 1982) studied how subjects made decisions about fictitious diseases; they found that correlated symptoms were given greater weight than uncorrelated symptoms, even when there were more uncorrelated symptoms. Whether advantageous or not, clinicians are likely to place more importance on symptoms that "hang together" or make conceptual sense.

How correlated should inclusion criteria be? Obviously, if high correlations are achieved, then item redundancy is unduly complicating diagnosis. Alternatively, if symptoms are uncorrelated, then it is difficult to argue that they constitute a single entity, such as a syndrome or disorder. To complicate matters, the current emphasis of polythetic diagnosis (e.g., any combination of three inclusion criteria are equivalent to any other three inclusion criteria) asks clinicians to assume the interchangeability of inclusion criteria (see Rogers et al., in press). From this perspective, high correlations and item redundancy would likely appear beneficial. I suggest that we have not come to grips with what constitutes the optimal level of intercorrelations and the ramifications for diagnosis.

Should intercorrelated symptoms that constitute the core characteristics of a particular syndrome/disorder be distinguishable from other syndromes/disorders? Ideally, the inclusion criteria should express a principle or conceptual coherence that explains the interconnections of symptoms (Schwartz & Wiggins, 1986). Not achieving that ideal, the current model of categorical diagnoses is postulated on the bimodality of symptoms with the presence of specific symptoms limited to particular diagnosis. Interestingly, Cloninger et al. (1985) attempted to establish the bimodality of symptoms for schizophrenia. They found a discontinuity of symptoms between schizophrenic and nonschizophrenic patients that was composed of the following: persecutory delusions, delusions of control, firmly fixed mood-incongruent delusions, auditory hallucinations, and the absence of manic spending sprees.[3]

---

[3]Please note that many of the *DSM-III* inclusion criteria either did not achieve this bimodality or were not included in the analysis.

How do we establish the inclusion criteria for a mental disorder? Broughton (1990) has made a compelling argument for the use of prototypical analysis to establish the central features of mental disorders. Based on the work of Rosch (1973, 1978; also see Osherson & Smith, 1981), categories such as diagnoses can be established with the most representative or cardinal features surveyed systematically. Livesley (1985a, 1985b, 1986) has championed this approach to diagnosis and conducted an extensive, if partially flawed,[4] survey of North American psychiatrists (Livesley & Jackson, 1986; Livesley, Reiffer, Sheldon, & West, 1987). A singular advantage of prototypical analysis is its simplicity in establishing prototypic symptoms and examining their underlying factors. With reference to the earlier discussion of APD, Rogers and his colleagues (Rogers et al., in press; Rogers, Duncan, Lynett, & Sewell, in press) found three relatively stable factors that appear central to APD diagnosis. For each factor, specific non-redundant symptoms can be identified to assess core features of APD. Extensive research is needed to test (a) which symptoms/dimensions are core features of a particular disorder, and (b) whether these features are unique to the disorder in question. As an example of inappropriate overlap, Trull, Widiger, and Frances (1987) found unacceptably high correlations between inclusion criteria for avoidant and dependent personality disorders.

Common features of a mental disorder may not reflect core characteristics. As a case in point, "social withdrawal" characterizes many diagnoses, including schizophrenic disorders, schizoid and avoidant personality disorders, depression and dysthymic disorders, social phobias, and agoraphobias. Despite their common occurrence, such symptoms do not represent the core characteristic of a specific disorder and, thus, have limited value as inclusion criteria.

Millon (1991) observed that factor analytic procedures may assist in establishing the central features of a disorder. Studies have yielded mixed findings on this point, since factors often appear to bridge disorders. As an example from Clark and Watson (1991), factor analytic studies of anxiety and depression often yield a nonspecific distress dimension as their first factor, although other dimensions more closely related to the respective disorders can also be found. Further to this point, Livesley and his colleagues (Livesley, 1991; Livesley, Jackson, & Schroeder, 1992) also found general factors underlying personality disorders that appeared to have very limited agreement with specific *DSM-III-R* disorders.

Exclusion Criteria

The foregoing discussion of unique factors and prototypic characteristics leads naturally to a discussion of exclusion criteria. Without exclusion criteria the establishment of a particular disorder as a distinct entity cannot be realized. In other words, diagnosticians must be able to competently classify a disorder by what it is (inclusion criteria) and what it is not (exclusion criteria).

An undue emphasis has been placed on inclusion criteria in *DSM-III-R* and *DSM-IV*. By comparison, relatively little attention has been paid to exclusion criteria. Most exclusion criteria in the *DSM-IV* are based on demographic data, such as age, or the co-occurrence of another mental disorder. For

---

[4]Despite the large sample of North American psychiatrists, the total symptoms/ characteristics used for each diagnosis greatly outnumbered the subjects involved in prototypical ratings.

example, *DSM-III* limited the diagnosis of schizophrenia to patients whose first episode occurred prior to the age of 45. With subsequent research (see Jeste, Harris, & Zweifach, 1988), this exclusion criterion was deemed to be unduly narrow and was deleted from *DSM-III-R* and *DSM-IV*. Age also plays a crucial role in the differentiation of "developmental" from adult disorders, such as conduct disorder from APD and identity from borderline personality disorders. As discussed by Lewis (1986), most personality disorders are seen as having their roots in childhood disturbances, although certain adolescents with developmental disorders do not later warrant the parallel adult diagnoses (e.g., not all oppositional disorders result in *DSM-III-R* passive-aggressive disorders). Whether age forms a natural discontinuity that demarcates one disorder from the other, or, as in the case of conduct disorders, likely reflects social policy considerations, the matter is worthy of our consideration.

The most frequent use of exclusion criteria occurs with so-called *functional disorders* in the presence of known etiology. The implicit assumption of such exclusion criteria is the rather tenuous supposition of unicausality. Whether this assumption is justifiable must be determined on a case-by-case basis. Certainly, a convincing argument can be made that alcoholic hallucinosis is etiologically related to chronic alcohol abuse (Mirin & Weiss, 1983). On the other hand, certain organic delusional disorders are likely to be multidetermined, with "functional" and other predispositional factors playing an important although unexplained role.

DSM-IV has accentuated this diagnostic use of differential etiology by the introduction of *substance-induced* disorders. For example, substance-induced anxiety disorder (APA, 1994, p. 443) must demonstrate either a temporal relationship (i.e., symptoms develop within a month of substance intoxication or withdrawal) or an etiological relationship. With chronic drug users, the first subcriterion appears to be difficult, if not impossible, to apply. The second subcriterion ("known" etiology) appears to beg the question it purports to answer. Further attempts to specify substance-induced anxiety (see Criterion C) also involve temporality (i.e., symptoms precede drug use or continue after acute withdrawal) and likewise pose a daunting task in cases of chronic drug use.

Quasietiological explanations have occasionally been employed to exclude certain diagnoses. For example, the *DSM-III* excluded APD as a disorder when "due to" severe mental retardation, schizophrenia, or manic episodes (APA, 1980, p. 321); the *DSM-III-R* excluded antisocial behavior which occurred "exclusively during the course of schizophrenia or manic episodes" (APA, 1987, p. 346). Do acts of social deviance arise from, or are they caused by, episodes of major mental illness? As observed by Rogers and Dion (1991), the *DSM-III-R* exclusion criteria for APD are likely to be ineffective, since APD symptoms typically emerge in midchildhood, much earlier than the age of modal onset for schizophrenia.

Hierarchic exclusion criteria are uncommon in *DSM-IV* diagnoses. One notable exception occurs within the schizophrenic spectrum. Both schizoid and schizotypal personality disorders are excluded in the presence of schizophrenia. Do such hierarchic exclusions impose artificial constraints on our understanding of these disorders? Alternatively, do they classify patients into meaningful categories on the basis of external correlates, etiological factors, and treatment response? We will address this matter from the vantage point of outcome criteria.

Much more could be accomplished if exclusion criteria were more widely specified at the symptom level. *DSM-III-R* examples of symptom-level exclusions include: (a) prominent hallucinations as an exclusion criterion for delusional disorders, and (b) predominating mood-incongruent delusions and hallucinations as an exclusion criteria for manic and depressive episodes.[5] In the *DSM-IV*, exclusions are sometimes less formalized. For example, mood-incongruent delusions and hallucinations are not exclusion criteria for manic and depressive episodes, but symptoms "clearly due" these psychotic features are not to be considered. In this same vein, Cloninger et al. (1985) found that the absence of manic spending sprees provided one of the highest standardized canonical coefficients for the classification of schizophrenic patients. Introduction of such exclusion criteria would likely improve the homogeneity of mental disorders. In addition, sophisticated exclusion criteria might utilize discriminating variables that do not appear to be related to differential diagnosis. As a case in point, Johnson, Margo, and Stern (1986) found that certain affective symptoms reported on the Beck Depression Inventory appeared to differentiate paranoid and nonparanoid schizophrenia.

Use of symptoms as exclusion criteria would probably decrease the number of diagnoses per patient currently found with our present multiaxial diagnosis. I would argue that the resulting simplification of the multiple diagnoses would be advantageous. For instance, studies (e.g., Blashfield, 1992; Nussbaum & Rogers, 1992; Skodol, Rosnick, Kellman, Oldman, & Hyler, 1988) have typically found that substantial numbers of clinical samples warrant four or more Axis II disorders. Within the domain of personality disorders, Blashfield (1992) found that less than one percent qualified for a single diagnosis. Given the frequency of Axis I and Axis II interactions (Widiger & Hyler, 1987), a welter of multiple diagnoses are likely to occur. From a validity perspective, the establishment of specific outcome criteria is compromised by multiple diagnoses. Simply put, how can we establish the antecedents and the course of the disorder as well as its treatment response, when multiple diagnoses are the norm?

Outcome Criteria

The longitudinal dimension, encapsulated here in the concept of outcome criteria, is the *sine qua non* of diagnosis. If the course of a disorder cannot be accurately charted, then its validity as a useful clinical entity is unavoidably vitiated. Description for description's sake says next to nothing about etiology or pathogenesis. Likewise, treatment efficacy can be understood only from a longitudinal perspective.

I will examine outcome criteria from four related perspectives: chronicity, course of the disorder, etiology, and treatment response. I will illustrate the

---

[5]Unfortunately, these exclusion criteria require a series of complex judgments; clinicians must determine (a) whether they occur in the absence of an affective syndrome, (b) whether they dominate the clinical picture, and (c) whether two of them (i.e., delusions and hallucinations) constitute a "preoccupation."

discussion with examples drawn primarily from schizophrenic disorders and APD.

Chronicity. One somewhat unwieldy measure of outcome criteria is the chronicity of a disorder. In differentiating schizophreniform from schizophrenic disorders, recovery becomes the retrospective discriminator between the two disorders. As described by Tsuang and Loyd (1985), this differentiation is an exercise in circularity with an unfortunate confusion of inclusion and outcome criteria. As noted in *DSM-III-R*, several symptoms (i.e., confusion, acute onset, and emotional turmoil) are associated with schizophreniform disorders (e.g., see Robins & Guze, 1970); perhaps these indices could be pressed into service as inclusion criteria. *DSM-IV* has made some progress in this direction by utilizing these symptoms for subtyping of "good prognostic features."

A similar problem occurred in *DSM-III-R* in distinguishing schizotypal personality disorder from schizophrenia. What separated schizotypal personality disorder from the prodromal phase of schizophrenia? Again, the answer is time, since the inclusion criteria were parallel, with the only distinction being that some patients will enter the active phase of schizophrenia at some later point in their lives. The solution to this problem in *DSM-IV* is less than satisfactory. The parallelism of the prodromal phase of schizophrenia and schizotypal personality disorder is simply obscured by eliminating the specific subcriteria in *DSM-IV* for prodromal symptoms of schizophrenia.

Use of chronicity as an outcome measure is not limited to the schizophrenic spectrum. Within dysthymic and cyclothymic disorders, a 2-year minimum is imposed as an inclusion criteria. Once again, this amalgamation of inclusion and outcome criteria is problematic for diagnosticians. When the onset ocurred within 2 years, psychologists must wait for the outcome criteria to be satisfied before diagnosing the disorder.

Chronicity of a disorder is an important dimension of outcome criteria. With the amassing of diagnostic studies, our diagnostic nomenclature would be immensely enriched with the explicit addition of outcome criteria as a formal component of psychiatric diagnosis. At present, the intrusion of chronicity into the inclusion criteria is likely to obscure rather than elucidate the core characteristics of mental disorders.

Course of the Disorder. Schizophrenic disorders are the best delineated in terms of the course of the disorder, with three well-defined phases: prodromal, active, and residual. Indeed, this longitudinal model for course of schizophrenia could serve as a model for other mental disorders. At present, core characteristics for schizophrenia do not appear to predict the course of the disorder (Endicott, Nie, Cohen, Fleiss, & Simon, 1986). Perhaps the explanation for this lies in four distinctive patterns that have emerged to describe the course of schizophrenia (Kendell, 1985): (a) one episode with full recovery, (b) multiple episodes with full recovery between episodes, (c) multiple episodes with residual impairment between episodes that becomes more pronounced, and (d) continuation of an episode with a chronic and deteriorative pattern. If we were to remain true to the Syndeham criteria, then subtypes of schizophrenia should be based on outcome criteria, such as the course of the disorder. In this instance, symptoms associated with a particularly good outcome (e.g., those mentioned previously for schizophreniform disorders; see Valliant, 1964) and associated with a chronic and deteriorative pattern (e.g., low intelligence and emotional blunting; see Stephens, Astrup, & Mangrum, 1966) would likely enhance our current typology. Moreover, the choice of outcome criteria (e.g., long-term stability) may affect the performance of inclusion/exclusion criteria (see Kendler, 1990).

Defining the course of the disorder is particularly troublesome for personality disorders, since risk factors for most Axis II disorders are general and an invariant trait model has been posited (Panzetta, 1974). One exception is APD, for which it has been assumed that an antecedent condition, namely, a conduct disorder, constitutes an early and necessary phase. Investigators have found that many conduct-disordered youth do not subsequently develop APD (see Robins, 1966; Rogers & Zinbarg, 1987). From the perspective of outcome criteria, the differentiating characteristics between conduct-only and conduct-APD disorders would appear to be a very useful typology. For example, Hamparian (1987) found that age of onset, violence, and chronicity of juvenile offenses were effective predictors of adult criminal behavior. Perhaps additional inclusion criteria could be garnered from the existing literature. Diagnosticians must be careful not to assume facilely a linear relationship between the "severity" of conduct disorders and subsequent aggression among those who qualify as APD (Forth, Hart, & Hare, 1990, partially address this point).

Further outcome criteria could be established to predict which individuals with APD will experience a remission or "burn out" of symptoms by the age of 40 (see Hare, McPherson, & Forth, 1988; Robins, 1966, 1985). If discriminating variables could be established as inclusion criteria, then a useful distinction could be made between active and residual APD in middle-aged patients. Again, the effectiveness of a diagnosis lies in its ability to predict accurately the course of a disorder or some other longitudinal dimension.

Etiology. The origin or "cause" of mental disorders also provides a longitudinal dimension. If the etiology of a particular disorder can be reliably demarcated and this disorder has an identifiable course, then the validity of a disorder appears to be well established (Cloninger et al., 1985). The problem with etiology lies in the multiplicity of factors that appear to play small but significant roles in the pathogenesis of mental disorders. As noted by Coie et al. (1993), risk factors are multifaceted based on (a) their manifestations in multiple dysfunctions, (b) cumulative effects, and (c) salience at different developmental periods. Because of this complexity, etiological explanations are often discussed under simpler but related constructs, such as biological markers and risk factors.

Trait markers provide a measurable variation in structure or performance prior to the first episode, between episodes, or among higher-risk relatives. Schuckit (1985) described useful trait markers as those that (a) are reliably and easily measured, (b) are present in those with the disorder and absent in others, and (c) predict future risk. With reference to schizophrenia, familial, adoption, and twin studies suggest a genetic influence (Schuckit, 1985). More recently, investigators (e.g., Cromwell, 1988; Holzman, Kringlen, & Mathysse, 1988) have suggested that certain cognitive functions, such as attention and information processing, may be genetically linked and serve as trait markers for schizophrenia.

Although a genetic role has been clearly implicated in the pathogenesis of schizophrenia (McBroom, 1980), the current status of this work does not allow for the reliable identification of future schizophrenic patients.

Risk factors reflect the established probabilities that a disorder will occur based on well-defined characteristics. From this perspective, trait markers for which prevalence and lifetime prevalence are available constitute a subset of risk factors. In the instance of schizophrenia (see Murphy & Helzer, 1985), increased risk has been established based on family history of schizophrenia, perinatal factors (e.g., birth complications and seasonality), age (i.e., higher risk between 15 and 45 years), and sex (greater risk for males). With reference to APD, risk factors include sex (6:1 ratio of males to females), urbanization (2.4:1 ratio of urban to rural), and age (see Robins, 1985).

The etiology of certain disorders has been well established in a few instances and implicitly assumed in others. In some instances, compromise of cognitive functioning can be clearly linked to a single etiological factor, such as mental retardation resulting from Down syndrome or dementia secondary to encephalitis (APA, 1987, 1994). In other cases, the etiology is implicit in the diagnosis. For example, post-traumatic stress disorder (PTSD) and brief reactive psychosis both assume that the disorder would not have occurred without the trauma. These diagnoses elude the troubling issue of why certain individuals become symptomatic and others do not.

Treatment Response. To employ treatment response as an outcome criteria, investigators must demonstrate a specific response by subjects with a particular disorder that can be differentiated from other subjects. Otherwise, we cannot hope to establish the uniqueness of the particular disorder on a longitudinal dimension. Since psychosocial treatments tend to be relatively effective (or ineffective) with a wide range of disorders, we must turn our attention to biological treatments. However, attempts to use treatment response to drugs designed to treat specific disorders are also thwarted. Kaplan and Sadock (1988) observed that drugs from a specific class often alleviate symptoms from other disorders (e.g., lithium for impulse disorders), and tend to be effective across disorders. While differentiating response rates are found across diagnoses (e.g., ECT and major depression), research has generally lacked a disorder-specific response to the degree that such findings could be used in the longitudinal validation of a disorder.

Longabaugh and his colleagues (Longabaugh, Fowler, Stout, & Kriebel, 1982; Longabaugh, Stout, Kriebel, McCullough, & Bishop, 1986) have argued for a problem-oriented approach to assessment as offering clear advantages over diagnosis-based treatment outcome. For example, in a study of 695 psychiatric patients, Longabaugh et al. (1986) found that a problem-oriented approach (i.e., a focus of specific symptoms and social behaviors) was (a) equally effective at predicting treatment response to medication and (b) more successful in predicting outcomes of psychosocial interventions (e.g., psychotherapy, vocational interventions and behavioral programs) than diagnosis alone. Although integration of problem-oriented assessment with diagnosis yields superior predictions, the presence of a competing model in the problem-oriented approach raises questions about the validation of certain diagnoses vis-a-vis outcome criteria. In other words, if specific problems (e.g., homelessness or delusions irrespective of diagnosis) predict treatment outcome better than any formal diagnosis, then it is difficult to argue for a singular if not unique course to a particular disorder, at least in terms of treatment response.

Commentary on Syndeham Criteria

Where does the foregoing discussion leave us? My sincerest hope is that psychologists will neither categorically discard or indiscriminately embrace our current diagnostic nosology. Rather, diagnostic validity must be considered with reference to specific disorders and subsequent interventions. The importance of this discussion to diagnostic and structured interviewing is that the validity of diagnostic methods is necessarily limited by the diagnoses themselves. Put simply, if the diagnosis is suspect (e.g., factitious disorders with psychological symptoms; see Rogers, Bagby, & Rector, 1989), then the diagnostic method, no matter how psychometrically sound, is also suspect.

We will examine in subsequent chapters the usefulness of diagnostic interviews in accurately classifying mental disorders. In each case, psychologists are compelled to question the diagnostic validity and its clinical relevance to the assessment issues. For example, the APD section of the SADS has good reliability, but what is its relationship to the *DSM-IV* diagnosis of APD? Furthermore, is the use of APD justified in psycholegal issues (see Rogers & Lynett, 1991), such as indeterminate sentencing?

DSM-III-R and *DSM-IV* Diagnostic Models

The integral elements of the *DSM-III-R* and, more recently, the *DSM-IV* nosology are their combined emphasis on a polythetic, categorical, and atheoretical diagnostic system. In addition, both *DSM-III-R* and *DSM-IV* posit a multiaxial system that attempts to integrate Axis I and Axis II disorders with medical conditions (Axis III) and quantifiable ratings of psychosocial stressors and global impairment (Axes IV and V). Although elegant discussions of these elements are available (see Barlow, 1991), I will distill and discuss briefly the most salient features of the *DSM-III-R* and the *DSM-IV*.

Polythetic Diagnosis

Diagnosis based on polythetic models rests on the intrinsic assumptions that inclusion criteria should be accorded equal weight and that any combination of symptoms that exceeds a predetermined cutoff is sufficient to warrant the mental disorder in question. With reference to major depression, repeated suicidal attempts and life-threatening weight loss are diagnostically equivalent to chronic fatigue and indecisiveness.[6]

An untoward effect of the polythetic model is a conceptual blurring of what constitutes the prototypic features of a mental disorder. In this respect, a myriad of diagnostic combinations occur with no notion of what constitutes a classic or prototypical example. As observed by Rogers and Dion (1991), these diagnostic variations can be truly number-numbing, with 29 trillion possibilities for APD.

---

[6]After the diagnosis is generated, these symptoms will have a differential effect on estimates of severity.

Lest psychologists view APD as simply a solitary outlier, other disorders such as schizophrenia also yield unwieldy numbers. When considered across prodromal, active and residual phases, the diagnostic variations of schizophrenia exceed nine million for the *DSM-III-R* and are gargantuan but unknowable for the *DSM-IV*.

I would argue that diagnostic simplification is essential to diagnostic validity. For example, if the prodromal and residual criteria of schizophrenia could be reduced by eliminating redundant and nondiscriminating symptoms with an increased stringency in the minimum criteria, then these endless variations could be curtailed. For instance, greater diagnostic homogeneity could be achieved if prodromal/residual symptoms could be reduced to six and the cutting score raised to three. Alternatively, subtyping (negative vs. positive symptoms) might be conceptually justifiable and achieve the same end.[7] However, the *DSM-IV* alternative of not specifying prodromal/residual symptoms is not a solution and may ironically lead to even more diagnostic variations.

Categorical Diagnosis

Diagnosis within the *DSM* paradigm is categorical and is based on nominal measurements (presence or absence) of inclusion and exclusion criteria. The chief advantage of categorical diagnosis is that clinical attention is paid to the patient's most salient characteristics, which allows for the rapid assessment of many diverse patients (Millon, 1991). Interestingly, the *DSM-III-R* disavows the very basis of a categorical model (APA, 1987): "There is no assumption that each mental disorder is a discrete entity with sharp boundaries (discontinuity) between it and other mental disorders, or between it and no mental disorder" (p. xxii). This view is echoed in the *DSM-IV* (p. xxii). Indeed, the very basis of the categorical model is discrete categories formed by differentiating criteria.

The chief alternative to the categorical model is dimensional diagnoses in which severity ratings (most likely ordinal measurements) are theoretically or empirically derived to compose diagnoses. An obvious advantage of dimensional diagnosis is that discontinuity is not a necessary precondition to diagnostic validation. Moreover, the *DSM-III-R* and *DSM-IV* models are not purely categorical, but also include dimensional components in several forms: (a) direct quantification as in the case of mental retardation, (b) explicit subtyping of certain disorders on the basis of severity, and (c) presentation of distinct severity ratings for Axes IV and V.

Frances (1982, 1985) provided a useful introduction to dimensional diagnosis. From his perspective, dimensional diagnosis provides more accurate descriptions of psychopathology and minimizes the pressure to force an atypical patient into one or another diagnosis. He worries, however, that the very complexity of dimensional diagnosis may be its undoing. Could clinicians make meaningful decisions when faced with an array of dimensional ratings? As noted by Millon (1991), additional advantages of the dimensional approach include the capturing of more precise information and the representation of psychopathology as continua from normality to abnormality. I believe that a further

---

[7]Four symptoms could be construed as "negative": social isolation, decreased vocational efforts, blunted affect, and decreased initiative.

advantage of dimensional models is that they are amenable for the testing of diverse models of psychopathology. Interesting developments, for example, have been made in defining diagnostic-specific interpersonal styles (Pincus & Wiggins, 1990; Widiger & Frances, 1985) and circumplex models of enduring traits associated with particular disorders (Kiesler, 1983, 1986). Such multidimensional perspectives of diagnosis are likely to enrich both our descriptive as well as explanatory models of mental illness.

Psychologists are often more comfortable with the dimensional model of diagnosis, because it serves as the structural basis for most psychometric measures. Blashfield and Livesley (1991) have described the political aspects of the categorical-dimensional debate, with psychiatry allied more closely with categorical models and psychology with dimensional models. While acknowledging these tensions, I believe that the answer lies not in interprofessional rivalry, but rather in the empirical testing of competing models. At present, I cannot endorse the dimensional model, since it has not been systematically tested with respect to outcome criteria and has not been shown to be superior to simpler categorical diagnoses. Like Frances, I am concerned that the diagnostic permutations of this admittedly more sophisticated approach may thwart even the most valiant efforts at diagnostic validity. Moreover, as noted by Skinner and Blashfield (1982), many of the multivariate approaches to diagnosis have neglected external validation studies to demonstrate the clinical usefulness of dimensional models.

Atheoretical Diagnosis

The *DSM-III*, *DSM-III-R*, and *DSM-IV* have attempted to circumvent strongly held and potentially divisive theoretical underpinnings (as exemplified by psychoanalytic and biological schools) by promoting a common language and sidestepping theoretical considerations. As discussed by Faust and Miner (1986), the theoretical debates are more submerged than subsided, and continue to inform diagnosis. Whether the *DSM-III-R* or the *DSM-IV* has actually achieved its atheoretical stance appears to be a matter influenced by professional affiliation. Maser, Kaelber, and Weise (1991) found nearly all psychiatrists (91%) thought that the *DSM-III-R* had done at least a fair job of achieving its atheoretical goal, as compared to 72% of psychologists.

Morey (1991a) has made cogent arguments for the retention of theory in our current nosology. According to Morey, theory provides the underlying principles that, if empirically tested, may inform diagnosis as well as an understanding of common properties underlying different but related disorders (also see Murphy & Medlin, 1985). Morey cautioned against equating theory with etiology and suggested that theory may play other important roles, such as specifying determinants of treatment responsiveness. As noted by Carson (1991), the current atheoretical stance is likely a backlash against "the almost regal and at times arrogant dominion enjoyed by psychoanalysis in the approximately three decades after World War II" (p. 306).

To ignore theory is to be ignorant of it. The placement of each disorder in the *DSM-III-R* and the *DSM-IV* implies a conceptual framework with implicit etiological factors. Recent debates over the determinants of factitious disorders with psychological symptoms (FDPS; see Cunnien, 1988; Rogers, Bagby, & Rector, 1989) centered on the production of Ganser-like symptoms. In the end, Ganser syndrome was moved from its FDPS placement in *DSM-III* to dissociative disorders in the *DSM-III-R* and the *DSM-IV*. Likewise, the theoretically defensible home for posttraumatic stress disorder (PTSD) is open to question with nosological candidates of anxiety, depressive, and dissociative disorders (Davidson & Foa, 1991).

In our subsequent review of diagnostic and structured interviews, we will address, where feasible, the theoretical underpinnings and implications as they relate to professional practice. Our conceptual framework dictates both the nature and parameters of structured interviewing and cannot, therefore, be ignored.

Multiaxial Diagnosis

DSM-IV classifies all mental disorders on Axes I and II. Axis II disorders are distinguished from Axis I largely on the basis of early onset and a stable but chronic course of the disorder. Within this framework, developmental and personality disorders are deemed to be Axis II and all other clinical syndromes, Axis I. From an empiricist perspective, this framework demands validation. If we accept, for the sake of argument, that onset and course are the preeminent features of mental disorders, then large clinical samples could be sorted by the three principal variables (age of onset, chronicity, and stability of the syndrome) through cluster-analytic techniques (for an overview of cluster analysis and classification, see Sokal, 1974). I seriously doubt whether the resulting Axes I and II disorders would approximate our current categorization.

An important consideration is whether the four most relevant Axes (I, II, IV, and V)[8] constitute discrete dimensions of diagnosis. Would nonoverlapping criteria from each Axis form orthogonal dimensions when large clinical samples are subjected to factor analyses rotated to varimax solutions? Do these dimensions predict outcome criteria? We might also speculate regarding the interrelationships among these Axes. For example, I would hypothesize that episodes of Axis I disorders, congruent with the prevailing stress-diathesis model, are likely to be more closely related to Axis IV's psychosocial stressors than are long-standing Axis II disorders. Moreover, it would be interesting to predict overall impairment by regressing severity ratings on Axes I, II, and IV against Axis V. Implementing a longitudinal perspective would be most useful in demarcating the relative contributions of these axial ratings to Axis V impairment during subsequent episodes.

Axis IV attempts to define psychosocial stressors on four dimensions: (a) relationship to mental disorders, (b) severity of the stressor, (c) duration, and (d) type of stressor. The resulting definition of psychosocial stressors is a curious admixture of idiographic and nomothetic elements. Stressors are identified that may have played a contributory role in the development of a mental disorder, recurrence of a prior mental disorder, or exacerbation of an existing disorder. Judgments of this kind are clearly idiographic, since similar stressors may precipitate a mental disorder in one person and have no observable effect in another. In

---

[8]The precise role of Axis III in the diagnosis of mental disorders, while obviously relevant, remains to be explicated. Indeed, *DSM-III-R* devoted one short, solitary paragraph to the description of Axis III.

contrast, judgments regarding the severity of a stressor are largely nomothetic; prototypic examples suggest that the death of a spouse is "extreme" and the death of a child is "catastrophic." Such differences are apparently based on group comparisons and do not take into account an individual's particular response to the stressor. In the *DSM-IV*, emphasis is diverted from the severity of the stressors to a description of their source (occupational, educational, housing, etc.). While side-stepping the arbitrariness of the *DSM-III-R*, the *DSM-IV* does not allow for severity ratings.

The time dimension of Axis IV in the *DSM-III-R* is also intriguing, with its attempt to dichotomize stressors into acute (less than 6 months) and enduring (greater than 6 months). The role of adaptation in the face of prolonged stressors and its direct relationship to increased impairment is simply too complex to make meaningful distinctions based on duration. Paradoxically, psychosocial stressors may be rated in their absence. According to the *DSM-III-R*, the anticipation of a stressor (e.g., retirement) may be rated as a stressor. An alternative view is that cognitions and concomitant emotions are not exogenous, even when they anticipate actual environmental changes, and should not be treated as such. The *DSM-IV* entirely skirts the issue of chronicity.

Axis V is designed to measure global impairment, irrespective of the particular diagnosis or its clinical presentation. *DSM-IV* has presented Global Assessment Functioning to assess overall dysfunction; this global rating scale has been borrowed, almost verbatim, from the Global Assessment Scale (GAS; Endicott, Spitzer, Fleiss, & Cohen, 1976). Although intended as a nonspecific measure of impairment, certain themes are apparent, with psychosis and violence (self- and other-directed) representing key criteria for those with severe impairment. In addition, Appendix B of the *DSM-IV* includes provisional global ratings for the assessment of relationships and social-occupational functioning.

The notion of impairment, which is implicit to nearly all diagnoses, may be conceptualized from multiple perspectives. As previously noted, Axis V has taken a symptomatic viewpoint in which certain symptoms are perceived as critical. This approach appears to obscure important facets of symptomatology, such as severity and frequency of symptoms. Obviously, a dimensional approach to Axis V would allow diagnosticians to capture more information about impairment. An apparent disparity in the assessment of impairment occurs with Axis II disorders. According to the *DSM-IV*, personality disorders can be diagnosed in the absence of impairment, if the patient reports subjective distress. In other words, a patient could be completely well-functioning in all areas of his/her life but be unhappy about certain symptoms or characteristics and, therefore, be defined as mentally ill.

What constitutes impairment resulting from a mental disorder? I believe that impairment extends well beyond the *DSM-IV* model. Table 1.2 provides a distillation of the multiple perspectives associated with impairment.

An Overview of Structured Interviews

Structured interviewing attempts to maximize the reliability and validity of its measurements by systematizing the assessment process. A major emphasis is the reduction of diagnostic disagreement by exerting control over information

Table 1.2
Multiple Perspectives on the Definition of Impairment

Retrospective view
    Deterioration: The patient has evidenced an observable decline since the
    onset of the disorder.

Prospective view
    Expectations: The patient or the patient's family anticipated that he/she
    would be better adjusted or have greater accomplishments.

    Potential: Earlier observations (e.g., intelligence or achievement testing in
    early grades) suggest that the patient has not optimized his/her
    abilities.

Normative view
    Deficit: On standard comparisons, the patient falls short of the average or
    some other accepted standard.

Individualistic view
    Distress: The patient experiences negative affect regarding his/her current
    abilities and adjustment.

and criterion variance. As reviewed in Table 1.1, lack of standardization in
clinical inquiries (information variance) and the idiosyncratic transformation of
patient responses into clinical criteria (criterion variance) are enduring problems
addressed by structured interviewing.

Organization and Format of Structured Interviews

Nearly all structured interviews are confronted with the "breadth-versus-
depth" dilemma, otherwise known as the "bandwidth-fidelity" issue (Widiger &
Frances, 1987). For example, the SADS provides in-depth coverage of schizophrenic and mood disorders, often devoting several questions to each rating.
Even more focused are the single-disorder structured interviews, such as the
Psychopathy Checklist (PCL), which provide comprehensive coverage, but with
a very narrow focus. In stark contrast, the SCID covers nearly all diagnoses but
generally limits its inquiry to the minimum number of one question per inclusion
criteria. In choosing among structured interviews, psychologists will need to
weigh competing demands for depth and breadth in the selection of the most
appropriate measure.

Structured interviews share many common features, several of which have
been implemented to facilitate the ease of interpretation and the rendering of
diagnoses. As summarized in Table 1.3, most structured interviews, with the
exception of those which are highly focused, tend to organize their measure by
syndrome/disorders (i.e., symptom clustering) and to have unidirectional
scoring. By topical organization, clinicians can readily observe whether a diagnosis is likely to be warranted and make an informed decision on how thoroughly to investigate a particular disorder. By the same token, unidirectional
scoring (i.e., endorsement is nearly always a sign of psychopathology) expedites
the scoring and diagnostic decision-making. These attempts to simplify the diagnostic process, as summarized below, have important implications for clinical
presentation and response styles.

Table 1.3
Components of Structured Interviewing

Component	Representative measure				
	SADS	SCID	DIS	PCL	SIRS
Symptom clustering	yes	yes	yes	no	no
Unidirectional items	yes	yes	yes	no	no
Inclusion of neutral questions	yes	no	no	yes	yes
Symptoms constitute criteria	no	yes	yes	no	no
Cross-checking of symptoms	indirect[a]	no	no	indirect[a]	yes

Note. SADS = Schedule of Affective Disorders and Schizophrenia (Spitzer & Endicott, 1978a); SCID = Structured Clinical Interview for *DSM-III-R* Diagnosis (Spitzer, Williams, Gibbon, & First, 1990b); DIS = Diagnostic Interview Schedule (Robins, Helzer, Cottler, & Goldring, 1989); PCL = Psychopathy Checklist (Hare, 1991); SIRS = Structured Interview of Reported Symptoms (Rogers, Bagby, & Dickins, 1992).
[a]Indirect cross-checking of symptoms involves a review of symptom consistency across prior episodes for the SADS and explicit rules for use of collateral sources with the PCL.

Structured interviews vary in how extensively they evaluate reported symptoms and presenting problems. Most measures have at least two types of questions: "standard questions" and "optional probes." As summarized in Table 1.4, standard questions are routinely asked of every patient, while optional probes are used to clarify ambiguities. In both cases, the questions are asked verbatim. More extensive diagnostic interviews often employ "branching questions," a variant of standard questions that enables the clinician to screen for specific mental disorders without comprehensively reviewing symptomatology.

An important distinction is created between structured and semistructured interviews. In structured interviewing, only verbatim inquiries are permitted. In semistructured interviewing, clinicians are allowed to fashion their own "unstructured questions" to supplement, but not replace, the standard questions and optional probes. While the introduction of unstructured questions unavoidably reduces the standardization, their use is sometimes justified by the recognition that no set of prespecified questions can anticipate the heterogeneity of responses.

Structured interviewing also varies with respect to its diagnostic focus. Broad-scoped inventories typically provide diagnostic information regarding Axis I disorders, but vary in the extent to which they evaluate patients' prior histories. As summarized in Table 1.5, the SADS alone attempts to organize data from prior episodes. In contrast, the Diagnostic Interview Schedule (DIS; Robins, Helzer, Cottler, & Goldring, 1989) and the SCID examine only the lifetime prevalence of mental disorders. The SADS is also distinguished from its alternatives by its emphasis on the severity of symptoms and additional symptoms associated with specific disorders. However, The DIS and SCID also have respective strengths. For example, the DIS has a strong cross-cultural emphasis while the SCID, in conjunction with the SCID-II, allows for a combined evaluation of Axis I and II disorders. Thus, even among similar measures, important differences emerge.

Table 1.4
Types of Clinical Inquiries Used in Structured Interviews

Type of inquiry	Definition	Sources
Standard questions	Key questions asked of all respondents	all
Branching questions	Key questions that are asked of respondents who meet an established threshold	SADS, SCID
Optional probes	Clarifying questions that are asked if ambiguity occurs in how responses meet criteria	SADS, SIRS, PCL
Unstructured questions	Nonstandardized questions that are formulated by the psychologist to assist in the rating of responses	SADS, PCL

Note. Under sources, examples of representative structured interviews are listed. SADS = Schedule of Affective Disorders and Schizophrenia (Spitzer & Endicott, 1978a); SCID = Structured Clinical Interview for *DSM-III-R* Diagnosis (Spitzer, Williams, Gibbon, & First, 1990b); SIRS = Structured Interview of Reported Symptoms (Rogers, Bagby, & Dickens, 1992); PCL = Psychopathy Checklist (Hare, 1991).

Table 1.5
Clinical Features of Diagnostic Interviews

Clinical feature	Representative measure		
	SADS	DIS	SCID
Current diagnosis	yes	yes	yes
Prior episodes	yes	no	no
Lifetime prevalence[a]	yes	yes	yes
Severity of symptoms	yes	no	no
Associated symptoms	yes	no	no
Axis II disorders	no	no	yes
Cross-cultural research	no	yes	no

Note. SADS = Schedule of Affective Disorders and Schizophrenia (Spitzer & Endicott, 1978a); SCID = Structured Clinical Interview for *DSM-III-R* Diagnosis (Spitzer, Williams, Gibbon, & First, 1990a); DIS = Diagnostic Interview Schedule (Robins, Helzer, Cottler, & Goldring, 1989).
[a]Lifetime prevalence refers to clinical data about whether the respondent ever had the disorder, without attempting to identify any specific episode.

Information and Criterion Variance in Structured Interviews

Discrepancies in Clinical Data

Psychologists are often confronted with seemingly inconsistent and discrepant clinical data. With traditional interviews, the problem lies in how to interpret these inconsistencies and discrepancies. Do they represent imprecision in the form and types of questions asked? Do they represent inaccuracies in the recording of responses? Do they represent deliberate attempts to distort the clinical presentation? Do they represent a fluctuating clinical state?

Standardized clinical inquiries can substantially reduce information variance: (a) within one clinician's evaluation of a particular patient, (b) across several clinicians' evaluations of the same patient, and (c) across many clinicians' evaluations of different patients. As an overview to structured interviewing, we must examine the nature of these standardized clinical inquiries.

Clinical Presentation and Response Styles

A long-standing concern of psychologists is that the clinical inquiries elicit accurate and complete information. We are concerned about patients who deliberately distort their presentations (see Rogers, 1988), either by fabricating symptomatology (malingering and factitious disorders) or denying the existence of psychological problems (defensiveness). Moreover, many patients either overemphasize or underplay their symptoms and the consequences (impairment and distress) arising from these symptoms. Early literature (e.g., Liberty, Lunneborg, & Atkinson, 1964) suggested that patients could be divided into two groups on the basis of their willingness to acknowledge psychological problems to themselves and others: repressors (high threshold) and sensitizers (low threshold). In such cases, the notion of deliberateness becomes obtenerated.

Other response styles may affect the accuracy and completeness of patients' self reports. Much research interest has been generated in the examination of social desirability and acquiescence (e.g., Couch & Keniston, 1960; Wiggins, 1962) which suggests that patients are less likely to be forthright when seeking social acceptance or approval. Interestingly, when subjects are asked to be honest, they may show less willingness to disclose their symptoms and psychological problems (Goldberg & Miller, 1966). Finally, some patients may foil the assessment process by assuming a role (e.g., a marginally-employed male patient may try to present himself as a successful businessman) which may distort the clinical presentation in subtle but important ways (see Kroger & Turnbull, 1975).

Minimizing the Effects of Response Styles

An important issue arises regarding the face validity of clinical inquiries and their order of presentation in the structured interview. Questions with high face validity have an increased liability for distortion because patients can recognize the intent of questions and, consequently, manipulate their responses. Ideally, standardized clinical inquiries should not be susceptible to social desirability. If inquiries promote a response bias, then their standardization may unwittingly promote systematic disinformation.

Most diagnostic interviews are designed to be unidirectional. As previously noted, endorsement of nearly every question signifies psychopathology. The problem with this approach is that patients can easily fall into response set (e.g., denial of most psychological problems). Counterbalancing questions so that both negative and positive answers are indicative of psychopathology is one logical method of addressing response sets, such as those found with acquiescence and social desirability.

Clinical inquiries can be written so as to minimize the potential for distortions. For example, *neutral questions* (e.g., "How have you been feeling? . . . Describe your mood.") are vastly superior to leading queries (e.g., "Are you depressed?"). In addition, *counter-poised questions* may be constructed which ask for the same information from very different perspectives. For example, queries about the presence of auditory hallucinations might be framed as "Do you have a heightened sense of hearing?" and "Do you hear voices that other people don't seem to hear?" In reviewing diagnostic and structured interviewing, attention must be paid to the sophistication of the questions themselves and whether a concerted effort is made to introduce neutral and counter-poised questions.

The organization of questions may also play an important role in the accuracy of patients' self reports. In particular, many diagnostic interviews are arranged by symptom clustering. In these cases, symptoms associated with a specific disorder are presented together. This format has been described by Nussbaum and Rogers (1992) as "clinician-friendly." As previously described, the clustering of symptoms allows for an easy interpretation of clinical data and formulation of a diagnosis. The liability of this approach is that patients can manipulate their presentations with relative ease.

Table 1.3 provides a summary of the previously described features of structured interviewing that help to address common response styles. In addition, some structured interviews include measures of symptom consistency (e.g., Structured Interview of Reported Symptoms [SIRS; Rogers, Bagby, & Dickens, 1992]) or multiple sources for the same symptoms (Psychopathy Checklist–Revised [PCL; Hare, 1991]). An important factor in the selection of structured interviews is the sophistication of the clinical inquiries and their organization.

Use of corroborative data to augment the patient's self-reporting is a common feature of many structured interviews. Unfortunately, no systematic rules exist on how to integrate collateral and interview data. Available methods may be either standardized or nonstandardized. For example, the SADS may be administered to a spouse by asking for his/her perspective of the patient (see Rogers & Cunnien, 1986); standard questions are asked and direct comparisons are made with the patient's self-report. In contrast, other measures, such as the PCL, ask that record material be routinely reviewed but do not provide any systematic method for doing so.

How are discrepancies between self-reporting and corroborative sources resolved? I believe that some psychologists give greater weight to reports from clinical staff than from the patients themselves. The danger of this practice is the perpetuation of misinformation. Indeed, if the psychologist routinely accepts the professional version, we might ask what purpose is served by the psychologist reevaluating the patient. Similarly, informants (e.g., family members) are sometimes viewed as more credible, particularly when the patient is an adolescent or is involved in legal proceedings. The implicit and sometimes inaccurate assumption is that family members can be objective and do not have "their own ax to grind."

Psychologists must make decisions about discrepant material on a case-by-case basis. They are confronted with three basic alternatives. First, the psychologist may judge one version to be so lacking in plausibility that it is readily discarded. Second, the psychologist may seek further information and clarification from some combination of sources including the patient, the informant, and others who know the patient. Third, the psychologist may interpolate between the two versions and assume some intermediary position (e.g., when both patient and informant describe a loss of appetite and decreased eating, but report different levels of food intake). In the absence of guidelines from structured interviewing, psychologists must (a) be explicit about how they resolve discrepancies, and (b) be able to justify their clinical conclusions to colleagues.

Reducing the Criterion Variance

Structured interviews typically include standardized ratings for reducing criterion variance. For instance, the SADS offers ratings that include descriptors and prototypic examples. Sometimes the descriptors are simply a gradation of severity (e.g., "mild," "moderate," "severe," or "extreme"); at other times, they offer either a brief characterization (e.g., "frequent obsessions or compulsions with some impairment in social or occupational functioning or daily routine") or some form of quantification (e.g., concerning weight loss, "5–10 lb," "10–15 lb," "15–25 lb," or "over 25 lb"). Problems occur both with inferential ratings based on severity as well as more descriptive ratings. With the former, reliability may be constrained by complicated judgments of severity. In the latter, psychologists are asked to make overly precise and sometimes arbitrary judgments (e.g., Given daily fluctuations in weight and nonsystematic sampling, how do we know for sure whether the patient lost 12 or 15 lb? Moreover, the same weight loss has a very different meaning for an anorexic vs. an obese patient). My point is that the standardized ratings of structured interviews are constructed on a continuum from highly inferential to very specific, each of which has its limitations. Irrespective of the form, standardized ratings are likely to improve reliability and assist in clinical judgments (Dawes, 1979). In addition, the use of prototypic examples is likely to improve the assessment process (Blashfield, 1992).

Structured interviews also vary in the simplicity of diagnostic decision making. The SCID was designed as an adjunct to the *DSM-III-R* with a one-to-one translation of its ratings to diagnosis. In contrast, the SADS was developed in relationship to the Research Diagnostic Criteria (RDC; Spitzer, Endicott, & Robins, 1978; Zwick, 1983). Given the close relationship between RDC and the *DSM-III-R*, the process of rendering a diagnosis is relatively straightforward, *if* the psychologist collects supplementary information. Similarly, the Comprehensive Assessment of Symptoms and History (CASH; Andreasen, Flaun, & Arndt, 1992) requires further interviewing to establish *DSM-IV* diagnoses. In this respect, the SCID has a singular advantage in reducing criterion variance by paralleling *DSM* criteria.

Psychometric Characteristics of Structured Interviewing

Preceding sections have provided a good introduction to diagnostic and structured interviewing that includes (a) their advantages over traditional interviews, (b) their general organization and format, and (c) their standardization of clinical inquiries and ratings. In this section, we will elaborate on several facets of structured interviewing that encompass their reliability and validity. The purpose of this section is to provide a very brief introduction to the terms used in subsequent chapters.

Reliability

Almost without exception, each structured interview provides estimates of its consistency. The most common estimates include the following:

Interrater Reliability. Interrater reliability forms the most fundamental reliability measure for structured interviews. If independent clinicians cannot achieve comparable results in applying a standardized interview to the same patients, then the whole assessment is in jeopardy. How is interrater reliability established? Most commonly, two or more clinicians observe the same interview, live or through videotapes, and make independent ratings of the patient. With some measures (e.g., the PCL), case materials are distilled and made available to these clinicians; this procedure may inflate the level of agreement, since such documentation is not typically available in clinical practice.

Satisfactory estimates of interrater reliability may be more difficult to achieve for categorical decisions regarding diagnosis than for dimensional ratings of psychopathology (Heumann & Morey, 1990). One potential limitation for establishing diagnostic reliability is the choice of statistics available for measuring nominal agreement. Kappa coefficients (Cohen, 1960) are the most commonly used; this statistic measures the proportion of agreement corrected for observed base rates. The correction may lead to highly variable kappas; for example, Grove, Andreasen, McDonald-Scott, Keller, and Shapiro (1981) demonstrated that a drop in base rates from 50% to 1%, when both sensitivity and specificity are very high (i.e., 95%), resulted in a dramatic decrease in kappa from .81 to .14. Spitznagel and Helzer (1985) recommended the use of Yule's Y for cases, such as psychiatric diagnosis, where the base rates are generally low.[9] Although not entirely independent of base rate, Yule's Y has greater stability over kappa with low to medium base rates. As a counterargument, Shrout, Spitzer, and Fleiss (1987) point out that Yule's Y is a nonlinear function which constrains its interpretability. Given the limits of both statistics, we do not appear to have an adequate measure of reliability for rare disorders.[10]

Intraclass coefficients are also commonly used as a measure of diagnostic reliability (see Andreasen et al., 1981; Keller, Lavori, et al., 1981); these coefficients are calculated on the basis of total variance in clinical ratings that is attributable to differences among clinicians. According to Fleiss and Cohen (1973), intraclass coefficients are equivalent to weighted kappas when used with substantial samples.

---

[9]According to Spitznagel and Helzer (1985), Yule's Y becomes an unstable statistic when the base rate exceeds 50%.

[10]A third rarely employed alternative is the Random Error Coefficient of Agreement (RE; Maxwell, 1977).

Test-Retest Reliability. Test-retest reliability involves the readministration of structured interviews after a specified interval by different clinicians. This form of reliability is far less common than interrater reliability in the validation of structured interviews (Endicott & Spitzer, 1978), but has a singular advantage of estimating the consistency across styles of questioning (i.e., information variance) as well as ratings (i.e., criterion variance). Robins (1985) reviewed test-retest reliability studies with the DIS and criticized the use of test-retest reliabilities, since some subjects may attempt to be overly consistent while others may seek to offer novel information. Since most clinical samples, especially inpatients, are repeatedly questioned about their symptomatology, I would argue similar influences may occur independent of the assessment method. Probably the strongest evidence of reliability is consistently high reliability estimates across interrater and test-retest designs.

A related issue for some diagnoses is "temporal stability." For example, personality disorders posit a chronic unremitting course. In such cases, the temporal stability of the diagnosis bridges test-retest reliability (i.e., consistency of measurement) and predictive validity (i.e., the hypothesized chronicity of the disorder).

Internal Reliability. Estimates of internal consistency are most often represented as alpha coefficients which estimates the homogeneity of items on a scale (Golden, Sawicki, & Franzen, 1984). Whether high alpha coefficients are desirable depends on the purpose of the structured interview and concomitant scales. With the SADS, the summary scales are intended to measure important dimensions of psychopathology. In this case, moderately high alpha coefficients are advantageous.[11] In contrast, briefer measures (e.g., Schedule of Affective Disorders and Schizophrenia–Change Version [SADS-C; Spitzer & Endicott, 1978b]) are intended to sample different dimensions of psychopathology and have low to moderate alpha coefficients. Given the paramount concerns with information and criterion variance, I do not believe that internal reliability, by itself, is a sufficient measure of consistency for structured interviews.

Validity

Basic forms of validity are composed of content-related, construct-related, and criterion-related validity (Anastasi, 1988). My intent is not to review the vast literature on test validation, but to provide a succinct overview of how structured interviewing has attempted to address this issue with particular reference to diagnostic validity.

Diagnostic validity within the Syndeham framework is based on inclusion and exclusion criteria, with the true test of diagnostic legitimacy being the longitudinal dimension of diagnosis, namely, the outcome criteria. Within this framework, many structured interviews attempt to establish criterion-related validity against an established diagnostic standard. Although many have employed *DSM* (e.g., DIS and SCID), others, such as the SADS, have used different standards (i.e., RDC). Validity is often described from this perspective as the accuracy of the measure to approximate the diagnostic standard. Terms used to describe this accuracy are presented in Table 1.6.

---

[11]Endicott and Spitzer (1978) found a median alpha coefficient of .80.

Table 1.6

Diagnostic Validity: Terms Used to Describe the Accuracy of Structured Interviews in the Classification of Mental Disorders

Term	Description
Sensitivity	The number of patients correctly classified by SI with a specific disorder, divided by the total number classified by SI with that disorder.
Specificity	The number of patients correctly classified by SI as not having a specific disorder, divided by the total number classified by SI as not having the disorder.
Positive predictive value	The number of patients correctly classified by SI with a specific disorder, divided by the total number classified by DS with that disorder.
Negative predictive value	The number of patients correctly classified by SI as not having a specific disorder, divided by the total number classified by DS as not having the disorder.
Hit rate	The total number of correct classifications divided by the total number of classifications.

Note. SI = structured interview; DS = diagnostic standard.

Structured interviews occasionally employ other forms of test validity. For example, Johnson, Magaro, and Stern (1986) employed convergent and divergent validity to examine the predicted relationships between the SADS-C and other psychometric measures. As part of the validation for the SIRS, Rogers, Bagby, and Dickens (1992) utilized discriminant validity to establish its classificatory accuracy.

Organization of the Chapters

A relatively uniform structure will be imposed upon the remaining chapters to assist psychologists in (a) understanding the clinical and psychometric characteristics of structured interviewing, and (b) making comparisons across specific structured interviews. The typical format for these chapters is summarized in Table 1.7.

The initial two sections of each chapter (description, development, and rationale) provide the overview to each structured interview, including its purpose, description, and development. The next two (and sometimes three) sections are devoted to validation with an examination of the principal psychometric characteristics (i.e., reliability, validity, and generalizability). The final section, clinical applications, addresses the practical relevance of each structured interview in clinical settings.

Table 1.7
Typical Format of Chapters on Structured Interviewing

Overview
   Description of the structured interview
   Development and rationale

Validation
   Reliability
   Validity
   Generalizability and cross-cultural research (optional)

Clinical applications

Part I

Differential Diagnosis for Axis I Disorders

2

Mental Status Examinations (MSEs)

A time-honored tradition of psychiatric training is the clinical use of the mental status examination (MSE), which was first introduced into American psychiatry by Adolf Meyer in 1917 (Tilley & Hoffman, 1981). Despite its long-standing tradition, what actually constitutes an MSE varies widely; it may even be composed largely of unstructured observations and interviewing (Bell & Hall, 1977; Othmer & Othmer, 1989). In a survey of 60 psychiatric training programs, Engel (1979) reported marked variability among the 56 MSEs currently used, both in their organization and content. For the purposes of this chapter, we will consider only what has been construed as "formal" MSE, that is, those procedures which have been standardized and empirically tested.

Even within the parameters of formal MSEs, marked variations occur. As described by Kaplan and Sadock (1988), the typical MSE includes the following content: (a) general presentation (appearance, behavior/psychomotor activity, attitude toward the clinician, and speech); (b) mood, feelings, and affect; (c) perceptions; (d) thought process (disturbances in the form and content of thinking); (e) sensorium (consciousness, orientation, concentration, cognition, memory, intelligence; and general fund of knowledge); (f) judgment; (g) insight; and (h) reliability. Broadly construed, some clinicians (e.g., Tancredi, 1987) view MSEs as encompassing standardized diagnostic interviews like the SADS. Alternatively, many other clinicians view MSEs much more narrowly as a measure of cognitive dysfunction. An example of the latter would be the substantial body of research on the Mini-Mental Status Examination (MMSE; Folstein, Folstein, & McHugh, 1975). As outlined by Donnelly, Rosenberg, and Fleeson (1970), part of this divergence may be explained by the different purposes of MSEs: assessment of psychopathology, recording of process issues, and clinical documentation.

Rodenhauser and Fornal (1991) examined the current usage of MSEs in a small survey of psychiatric residents and faculty. They found that both groups tended to rank the MSE as a necessary component of psychiatric evaluation, roughly the equivalent of a physical examination in medicine. Interestingly, residents in particular were less positive in their assessment of MSE's reliability and validity for evaluating memory, concentration, and abstract thinking. The survey also suggested that more-experienced clinicians were less inclined to employ standardized forms of the MSE. An earlier survey of Canadian psychiatric residents found that the MSE is an essential component of psychiatric evaluations, while suggesting the need for more formal training in its implementation (Ross & Leichner, 1984, 1988).

The primary advantage of formal MSEs is their substantial improvements over unstructured evaluations in controlling information variance. For example, Palmateer and McCartney (1985) found that nurses on a geriatric unit overlooked most cognitively impaired patients (72.3%) when they relied on clinical observations. Bailine, Katzoff, and Rau (1977) determined that systematic data from the MSE facilitated diagnosis more than other hospital records. In this light, Ruegg, Ekstrom, Dwight, and Golden (1990) found that the implementation of a detailed MSE improved the assessment and recording of observational data (appearance, movements, and speech), orientation, concentration, memory, thinking, and psychotic symptoms. As they noted, however, the chief difference was that MSEs recorded negative findings (e.g., absence of hallucinations); a more stringent test would be systematic comparisons of positive findings, since treatment decisions are usually formulated on the basis of diagnosis and prominent symptomatology. From this perspective, Weitzel, Morgan, Guyden, and Robinson (1973) found that standardized MSEs recorded more than three times more symptoms than unstructured MSEs.

Several commentators have expressed their strong reservations over the use of MSEs. Yager (1989) observed that MSE evaluations are often mechanical and insensitive in their presentation. Rosenthal (1989) was particularly concerned that the structured format of the MSE with its "preprogrammed agenda" (p. 208) might impede the professional relationship. He also questioned the discriminant validity of the MSE's components, such as the use of serial-sevens (also see Rosen & Fox, 1986) and their potential misuse by clinicians. Tancredi (1987) raised doubts regarding the validity of MSE. He found the clinical interpretation of negative findings especially problematic, since the relationship of these findings to brain pathology and diagnosis is often equivocal. He also argued that the underlying premise of many MSE questions was the "correctness" of highly conventional responses, which unduly penalizes creativity and cultural diversity (also see Rapp, 1979).

The two main objectives of this chapter are to provide an overview of available MSEs and to present a detailed investigation of MSEs focused solely on cognitive dysfunction. "Comprehensive" MSEs, designed to measure both cognitive impairment and psychopathology, generally provide a conceptual framework but little validation. Because of this paucity of research data, I provide descriptions of several comprehensive MSEs with only limited discussions of their validity. Comprehensive MSEs include the Mental Status Evaluation Record (MSER; Spitzer & Endicott, 1970), the Missouri Mental Status (MMS; Sletten, Ernhart, & Ulett, 1970); MSE Checklist (E. Othmer & S. C. Othmer, 1989), and the North Carolina MSE (NC-MSE; Ruegg, Ekstrom, Dwight, & Golden, 1990).

Unlike comprehensive MSEs, "cognitive" MSEs provide a standardized evaluation of memory and other intellectual functions, often with substantial validation (Gregory, 1987; Yazdanfar, 1990). Cognitive MSEs include the Mental Status Questionnaire (MSQ; Kahn, Goldfarb, Pollack, & Peck, 1960), the Short Portable Mental Status Questionnaire (SPMSQ; Pfeiffer, 1975), the MMSE (Folstein et al., 1975), the Cognitive Capacity Screening Examination (CCSE; Jacobs, Bernhard,

Delgado, & Strain, 1977), the Cambridge Cognitive Examination (CAMCOG; Roth et al., 1986), and the Neurobehavioral Cognitive Status Examination (NCSE; Schwamm, VanDyke, Kieran, Merrin, & Mueller, 1987).

Description of Comprehensive MSEs

Early forms of the comprehensive MSE, such as the MSER and MMS, were devised in conjunction with state mental health systems as methods of standardizing relevant clinical data. Despite large-scale efforts, the MSER and MMS have not achieved wide-spread acceptance among psychiatrists and other clinical staff. Interestingly, a new generation of comprehensive MSEs has been proposed, of which the MSE Checklist and the NC-MSE are good examples. Developed as clinical tools for practitioners, these more recent measures often lack any systematic attempts at formal validation. A summary of comprehensive MSEs is presented in Table 2.1.

Mental Status Evaluation Record (MSER)

Spitzer and Endicott (1970) developed a comprehensive MSE designated as the MSER. Its primary emphasis was the systematic reporting of clinical data. In this respect, the MSER does not standardize the clinical inquiries, but rather provides operational definitions of the criteria and concomitant ratings of symptomatology on 5 gradations: none, slight, mild, moderate, and marked. Of these clinical ratings, 50 are deemed essential for all patients and are presented in bold print. Altogether, clinical judgments address a total 392 descriptors organized into 172 clinical characteristics.

A distinguishing characteristic of the MSER is its emphasis on observational data. Nearly one-half of the MSER can be completed simply through detailed clinical observations. For example, clinical ratings address: apparent physical health (e.g., physical deformities, problems in walking, deviations in height and weight), psychomotor behavior (e.g., tremors, tics, and posturing), dressing and grooming, posture, facial expressions, and eye contact. Similarly, verbal behaviors are reviewed, such as speech and thought disturbances (e.g., volume, rate, productivity, incoherence, circumstantiality, loosening of associations, and concreteness). Observations of mood and affect are also considered, both in terms of type (depression, anxiety, etc.) and quality (e.g., flatness, inappropriateness, and lability).

The MSER is designed to provide systematic ratings of psychopathology with an emphasis on psychotic symptoms (delusions and hallucinations, bizarre or atypical ideation), somatic functioning and concerns, and interpersonal characteristics (overall attitude and behavior). Symptoms of mood disorders are embedded in a variety of categories, including nonpsychotic thoughts, somatic functioning, and mood and affect. Comparatively less attention is paid to cognitive deficits, although the sensorium (e.g., orientation, recent and remote memory, and clouding of consciousness), attention, distractibility, and a gross estimate of intellectual functioning are evaluated. Consideration is also given to violent and suicidal behavior, including overt expressions of anger and any prior suicidal attempts.

Endicott, Spitzer, and Fleiss (1975) examined the psychometric properties of the MSER on 2,001 inpatients. They inspected the MSER's factor structure for 152 clinical variables and extracted a total of 20 factors which covered a broad spectrum of psychopathology. The factor loadings, variance accounted for, and eigen values are not reported for each factor. Moreover, 6 of the 20 factors appear to have poor representation, with three or fewer items. Despite these constraints, the factors were labeled as scales and formed the basis of subsequent research.

Table 2.1
A Description of Comprehensive MSEs That Addresses Both Cognitive Functioning and Current Psychopathology

Mental Status Evaluation Record (MSER; Spitzer & Endicott, 1970)

Description: The MSER is a 172-item MSE in which 50 clinical ratings of each patient are made, with supplementary ratings as warranted. Ratings use a 5-point scale: none, slight, mild, moderate, and marked. Major categories are composed of the following: (a) reliability and completeness of information, (b) appearance, (c) motor behavior, (d) general attitude and behavior, (e) mood and affect, (f) quality of speech and thought, (g) content of speech and thought, (h) somatic functioning and concern, (i) perception, (j) sensorium, (k) cognitive functions, (l) judgment, (m) potential for suicide or violence, and (n) insight and attitude toward illness.

Reliability: Moderate interrater reliability estimates are reported for MSER scales (median ICC = .75, range = .36 – 1.00); interrater reliability is generally poor (median ICC coefficients across three studies of .35, .36, and .50).

Validity: Endicott et al. (1975) summarized several studies which evidenced group differences based on clinical status (inpatient vs. discharged), response to treatment, and certain diagnoses. No attempt was made to establish and validate specific cutting scores for these clinical issues.

Missouri Mental Status Examination (MMS; Sletten, Ernhart, & Ulett, 1970)

Description: The main items of this 120-item MSE are composed of multiple clinical characteristics rated on a 4-point scale (absent, mild, moderate, and severe). The MMS is organized into 10 sections: general appearance, motor activity, speech, interview behavior, flow of thought, mood and affect, thought content, sensorium, intellect, and insight and judgment.

Reliability: Seventeen psychiatric residents rated 18 videotaped MSEs of psychiatric inpatients. Marked variations were found in the intraclass coefficients, with the majority of ratings suggesting poor agreement (< .40).

Validity: The MMS has been widely employed in Missouri with more than 10,000 patients; less information exists, however, on its specific validity. Sletten et al. (1970) reported a 69% agreement on *DSM-II* diagnoses for psychiatric residents who used the MMS in the videotaped reliability study. Other studies, presented in the text, suggest good predictive validity of specific MSE items, but not for the measure as a whole.

Table 2.1   (continued)
A Description of Comprehensive MSEs That Addresses Both Cognitive Functioning and Current Psychopathology

MSE Checklist (E. Othmer & S. C. Othmer, 1989)

Description: On this 61-item MSE, most items consist of multiple subcomponents, each rated for presence or absence. The MSE Checklist addresses the following clinical issues: appearance, consciousness, psychomotor behavior, attention and concentration, speech, thinking, orientation, memory, affect, mood, energy, perception, content of thinking, somatic symptoms, conversion symptoms, multiple personality, paroxysmal attacks, and insight.

Reliability: Unreported.

Validity: A minority of items are based on empirical studies by other investigators; no reported validation exists for the Checklist as a single measure.

North Carolina MSE (NC-MSE; Ruegg, Ekstrom, Dwight, & Golden, 1990)

Description: Thirty-six items are recorded on a 3-point scale (not present, slight or occasional, marked or repeated) on the following clinical issues: physical appearance, behavior, speech, thought process, thought content, mood, affect, cognitive functioning, orientation, recent memory, immediate recall, and remote memory.

Reliability: Unreported.

Validity: Content was derived from recognized authorities; however, no attempt was made to formally assess content validity.

Endicott et al. (1975) evaluated the internal consistency and reliability of the MSER. On the initial sample of 2,001 inpatients, a median alpha of .83 was established, with a comparable estimate of internal consistency (median $\alpha = .78$) on an additional sample of 1,000 psychiatric patients. Interrater reliabilities on these scales for a combined sample of 90 patients ranged from .36 to 1.00, with a median ICC of .75. Test-retest reliabilities for three closely related studies (total $N = 119$) were generally disappointing (range = –.41 – .82, with median ICC coefficients for the three studies of .35, .36, and .50). Endicott et al. suggested that changes in clinical status might explain these results, since patients were newly admitted and the retest periods extended up to 2 weeks. Three scales in particular (depressive ideation, suicide, and hallucinations) appeared to yield adequate to excellent reliability across both methods and samples.

Endicott et al. (1975) reported several validity studies. These investigators contrasted inpatients with discharged psychiatric patients and relatives of psychiatric patients who had never been hospitalized. Not surprisingly, they found differences on many of the 20 scales in the expected direction (i.e., more impairment in inpatients). More stringent tests of the MSER's clinical utility yielded meaningful differences between paranoid and nonparanoid schizophrenics and between organic and nonorganic elderly patients. Furthermore, Endicott et al. were able to document clinical changes in psychiatric patients following inpatient treatment.

In summary, the MSER provides a fairly comprehensive review of symptom-atology and clinical observations. Although we do not have data regarding indi-vidual symptoms, seven scales appear to have good internal consistency and interrater reliability. In addition, three of these seven scales have adequate test-retest reliability. Validity studies offer evidence of discriminant validity between various criterion groups. The clinical utility of the MSER, as with all measures, is highly dependent on the circumstances of its use and on the available alterna-tives. In clinical settings where the standard of practice has been idiosyncratic evaluations of varying quality, then the MSER may offer an incremental improve-ment in standardizing the assessment and offering a basis of comparison for diag-nosis and treatment outcome. The MSER does not compete, nor was it intended to, with comprehensive diagnostic interviews such as the DIS or SADS.

Missouri Mental Status (MMS)

Beginning in 1966, the Missouri mental health system began to standardize and automate a group of seven clinical measures that included the MMS (Sletten & Evenson, 1972). Conceptualized as an integrated system, the Missouri program followed the inpatient and outpatient interventions on more than 180,000 patients with computer-based approaches to psychological testing, patient histo-ries, treatment and community adjustment (Altman, Evenson, Hedlund, & Cho, 1978). Because of this focus on the comprehensive system, less attention was paid to the individual measures, such as the MMS.

The MMS was designed as a standardized, single-page MSE. Like the MSER, most of the attention was paid to the rating of symptomatology rather than the provision of clinical inquiries. As noted in Table 2.1, symptoms are graded according to their severity (absent, mild, moderate, and severe). The first four sections are devoted to clinical observations regarding appearance (e.g., facial expression and dress), motor activity (e.g., amount of activity, tremors and tics, repetitive acts), speech (e.g., amount, rate, and volume), and interview behavior (e.g., affective-based behavior toward the interviewer). One section is dedicated to mood and affect, while two others address disturbances in thinking as charac-terized by formal thought disorders (e.g., circumstantiality, perseveration, and loosening of associations) and thought content (e.g., suicidal ideation, obses-sions, sexual preoccupation, delusions, and hallucinations). Cognitive abilities are subsumed under two sections: sensorium (e.g., orientation, concentration, and memory) and intellect (e.g., serial-sevens, abstraction, vocabulary, and overall ability).

Sletten, Ernhart, and Ulett (1970) attempted to establish the interrater relia-bility of the MMS, with only modest success. The great majority of the individual ratings have poor intraclass coefficients (< .40), based on 18 videotaped inter-views. Moreover, given the MMS's lack of standardization for clinical inquiries, the videotaped format, with all questions being identical, is likely to provide an *overestimate* of the MMS's reliability. Moreover, Sletten, Ernhart, et al. regrouped MMS items into symptom clusters, a change which makes reliability estimates for specific MMS sections difficult to compute.

Hedlund, Evenson, Sletten, and Cho (1980) summarized 10 studies that employ the MMS in establishing psychiatric diagnosis, predicting response to treatment, and evaluating management problems. Of these, only one study (i.e., Sletten, Altman, Evenson, & Cho, 1973) relies exclusively on the MMS; most of the studies incorporate demographic and admission data. Diagnostic studies, such as Altman, Evenson, and Cho (1976), found classification rates with clinical diagnosis of 55% on a cross-validated study of 3,278 psychiatric outpatients; 13 MMS items contributed to this classification. These results are similar to earlier findings by Sletten, Ulett, Altman, and Sundland (1970). While limited by comparisons to *DSM-II* diagnoses,[1] these results do not support the clinical usefulness of the MMS in confirming psychiatric diagnoses.

Several studies (Altman, Evenson, & Sletten, 1973; Evenson, Altman, Sletten, & Cho, 1973b; Evenson, Altman, Cho, & Sletten, 1974a, 1974b; Sletten et al., 1973) have examined the usefulness of the MMS in assigning patients to drug trials. When given broad categories (i.e., major tranquilizers, minor tranquilizers, antidepressants, and no drugs), fairly high levels of agreement (62 – 84%) were reached. While these findings are encouraging, their clinical applicability seems unclear, since it is doubtful that discriminant models will ever supplant psychiatrists, and the classifications themselves were limited to broad categories.

An interesting use of the MMS is its application to the multivariate models for predicting hospital stay and problematic behavior. Altman, Angle, Brown, and Sletten (1972a), with a two-stage discriminant model, were able to predict 71% of patients who needed extended hospitalizations. More importantly, these same investigators (Altman, Angle, Brown, & Sletten, 1972b) with an expanded sample were able to predict which patients represented elopement risks with a similar classification rate. Finally, Altman and his colleagues (Altman et al., 1977; Hedlund, Sletten, Altman, & Evenson, 1973) attempted to evaluate aggressive behavior towards self and others on the basis of the MSS and other standardized measures. In a cross-validation on 2,762 patients, they were able to rule out suicidal attempts in nearly all cases (95.7%), but were less successful at identifying those with prior attempts (44.9%). From the MSS, suicidal thoughts, hypochondriasis, flat affect, and the absence of persecutory delusions contributed to these classifications. In a similar analysis, the researchers were able to rule out nearly all patients who did not have a past history of physical aggression (95.9%), but correctly identified only about one-third (34.4%) of aggressive patients. Items from the MSS that contributed to this prediction were assaultive ideas, angry outbursts, impulsive behavior, and nonacceptance of hospitalization.

In summary, the MSS appears to have relatively low interrater reliability, which limits its clinical applications. With more detailed clinical inquiries, the reliability of the MSS would undoubtedly improve. However, the hallmark of the MSS and related measures was the effort to comprehensively assess nearly all patients in the Missouri mental health system. Standardized data exist on several hundred thousand patients; although imprecise, the data provide an unprecedented view of symptomatology and response to treatment in unselected populations. This information has proven invaluable in scale development (e.g., Community Adjustment Profile Scales [Evenson, 1976]) and psychological testing (e.g., MMPI correlates [Gynther, Altman, & Sletten, 1973]).

---

[1]Given the limited reliability of *DSM-II* itself, higher reliability estimates may not be possible for the MMS.

MSE Checklist

E. Othmer and S. C. Othmer (1989) devised an extensive outline for MSE evaluations in the form of the MSE Checklist. E. Othmer and S. C. Othmer provide sample questions and operational criteria for the scoring of individual items, which are evaluated on a nominal scale (presence or absence). In addition, the MSE Checklist incorporates specific cognitive tasks and other standardized measures to test for aphasias and agnosia (e.g., the MMSE and a screening measure for intelligence [Kent, 1946]).

The MSE Checklist provides an extensive format for clinical observations (see Table 2.1). Clinical characteristics are also rated as present or absent; the MSE Checklist distinguishes itself from other MSEs by offering highly detailed definitions and descriptions of the included symptomatology. Criteria are also highly specific. For example, affect is assessed by intensity, range, attempts to control, and forms of expression (i.e., gestures, facial expressions, tone, pitch, and choice of words). In contrast, hallucinations and delusions are given relatively less attention.

The final section of the MSE Checklist ("Testing") focuses exclusively on cognitive functions. Clinicians are presented with standardized tasks to assess specific dysfunctions. For example, attention and concentration are assessed through digit span, serial-sevens, naming the months backward, and spelling words backward. Tasks are presented to screen for aphasia, agnosia, apraxias, and pseudoneurological problems. The question needing empirical testing is whether these brief inquiries and techniques have sufficient sensitivity and specificity to warrant their inclusion in an MSE. Moreover, several of the brief tasks for the assessment of cognitive abilities and memory impairment appear to be highly truncated imitations of standardized tests. E. Othmer and S. C. Othmer recommend a Paired Associates Test (Strub & Black, 1977) which strongly resembles a subtest of the Wechsler Memory Scale–Revised (Wechsler, 1987) by the same name, but consists of only four word pairs and two presentations.

The empirical validation for the MSE Checklist is unfortunately not forthcoming. More specifically, the MSE Checklist does not have established reliability, so that the reproducibility of ratings across psychologists is unknown. Moreover, clinicians do not have adequate data to know how to interpret deviant responses in terms of discriminant validity.

The greatest potential for the MSE Checklist is its coverage of organic and neurological symptoms. Selective review of these symptoms might signal to the evaluating psychologist the need for neurological consultation or neuropsychological evaluation. Toward this end, E. Othmer and S. C. Othmer suggest a number of screening items, although several (e.g., pseudo-neurological symptoms) are likely to be outside most psychologists' expertise.[2]

---

[2]For neuropsychologists with appropriate training, standardized neurological assessments are also available that appear to have substantial validation (e.g., Quantitative Neurological Examination; Brandt et al., 1984; David, Jeste, Folstein, & Folstein, 1987; Folstein, Jensen, Leigh, & Folstein, 1983).

North Carolina MSE (NC-MSE)

Ruegg et al. (1990) devised the 36-item NC-MSE to assess what they considered to be the essential features of mental status. They reported a review of three standard psychiatric textbooks for item generation in what appears to be an informal approach to content validity. Ruegg et al. did not report reliability data; instead, they described a reinspection of 15 patients' NC-MSE profiles as a high accuracy of data entry.[3]

Ruegg et al. found that 36 psychiatric residents produced more comprehensive recordings of mental status with the NC-MSE than with unstructured formats. However, a major difference was that unstructured approaches often did not report negative findings (e.g., the absence of hallucinations). As noted in the introduction, a more stringent test would be a comparison of positive findings.

In comparison to other comprehensive MSEs, the NC-MSE appears to have relatively little validation. In the absence of further research, I would recommend the MSER and MSS over the NC-MSE.

Conclusions Regarding Comprehensive MSEs

Today, comprehensive MSEs have more historical importance than clinical relevance. Both the MSER and the MSS have been subjected to extensive research as methods of standardizing the assessment of psychopathology and improving clinical diagnosis. Work on the MSER laid the crucial groundwork for the subsequent development of the SADS. Studies with the MSS and its family of assessment measures provided the most comprehensive pre-*DSM-III* view of diagnosis, treatment, and community adjustment for severe mental disorders.

When should comprehensive MSEs be used? The question is highly dependent on the clinical setting. I have found, for example, that the MSER offers an excellent format for the clinical description of psychiatric patients. In an outpatient assessment setting where line staff played an ancillary role in psychiatric evaluations, the MSER was a valuable tool for staff to standardize their observations.

The MSS and related measures from the Missouri system may still be useful for inpatient data management. Despite constraints on its reliability, the MSS would be strongly preferred over the unstandardized and idiosyncratic approaches found in many hospitals. Hospital systems would be wise to improve on an existing system rather than starting again. Given the MSS's pre-*DSM-III* development, the emphasis would not be on diagnosis but rather on symptom constellations and their usefulness in the patient treatment, management, and predictions of outcome.

Decisions regarding the clinical use of comprehensive MSEs are comparative. For example, the MSE Checklist is preferable to an idiosyncratic assessment of a patient's overall clinical status. Its standardization at least ensures that major areas of clinical inquiry are not completely overlooked.

---

[3]Their description is very abbreviated (Ruegg et al., 1990, p. 161); it appears that the investigators checked only the consistency of their data entry, but not the reliability of the NC-MSE itself.

Psychologists must also be aware that some psychiatrists hold comprehensive MSEs in high regard. In multidisciplinary settings, psychologists must balance their respect for professional differences with patients' needs for accurate assessments of their psychopathology. I have found a working knowledge of comprehensive MSEs and their occasional use to be very helpful in reducing interprofessional barriers and rivalry. Conversely, despite their psychometric limitations, wholesale attempts to categorically discredit comprehensive MSEs are both clinically unnecessary and professionally unwise. Rather, the comprehensive MSE may be seen as one of many data sources in the multidisciplinary evaluation of psychiatric patients.

Description of Cognitive MSEs

Cognitive MSEs were developed during the last three decades for the psychiatric screening of patients for possible cognitive dysfunction and organic involvement. This development is steeped in tradition; many test items are included more out of convention than for their diagnostic value. Before reviewing the cognitive MSEs themselves, I will explore studies on common components (e.g., orientation, serial-sevens, short-term memory) of these measures.

Common Components of Cognitive MSEs

Withers and Hinton (1971) compared three research versions for testing the orientation, concentration, and memory of 108 psychiatric patients. They found that patients were highly consistent when assessed across alternate versions for digit span (similar to the WAIS-R [Wechsler, 1981]), logical memory (similar to the WMS-R [Wechsler, 1987]), and long-term memory. When retested in less than 1 week, the results were more variable. Orientation (time, place, person) correlated between the two times at .70 for females and .63 for males. Likewise, digit span averaged .66 for females and .49 for males. Lower correlations were found for logical memory (averaged across immediate and 5-minute delays, correlations were .60 for females and .67 for males). With the exception of digit span for males, test-retest reliabilities appear to be in the moderate range.[4]

Sullivan, Sagar, Gabrieli, Corkin, and Growdon (1989) examined memory dysfunction in patients with Parkinson's disease (PD) and Alzheimer's disease (AD). Among the various test findings, digit span backwards appeared to consistently differentiate PD and AD patients from controls, even including those PD patients who otherwise appeared intact on MSE examination. This study would suggest the discriminant validity of digit span backwards as one possible screen for organic involvement.

Interpretation of proverbs is typically included in cognitive MSEs. The use of proverbs has been criticized because of their cultural dependence (Tancredi, 1987; Taylor, 1981) and lack of discrimination among criterion groups

---

[4]As observed by the authors, these subjects appear to be unusually bright (*M* WAIS IQ = 111.3) for psychiatric inpatients. This level of tested intelligence would suggest that they were cognitively intact; we might suspect that these reliability estimates would be lower in populations with greater impairment.

(MacKinnon & Yudofsky, 1986). As noted by Lancker (1990), an important dimension of proverb interpretation is familiarity; some impaired persons are able to give correct responses not as a measure of abstract thinking, but due to their memory of the proverb and the highly conventionalized, although correct, response. Indeed, the use of proverbs has been questioned even in comprehensive measures of intelligence (Gregory, 1987). Andreasen (1977) discouraged the use of proverbs in MSEs because of their poor interrater reliabilities (<.55). Interestingly, Reich (1981) also found that reliability estimates for individual proverbs were poor, but that the use of four proverbs and a standardized scoring based on Gorham (1956) produced satisfactory reliability (r = .82). If proverbs are to be used and interpreted in MSEs, then Reich's approach is recommended.

Use of serial-sevens was originated by Kraepelin in 1907 and has been incorporated into cognitive MSEs. Taylor, Abrams, Raber, and Almy (1980) established a high interrater reliability for serial-sevens (ICC = .89) for a sample of 25 psychiatric inpatients. As noted by Smith (1967), however, more than 40% of normals made at least one error, and approximately one-fourth (24.2%) made 3 to 12 errors. Keller and Manschreck (1981) have questioned the use of serial-sevens on the basis of their poor discriminant validity.

An important consideration in the use of cognitive MSEs is the interpretation of deficits in orientation, concentration, and memory. To assist in the assessment of dementia, Reisberg and his colleagues have devised several highly specific ratings for MSE items. For example, Reisberg, Schneck, Ferris, Schwartz, and De Leon (1983) developed the Brief Cognitive Rating Scale (BCRS) with five criterion-based ratings for concentration, recent memory, past memory, orientation, and day-to-day functioning. In elderly patients, these ratings evidenced a very high level of intercorrelations (rs range = .88 – .93) and moderate correlations (median = .64; range = .51 – .69) with the Guild Memory Test (Crook, Gilbert, & Ferris, 1980). Reisberg, Ferris, De Leon, and Crook (1992) also developed a stage model (i.e., the Global Deterioration Scale or GDS) for the description of degenerative dementia that incorporates psychometric and mental status data. Foster, Sclan, Welkowitz, Boksay, and Seeland (1988) established high interrater reliabilities for the BCRS (.76 – .97, median r = .92) and the GDS (r = .94). Together, these ratings, while not extensively validated, may provide at least a preliminary empirical basis for interpreting cognitively impaired MSEs among the elderly.

We will now turn our attention to a selective review of six cognitive MSEs (see Table 2.2). The original three MSEs (i.e., MSQ, MMSE, and SPMSQ) are very brief measures consisting of 10 or 11 items, with considerable item overlap. Nelson, Fogel, and Faust (1986) provide a masterful overview of their development and initial validation. A second generation of cognitive MSEs includes the CCSE, CAMCOG, and NCSE. These more extensive measures cover a wider range of cognitive functions. Of these, the CAMCOG has incorporated the MMSE as a component of its assessment.

Table 2.2 is intended to serve two useful purposes. First, it provides a direct comparison of the cognitive MSEs by juxtaposing their descriptions and validation. Second, the table affords a ready reference for quickly reviewing cognitive MSEs.

Table 2.2
A Description of MSEs Designed to Assess Cognitive Dysfunction

Mental Status Questionnaire (MSQ; Kahn, Goldfarb, Pollack, & Peck, 1960)

Description: This MSE is designed to assess cognitive impairment in the elderly using 10 items that are scored as correct or incorrect. Test items address orientation to time and place, knowledge of one's own birth date and age, and memory of current and past presidents.

Reliability: Foster et al. (1988) established a very high interrater reliability of .99. Lesher and Whelihan (1986) reported good internal consistency (α = .81), split-half reliability (r = .82), and test-retest reliability (r = .87).

Validity: Extremely low scores appear to be strongly associated with moderate to severe cognitive impairment. The MSQ tends to be highly correlated with other MSEs. Studies conflict over the efficacy of cutting scores for cognitive impairment.

Short Portable Mental Status Questionnaire (SPMSQ; Pfeiffer, 1975)

Description: Specifically designed to measure cognitive deficits in patients 50 years and older. These 10 items assess orientation, long-term memory (e.g., names of the two most recent presidents), and remote memory (e.g., place and date of birth, mother's maiden name). In addition, subjects are asked to carry out serial subtractions of three.

Reliability: Pfeiffer (1975) reported test-retest correlations of .82 and .83. Lesher and Whelihan (1986) reported good internal consistency (α = .83), split-half reliability (r = .95), and test-retest reliability (r = .82).

Validity: Studies consistently demonstrate that low scores are associated with dementia and other organic conditions. However, cutting scores are likely to miss one-third to nearly one-half of those patients with cognitive impairment.

Mini-Mental State Examination (MMSE; M. F. Folstein, S. E. Folstein, & McHugh, 1975)

Description: An 11-item MSE for the assessment of cognitive impairment with most items scored as correct or incorrect, the MMSE was designed to address orientation, registration, attention and calculation, and language.

Reliability: Excellent interrater and test-retest reliability data are presented in Table 2.3.

Validity: In impaired populations, low MMSE scores correlate with lower WAIS IQs and poorer prognosis. The MMSE appears reasonably accurate at identifying global and left hemisphere deficits but inaccurate with focal and right hemisphere lesions.

Cognitive Capacity Screening Examination (CCSE; Jacobs, Bernhard, Delgado, & Strain, 1977)

Description: Thirty items scored on a nominal scale assess cognitive impairment. The content of the CCSE includes orientation, digit span, serial-sevens, repetition, verbal concept formation, and short-term memory. The CCSE focuses more than other MSEs on numbers and calculations; for example,

Table 2.2   (continued)
A Description of MSEs Designed to Assess Cognitive Dysfunction

numbers are repeated forwards, backwards, and with a distractor. Verbal concept formation is composed of opposites and similarities.

Reliability: A preliminary test on six patients by three clinicians suggested a very high concordance (Jacobs et al., 1977). Foreman (1987) found that the CCSE had a high level of internal consistency (α = .97) in a study of 66 elderly patients. Haddad and Coffman (1987) reported excellent test-retest reliability (r = .87).

Validity: As summarized by Nelson et al. (1986), four studies have been conducted on the CCSE which offer criterion-related validity based on psychiatric and medical patients. In general, recent research has found that the CCSE has good sensitivity and excellent specificity.

Cambridge Cognitive Examination (CAMCOG; Roth et al., 1986)

Description: The CAMCOG incorporated 11 items from the MMSE with 43 additional items to address other elements of cognitive dysfunction. Although the authors do not describe this MSE in detail, it appears that the CAMCOG addresses orientation, language, memory, praxis, attention, abstract thinking, perception, and calculation.

Reliability: Interrater reliability was assessed on 40 patients with a moderate level of agreement on diagnosis (ϕ coefficient = .63). The individual phi coefficients for the CAMCOG were very high with a median of .90 (range = .30 – 1.00).

Validity: Roth et al. (1986), in a study of 92 elderly patients, found that the CAMCOG had 92% sensitivity and 96% specificity in classifying organic patients and differentiating them from normal and depressed elderly. The CAMCOG was significantly correlated with a standard measure, the Blessed Dementia Scale (r = –.70; Blessed et al., 1968) and clinical assessment of the severity of dementia (r = –.78).

Neurobehavioral Cognitive Status Examination (NCSE; Kiernan, Mueller, Langston, & Van Dyke, 1987)

Description: The NCSE is composed of 64 items of graded difficulty for the assessment of cognitive impairment in adults. These items are divided into 10 scales: consciousness, orientation, attention, comprehension, repetition, naming, constructions, memory calculations, similarities, and judgment. Each scale begins with a difficult screening item which is failed by approximately 20% of the normal population. If this item is failed, then the patient is administered the complete scale with test items of varying difficulty.

Reliability: Kiernan et al. (1987) did not report reliability data.

Validity: Schwamm et al. (1987) examined 30 patients with documented brain lesions and found that the NCSE accurately identified 97.3%, a far superior rate to the MMSE and CCSE. However, we do not have an accurate estimate of the NCSE's diagnostic accuracy since (a) these results were not cross-validated and (b) the absence of cognitively intact and psychiatric samples do not allow us to evaluate its specificity.

Mental Status Questionnaire (MSQ)

The first cognitive MSE to gain consistent recognition was the MSQ, which was developed by Kahn, Goldfarb, Pollack, and Peck in 1960. The MSQ was designed as a brief screening measure for elderly populations; original work on the MSQ was started in the 1950s in response to the growing realization of widespread organicity among the institutionalized elderly (Gurland, Cote, Cross, & Toner, 1987). This 10-item MSE focuses entirely on verbal responses to questions regarding orientation to time (date, month, year) and place (location name and address), and long-term memory of information, both personal (age, date, and year of birth) and public (current president and his predecessor).

Reliability. Foster et al. (1988) conducted an interrater reliability study of the MSQ with 40 psychiatric patients and found very high reliability ($r = .99$) for both psychiatrists and research assistants. Nelson et al. (1986) report an unpublished study of the MSQ's test-retest reliability (i.e., Wilson, Roy, & Bursill, 1973) which involved four administrations of the MSQ to 55 elderly patients and yielded relatively consistent results. Finally, Lesher and Whelihan (1986) administered the MSQ and seven other MSE measures to 36 nursing home residents in a test-retest design at 2- to 4-week intervals. They found that the MSQ had excellent overall reliability as evidenced by internal consistency ($\alpha = .81$), split-half reliability ($r = .82$), and test-retest reliability ($r = .87$).

Validity. Kahn et al. (1960) performed the original validation with a sample of 1,077 institutionalized patients from state mental hospitals, nursing homes, and homes for the aged. Nearly all patients with no errors on the MSQ had mild or no cognitive impairment; conversely, nearly all patients that completely failed the MSQ had moderate to severe impairment. However, middle-range scores were apparently less discriminating, although these percentages went unreported. With respect to validity, Fillenbaum (1980) reported a sensitivity of 55% and a specificity of 96% for diagnosis of organic mental disorder in a community sample of 83 elderly.

Several investigators (e.g., Baker, 1990; Lesher & Whelihan, 1986; Reid, Tierney, Zorzitto, Snow, & Fisher, 1991) have examined the reliability and concurrent validity of the MSQ in relationship to other cognitive measures. For instance, Lautenschlaeger, Meier, and Donnelly (1986) found high rates of agreement between the MSQ and the MMSE for severely impaired and completely unimpaired subjects in a sample of 48 elderly patients, but had poor agreement on moderately impaired individuals.[5] Lesher and Whelihan (1986) found a generally high correlation ($M r = .90$) between the MSQ and seven other MSE measures including the SPMSQ and lesser-known MSE measures.[6] As a further example, Reid et al. (1991) conducted a large clinical study of the MSQ with 162 demented patients (Alzheimer's, Parkinson's, and other etiologies) and 102 neurologically normal subjects. They found that the MSQ had a moderately high

---

[5]Overall concordance was 66.7%; no correlations are reported.

[6]These high correlations are not surprising given the large item overlap with the SPMSQ and other closely related measures (i.e., Extended Mental Status Questionnaire [Whelihan, Lesher, Kleban, & Granick, 1984]; and the Simplified Mental Status Questionnaire [Isaacs & Walkey, 1963]).

correlation ($r = -.79$) with the London Psychogeriatric Rating Scale (Hersch, Kral, & Palmer, 1978) and significantly predicted organic diagnosis.

Research on the MSQ raises several caveats which are likely to apply to other MSEs. As previously noted, Reisberg et al. (1982) found that the MSQ was ineffective at detecting mild cognitive deficits. Moreover, Ohta, Carlin, and Harmon (1981) found that hearing loss may confound the MSQ as a measure of cognitive decline. In a study of 27 nursing home residents, Ohta et al. observed that moderate hearing loss was often not considered in the assessment of mental status, although it often substantially impaired performance.

Research interest in the MSQ appears to have dwindled with the introduction of a slightly expanded version, the SPMSQ. Because of the greater availability of research data on the SPMSQ and its broader clinical appeal, we will now turn our attention to this modified version.

Short Portable Mental Status Questionnaire (SPMSQ)

Pfeiffer (1975) developed the SPMSQ as an overall measure of organic impairment in the elderly. Pfeiffer criticized the MSQ as being used chiefly with institutionalized populations and for lacking norms based educational attainment. The SPMSQ evaluates orientation to time (day of the week and date) and place (name of the place and street address), memory of personal and public information (birth date, age, telephone number, and mother's maiden name; current president and his predecessor), and concentration (serial-threes). The SPMSQ differs from the MSQ by the addition of three items: telephone number, mother's maiden name, and serial-threes. Pfeiffer (1975) proposed four classes of intellectual functioning on the basis of SPMSQ scores and educational levels: intact functioning, and mild, moderate and severe impairment.

Item difficulties were calculated by race. One cause for concern in the initial normative sample ($N = 939$) was pronounced differences in individual-item failure rates for Whites (1 – 44%; $M = 11.1$%) and African-Americans (2 – 75%; $M = 21.8$%). Similar differences were observed in a subsequent clinical study of 141 patients with three times more African-American than White patients having seven or more errors. To account for these differences, Pfeiffer proposed cutting scores that are one point lower for African-Americans than for Whites. Unfortunately, he does not offer an explanation for this scoring modification.[7]

Reliability. Pfeiffer (1975) conducted the original test-retest reliability study of the SPMSQ on two samples of elderly subjects ($ns = 30$ and 29). After an interval of 4 weeks, moderately high correlations of .82 and .83 were established. In the previously cited study, Lesher and Whelihan (1986) reported high overall reliability for the SPMSQ with respect to internal consistency ($\alpha = .83$), split-half reliability ($r = .95$), and test-retest reliability ($r = .82$). Similarly, Foreman (1987) reported a high internal consistency ($\alpha = .90$).

---

[7]The revised scoring results in 69% of Whites and 62% of African-Americans being classified as "cognitively intact," but 0% of Whites and 4% of African-Americans as "severely impaired." More to the point, the accuracy of these cutting scores must be determined through clinical investigations.

Validity. Pfeiffer (1975) administered the SPMSQ to two nonrandom samples: 141 elderly patients referred to the Duke University Center for the Study of Aging and Human Development, and 102 elderly subjects living in institutions. From the clinic population, most patients (92.3%) with moderate or severe impairment on the SPMSQ were diagnosed with organic brain syndrome (OBS), while approximately two-thirds (67.9%) of those with OBS received low scores on the SPMSQ. The SPMSQ was much less effective with the institutional sample; only 7 of 27 OBS patients (25.9%) had low scores on the SPMSQ.

Nelson et al. (1986) summarized the early validity studies with the SPMSQ (Fillenbaum, 1980; Wolber, Romaniuk, Eastman, & Robinson, 1984), which revealed differences in SPMSQ scores for cognitively intact and impaired subjects. Fillenbaum found that the SPMSQ did not differ from the MSQ in either sensitivity (55%) or specificity (96%). Wolber et al. (1984), in a study of 95 geriatric patients, revealed a moderate agreement of .76 with psychiatric diagnosis, and moderate correlations with the Bender-Gestalt (Bender, 1938) and the digit-span subtest of the WAIS.

Berg, Edwards, Danzinger, and Berg (1987) followed 58 elderly controls and 43 patients with mild Alzheimer's disease with retesting on SPMSQ and the Blessed Dementia Scale (BDS; Blessed, Tomlinson, & Roth, 1968) at 12- and 30-month follow-ups. They concluded that the SPMSQ was superior to the BDS in quantifying deterioration due to dementia.

Foreman (1987) examined the internal consistency, intercorrelations, and external validity of three MSEs, including the SPMSQ, on 66 elderly medical inpatients admitted to a medical-surgical unit of a teaching hospital; the sample was divided evenly into those who were cognitively intact and those with global cognitive impairment. All patients were administered the SPMSQ, MMSE, CCSE, and the Dementia Rating Scale (Lawson, Rodenburg, & Dykes, 1977). Results revealed a high correlation of the SPMSQ with the MMSE ($r = .83$) and moderate correlation with the CCSE ($r = .63$), and indicated a sensitivity of .73 and specificity of .91.

Erkinjuntti, Sulkava, Wikstrom, and Autio (1987) administered the SPMSQ and a neuropsychological test battery to 118 elderly community residents and 282 elderly medical inpatients. They found that a cutting score of three or more errors for cognitive impairment has reasonably good sensitivity for dementia (66.7% for community residents and 86.2% for inpatients) and superb specificity (100% and 99.0% for community residents and inpatients, respectively). Interestingly, they found no need for an education correction recommended by Pfeiffer. Christensen, Hadzi-Pavlovic, and Jacomb (1991) conducted a meta-analysis of three SPMSQ studies and found a mean effect size that was slightly lower than other MSEs (2.39 vs. 2.73) but superior to many neuropsychological tests and subtests (i.e., their *M* effect size = 1.84).

Smyer, Hofland, and Jonas (1979) examined SPMSQ scores for 103 institutionalized and 78 community subjects with respect to their day-to-day functioning. They found that the SPMSQ was accurate at making broad categorizations (i.e., intact/mildly impaired versus moderately/severely impaired), but was relatively poor at identifying mildly impaired individuals. A practical implication of these results is use of the SPMSQ as a screen only for moderate to severe cognitive impairment.

Several studies have underscored the limitations of the SPMSQ as a screening measure for organicity. For example, Dalton, Pederson, Blom, and Holmes (1987) reported in a study of 40 VA patients that performance on the SPMSQ did not correlate significantly with either clinical diagnosis (ϕ = .20) or neuropsychological data (ϕ = .24). More than one-half of those with a diagnosis of organic brain syndrome had one or zero errors on the SPMSQ. Skurla, Rogers, and Sunderland (1988) found differences based on the severity of dementia, and on the ability of nine Alzheimer's patients on a geriatric unit and nine community controls to carry out common activities of daily living. While the SPMSQ correlated with severity of dementia (r = .60), it appeared unrelated to daily living tasks (r = .14). In addition, Albert et al. (1991) examined the SPMSQ scores for 134 subjects with probable Alzheimer's disease in comparison to 333 subjects without. They found that the SPMSQ was limited by sensitivity as a screening measure, with very modest sensitivity (16.4% – 33.0%, depending on age), although excellent specificity was reported (88.8% – 96.2%). However, Edwards, Baum, and Deuel (1991) found that Alzheimer's patients in early stages of dementia often experience constructional apraxia, which is typically undetected by the SPMSQ.

Like the MSQ, the SPMSQ has relatively modest sensitivity and generally acceptable specificity. In other words, low scores on the SPMSQ typically signal organic impairment. In contrast, subjects with mild dementias or delirium are unlikely to be detected by the SPMSQ. As observed by Dalton et al. (1987), psychologists should avoid drawing conclusions from "normal" scores on the SPMSQ alone because of the very real possibility of undetected cognitive impairment.

Mini-Mental State Examination (MMSE)

M. F. Folstein et al. (1975) devised the MMSE for the quantitative assessment of cognitive performance. They described the MMSE as "mini" because of its exclusion of psychopathology, but believe the MMSE constitutes a thorough review of cognitive functions. They constructed the MMSE, based on earlier work (e.g., see Shapiro, Post, Lofving, & Inglis, 1956), in two sections with the first requiring only verbal responses and the second necessitating reading and behavioral responses. The MMSE consists of 11 items that entail the following: orientation (time and place), naming of objects, serial-sevens, remembering objects, following directions, writing a sentence, and copying a geometric figure. Rovner and M. F. Folstein (1987) provide detailed instructions on its administration.

Reliability. As summarized in Table 2.3, the overall reliability of the MMSE is consistently high. With one exception (i.e., Olin & Zelinski, 1991), studies of both interrater and test-retest reliabilities (Bird, Canino, Rubio-Stipec, & Shrout, 1987; Dick et al., 1984; M. F. Folstein et al., 1975; Foster et al., 1988; Uhlmann, Larson, & Buchner, 1987) exceed .80 when administered to neurological patients, psychiatric patients, and community samples. In addition, the Spanish version (see following discussion) also appears to have excellent reliability.

The notable exception is the research by Olin and Zelinski (1991), who found a very poor test-retest correlation for nondemented subjects at a 12-month interval. Moreover, the variations in scores did not reflect a decrement in functioning on either the MMSE or neuropsychological tests. While this negative finding is worthy of our attention, it may be explained by the very narrow range

Table 2.3
Reliability Studies of the Mini-Mental State Examination (MMSE)

Study	Agreement
M. F. Folstein, S. E. Folstein, & McHugh (1975) MMSE was administered to patients with dementia and/or mood disorders in a test-retest design, with 19 patients at a 1-day and 23 "clinically stable" patients at a 28-day interval.	Test-retest (1 day), $r = 83$ Test-retest (28 days), $r = .99$
Dick et al. (1984) MMSE was administered to 45 neurological inpatients in a test-retest design at a 24-hour interval, either by the same or a different clinician.	$r = .92$
Bird, Canino, Rubio-Stipec, & Shrout (1987) The Spanish version of the MMSE was administered twice on the same day; the format was random with lay interviewers compared to psychiatrists. A total of 60 community subjects and 129 outpatients were preselected to cover representative diagnoses.	Individual items, $\kappa = .57$ MMSE scale, ICC = .90
Uhlmann, Larson, & Buchner (1987) Test-retest reliability was established at a 12-month interval by different clinicians evaluating demented patients.	$r = .86$
Foster, Sclan, Welkowitz, Boksay, & Seeland (1988) Interrater reliability was studied for 40 psychiatric patients with a range of diagnoses; the same reliability was obtained whether the MMSE was administered by psychiatrists or research assistants.	$r = .99$
Olin & Zelinski (1991) Test-retest reliability for a community sample of 57 nondemented subjects (55 years and older) was assessed at a 12-month interval.	$r = .34$

Note. κ = unweighted kappas; ICC = intraclass coefficients. Except where otherwise noted, median statistics are reported.

of MMSE scores (first testing, $M = 28.08$, $SD = 1.70$; second testing, $M = 27.68$, $SD = 1.87$) and the systematic exclusion of cognitively impaired subjects. Put more simply, 82% of the sample had differences in testing of 1 or less than 1 point.

The MMSE was also included in the National Institute of Mental Health (NIMH) epidemiological studies as a component of the Diagnostic Interview Schedule (DIS; Robins, Helzer, Croughan, & Ratcliff, 1981). In a test-retest format at a 6-week interval, Helzer et al. (1985) found that 32 of 34 subjects continued to evidence impairment on the MMSE; no formal reliability estimates were presented. As evidence of generalizability across epidemiological studies, Robin et al. (1984) found comparable rates of severe cognitive impairment as measured by the MMSE for New Haven (1.3%), Baltimore (1.3%), and St. Louis (1.0%).

In summary, the MMSE evidences excellent reliability in clinical and community settings. Its reproducibility of results would recommend its clinical and research applications.

Validity. Nelson et al. (1986) summarized the early criterion-related validity studies. The original studies (Anthony, LeResche, Niaz, Von Korff, & M. F. Folstein, 1982; Dick et al., 1984; M. F. Folstein et al., 1975) suggest that the MMSE differentiates among criterion groups (dementia, nonorganic disorders, and normal), although the use of specific cutting scores may produce significant misclassifications. For example, the recommended cutting score (< 24) resulted in high numbers of false positives for those with less than an eighth-grade education (Anthony et al., 1982) and the very elderly (Bleeker, Bolla-Wilson, Kawas, & Agnew, 1988). In contrast, Jackson and Ramsdell (1988) studied 380 elderly outpatients and found that the less than 24 cutting score had an excellent hit rate, with a sensitivity of 85.0% and a specificity of 98.0%.

M. F. Folstein, Anthony, Parhad, Duffy, and Gruenberg (1985), as part of the NIMH epidemiological studies in Baltimore, examined the MMSE for 3,481 community subjects. Of these, 810 were reevaluated by psychiatrists and 34 subjects were referred for complete neurological assessments. They found no differences in MMSE performance on the basis of race or sex. Very few subjects without dementia or delirium scored in the impaired range on the MMSE. They concluded that the MMSE should be employed for screening patients rather that diagnosing them.

An interesting application of the MMSE has been in the predicting of treatment outcome. Folstein et al. (1975) documented changes in the MMSE for mood-disordered patients following treatment but found negligible changes for those with chronic organic disorders. In a study of elderly depressed patients, LaRue, Spar, and Hill (1986) found that low MMSE scores predicted a slower treatment response and need for antipsychotic medication. However, community follow-up found few differences in adjustment, perhaps because of improvements in the performance of the original low scorers on the MMSE. Fisk and Pannill (1987) observed that low MMSE scores predicted which Alzheimer's patients would be institutionalized at an 18-month follow-up, although the differences were not dramatic. Zubenko, Rosen, Sweet, Mulsant, and Rifai (1992) found that MMSE documented response to inpatient treatment for 120 Alzheimer's patients.

McHugh and Folstein (1988) have employed the MMSE to document the progressive cognitive deterioration which is the hallmark of Alzheimer's disease. On average, decrements in MMSE are relatively mild in the first year (MMSE scores of approximately 20) and typically decrease to less than 12 after 5 years.

Validation of the MMSE has also included evidence of neurological impairment and concurrent validity with cognitive measures. Studies have produced mixed results with respect to brain lesions and atrophy. For example, DePaulo and M. F. Folstein (1978) examined MMSE scores for 126 neurological patients and found that the cutting score (< 24) identified only a minority of patients with lesions. Tsai and Tsuang (1979) found that MMSE differentiated between 31 patients with positive (i.e., pathological) and 32 patients with negative computerized tomographic scans. On closer inspection, however, it is seen that the MMSE was effective when general cerebral atrophy occurred, but not with focal lesions alone. Patients with cerebral atrophy were distinguishable from others on their total MMSE scores, orientation, registration, and recall. Dick et al. (1984), in a study of 126 neurological patients and 17 additional patients with cognitive impairment, found that the MMSE differentiated approximately three-fourths (76%) of those with cerebral lesions but was consistently ineffective with right hemisphere lesions. Schwamm et al. (1987) established a sensitivity for the MMSE of 53.3% on 30 patients with confirmed brain lesions. Prohovnik, Smith, Sackeim, Mayeux, and Stern (1989) found a positive correlation ($r = .39$) between the loss of gray matter in demented patients and scores on the MMSE.

Rosen and Fox (1986) examined the discriminant validity of individual MMSE items on 31 demented, 104 depressed, 21 bipolar, 33 schizophrenic, and 55 substance abuse patients. Demented patients were clearly differentiated from others on orientation, spelling "world" backwards, words recalled, and serial-sevens. Although not specified, I would assume from the mean scores that the demented group fell in the moderate to severe range, which would therefore limit the generalizability of these results. Foreman (1987) found that the MMSE discriminated between cognitively intact and cognitively compromised elderly, with a sensitivity of .82, and a specificity of .80.

Several studies have correlated the MMSE with the WAIS. For example, M. F. Folstein et al. (1975), for a mixed sample of 26 patients, found correlations of the MMSE of .78 for Verbal IQ and .66 for Performance IQ. From a sample of Alzheimer's patients, Farber, Schmitt, and Logue (1988) found a correlation of .83 between the MMSE and the WAIS-R Full Scale IQ. In a study of 37 neurological patients, Dick et al. (1984) found somewhat lower correlations for Verbal ($r = .45$) and Performance ($r = .58$) IQs.[8]

Research on the MMSE in relationship to neuropsychological testing has been less encouraging. Faustman, Moses, and Csernansky (1990) employed the Luria-Nebraska Neuropsychological Battery as a criterion measure for evaluating the efficacy of the MMSE. They found in a study of 90 psychiatric inpatients that the MMSE identified only approximately 20% of patients with clear evidence of cognitive impairment. McBride-Houtz (1993) administered the MMSE and other MSE measures (i.e., CCSE and NCSE) to 52 geriatric patients with the Halstead-Reitan Neuropsychological Test Battery as the criterion measure. A moderate correlation of –.60 was found between the MMSE and the global performance score of the Halstead-Reitan (i.e., General Neuropsychological Deficit Scale [Reitan & Wolfson, 1988]). However, categorizations of impaired and unimpaired subjects by the Halstead-Reitan yielded a disappointing sensitivity of 20.0%. Consistent with earlier research, all mildly impaired patients were missed by the MMSE. One

---

[8]Patients with marked cognitive impairment were excluded from this component of the study, which may alter the correlations.

disadvantage of the study was that nearly every patient was impaired (50 of 52); therefore, estimates for specificity are inadequately represented.

Christensen et al. (1991) performed a meta-analysis on 12 studies of the MMSE. They found slightly higher mean effect sizes for the MMSE in differentiating between demented and nondemented subjects than several other MSEs and many neuropsychological measures. These data provide strong evidence of criterion-related validity for the MMSE, including ratings of severity (mild, mild–moderate, and severe).

Several conclusions can be drawn regarding the validity of the MMSE from studies on neuropathology and intelligence. First, the MMSE appears to be related to brain pathology, although the nature of this relationship is not well understood. Second, at least in cognitively impaired populations, the MMSE is correlated with intelligence.[9] With respect to documented brain damage, the MMSE does not appear to be clinically useful. Localized lesions and lesions in the right hemisphere are unlikely to result in impaired scores on the MMSE.

The MMSE is a brief and highly reliable screen for cognitive functions. While influenced by educational status (Uhlmann & Larson, 1991), validity data suggest that the MMSE may be effective in the assessment of patients with moderate to severe dementia. Although imprecise, the MMSE may also yield valuable information on course of dementia and treatment outcome. The danger with the MMSE, as with other first-generation cognitive MSEs, is the assumption that "normal" scores are, by themselves, evidence that patients are cognitively intact.

Modified MMSE. Mayeux, Stern, Rosen, and Leventhal (1981) expanded the MMSE to include additional items for language, memory, and praxis. They added digit-span, naming 5 presidents, identifying 10 picture objects from the Boston Naming Test (Kaplan, Goodglass, & Weintraub, 1976), an additional sentence, and a geometric figure. They found that the modified MMSE was correlated with the severity of Parkinson's disease ($r = -.43$). Potential confounds for the modified MMSE were depression, as measured by the Beck Depression Inventory ($r = -.33$), and years of education ($r = .36$). No reliability has been established for the modified MMSE. In summary, I see no advantage to this expanded version, which remains inadequately validated.

Other modified versions include a shortened version of the MMSE for epidemiological studies (Margaziner, Bassett, & Hebel, 1987) and clinical practice (Galasko et al., 1990). Teng and Chui (1987) added four test items to the MMSE and were able to achieve high consistency of interscorer agreement. As with the Mayeux version, these alternative versions have not been thoroughly tested and cross-validated. Clinicians should consider either the use of the original version or its inclusion in the CAMCOG, a well-validated, second-generation MSE described in a later section of this chapter.

Spanish MMSE. Several studies have investigated the clinical utility of Spanish versions of the MMSE. The MMSE was originally translated as part of the Epidemiological Catchment Area program (see Burnam, Karno, Hough, Escobar, & Forsythe, 1983; Karno, Burnam, Escobar, Hough, & Eaton, 1983). Escobar

---

[9]Because of the MMSE's ceiling effect, we would not expect this association with unimpaired subjects.

et al. (1986) administered the MMSE to 1,244 Mexican-Americans. They found that three orientation items (season, state, and county), two memory and calculation items (serial-sevens and spelling "world" backwards), and one language item (repeating a sentence) appeared ethnically biased.[10]

Bird, Canino, Rubio-Stipec, & Shrout (1987) conducted a large-scale Puerto Rican study of the MMSE. They modified the MMSE to make it more appropriate to the Puerto Rican culture; modifications included seasons of the year, orientation (i.e., Puerto Rico has no states or counties), and several linguistic changes.

Several studies based on the DIS, which incorporates the MMSE, suggest a moderate level of agreement for the MMSE as a general measure of cognitive impairment. For example, research by Burnam et al. (1983) suggested a high test-retest reliability for organic brain syndrome on Spanish-Spanish administrations ($\kappa = .88$) and English-English administrations ($\kappa = .79$), but low levels of agreement for Spanish-English administrations ($\kappa = .32$). These results reflect only indirectly on the MMSE, since other components of the DIS also address organicity. More germane is a study by Canino and her associates (Canino, Bird, Shrout, Rubio-Stipec, Bravo, Martinez, Sesman, Guzman, Guevara, & Costas, 1987) in which cognitive impairment was reevaluated (Spanish-Spanish administrations) with a moderate reliability ($\kappa = .69$).

Malingering on the MMSE. An important consideration in some clinical settings is whether the patient is distorting his/her presentation. Schretlen, Brandt, Krafft, and Van Gorp (1991) examined the MMSE scores of two patients suspected of feigning cognitive impairment. These patients exhibited an ability to produce impaired scores ($M = 21.0$) and were unlikely to be differentiated from cognitively impaired groups.

Powell (1991) asked 40 mental health workers to feign schizophrenia on the MMSE and compared their responses to an equal number of schizophrenic inpatients. She found that the majority of feigners scored 20 or less on the MMSE and were distinguishable on the basis on orientation, recall, and total scores. Malingerers appeared to make a greater proportion of errors on relatively easy items than did their inpatient counterparts. Powell devised a scoring procedure based on gross errors and absurd responses for differentiating the malingerers from schizophrenics on the MMSE. Despite its promise, this study of MMSE has limited clinical applicability since the response patterns of demented patients (e.g., confabulated answers) are not known.

Cognitive Capacity Screening Examination (CCSE)

Jacobs et al. (1977) developed the CCSE as a more extensive MSE than its predecessors (MSQ, SPMSQ, and MMSE). While the CCSE covered similar cognitive tasks (orientation, concentration, serial-sevens, repetition, verbal concept formation, and short-term recall), it places a greater emphasis on the recall of numbers (forwards and backwards) and simple calculations. Patients are questioned regarding antonyms (three simple items) and similarities (also three

---

[10]Items were deemed to be ethnically biased if Spanish-speaking respondents scored significantly lower than English-speaking subjects. Of course, other factors (e.g., unknown sampling biases) could contribute to these differences.

items). Although the CCSE is described as a 30-item MSE, sequential subtractions for serial-sevens are counted as six items. One major difference between the CCSE and other cognitive MSEs is that the CCSE does not include any items from long-term memory based on either personal history or common knowledge.

Reliability. The original study by Jacobs et al. (1977) did not include any formal estimate of reliability, but simply the overall concordance of three clinicians and six subjects. Haddad and Coffman (1987) reported excellent test-retest reliabilities ($r = .87$) on 49 elderly subjects at 1-week intervals. In a previously cited study, Foreman (1987) found a high internal consistency for the CCSE ($\alpha = .97$).

A brief report by Carnes, Gunter-Hunt, and Rodgers (1987) on 27 elderly patients documented variations in the CCSE when readministered by the same clinician after a 2-hour interval; nearly every subject manifested changes in scores on both short-term memory (88.9%) and calculation tasks (100.0%).[11] This lack of stability in CCSE scores, while possibly reflecting diurnal variations in the elderly, does raise questions regarding test-retest reliability. Carnes et al. do not provide any formal estimates of reliability.

Validity. In the original study, Jacobs et al. (1977) compared the performances on the CCSE for 24 patients with organic disorders to 25 psychiatric inpatients and 25 hospital staff. They found a high sensitivity (95.8%) and specificity (98.5%). Nelson et al. (1986) summarized three additional studies of the CCSE's validity. For example, Kaufman, Weinberger, Strain, and Jacobs (1979) examined 59 neurological inpatients and found good sensitivity (72.7%) and excellent specificity (92.3%). Omer, Foldes, Toby, and Menczel (1983) found that all organic patients scored below the cutting score (< 20), as did 28% of patients without organic disorders and 18% of community controls. Webster, Scott, Nunn, McNeer, and Varnell (1984), in a study of 62 VA patients, found that the CCSE had poor sensitivity (48.8%) and excellent specificity (91.3%). Consistent with research on the MMSE, they found the CCSE to be ineffective with right hemisphere lesions.

Recent research has provided empirical support for the CCSE. Haddad and Coffman (1987) studied 87 elderly psychiatric patients with significant differences between those who were cognitively impaired and those who were not; they established a sensitivity of 100% and specificity of 59.4%. Roughly two-thirds of patients with functional disorders also scored in the cognitively impaired range. Hershey, Jaffe, Greenough, and Yang (1987) evaluated 13 patients with vascular dementia, 19 who were marginal for the diagnosis, and 31 without dementia. They found for the CCSE both high sensitivity (84.6%) and specificity (87.1%) as well as a moderate correlation ($r = -.60$) with a measure of functional abilities (Functional Abilities Questionnaire [Pfeiffer, Kurosaki, Harrah, Chance, & Filos, 1982]). Meyers, Rogers, McClintic, Mortel, and Lofti (1989) provided indirect evidence of a relationship between changes in CCSE scores and concomitant changes in quantitative cerebral blood flow.

---

[11]Retesting by the same clinician may improve estimates of consistency; interestingly, changes were evenly divided between those who improved on short-term memory and calculations (50.1%) and those who deteriorated (49.9%).

Several studies have compared the diagnostic efficacy of the CCSE with that of other MSEs, often with inconsistent results. Folks and Rabin (1985) asserted that the CCSE was not superior to nonstandardized MSEs. Their conclusion was based on similar base rates in different samples and, therefore, offers no empirical justification for this assertion. Schwamm et al. (1987) found that the CCSE was inferior to the NCSE in accurately classifying 30 neurological patients (i.e., 43.3% vs. 93.3%). In contrast, Foreman (1987) concluded that the CCSE was superior to SPMSQ and MMSE in a previously reported study of 66 inpatients. Foreman found that the CCSE had perfect agreement with clinical diagnosis, with a sensitivity and specificity of 100%. Strain et al. (1988) evaluated 97 medical inpatients on the CCSE and the MMSE; their results suggested a strong correlation between the two measures ($r = .85$); the CCSE manifested a moderate sensitivity of 54% and good specificity of 85% when compared to psychiatric diagnosis.

McBride-Houtz (1993) conducted the only study of the CCSE in comparison to a neuropsychological test battery (Halstead–Reitan). In her previously cited study, she reported a moderate correlation of $-.62$ between the CCSE and a global measure of impairment on the Halstead–Reitan. As for the MMSE, she found a very modest sensitivity rate of 22.0%. A higher cutting score (≤ 24) improved the sensitivity to 56%.

In conclusion, the CCSE appears to be a worthwhile screening measure with validity comparable to that of the MMSE. The CCSE offers a broader sampling of verbal abilities than previously described MSEs, although these additional items do not appear to add incremental validity. Psychologists may feel comfortable using either the MMSE or the CCSE in a brief screen for cognitive impairment. As previously noted, the absence of observed deficits cannot be equated with normal functioning, given the very modest sensitivity rates.

Cambridge Cognitive Examination (CAMCOG)

Roth et al. (1986) devised the CAMDEX for the comprehensive assessment of the elderly through diagnostic interviews, collateral interviews, medical procedures, and a structured interview for cognitive dysfunction referred to as the CAMCOG (Cambridge Cognitive Examination). As summarized in Table 2.2, the CAMCOG supplements the MMSE with additional items to assess memory functions and the capacity to learn new information. Greater coverage is given to such cognitive abilities as language, abstract thinking, and calculation. One goal of the CAMCOG was the creation of a measure that could accurately evaluate mild dementias that are often missed by the earlier MSEs (see Reisberg et al., 1982).

Reliability. The original reliability study on 40 geriatric patients suggested high concordance rates for dementia (95.7%), with exceptionally high interrater reliabilities for individual items (median ϕ coefficient = .90). One notable exception was the CAMCOG item for naming different animals (ϕ coefficient = .30), which needs a refinement of its scoring. When fine distinctions are attempted with respect to subcategories of dementia, a moderate level of agreement (ϕ coefficient = .63) was achieved.

Hendrie et al. (1988) also found a high interrater reliability in a videotaped study of 40 elderly psychiatric patients and 15 age-matched controls. Phi coefficients for the CAMCOG ranged from .50 to 1.00, with the large majority (78.3%)

of individual items exceeding .75. The overall correlation between CAMCOG ratings was also high (r = .88).

Validity. The CAMCOG appears to be highly accurate in distinguishing demented patients from elderly depressives and controls (see Table 2.2). In the original validation, the CAMCOG showed evidence of convergent validity with a standardized dementia score and clinician ratings. An important but supplementary finding was that demented patients did not have an accurate appraisal of their memory dysfunction. O'Conner (1990) concluded that the CAMDEX, including CAMCOG, may be the measure of choice with mild dementia because of its diagnostic accuracy.

Hendrie et al. (1988), in the previously described study, compared CAMCOG scores to the Newcastle Dementia Scale (Blessed et al., 1968) and clinical diagnosis. The CAMCOG evidenced a moderately high correlation with the Newcastle score (r = -.77). They also found significant differences in CAMCOG scores among demented, depressed, and elderly controls.

The CAMDEX has been utilized in several epidemiological studies (Brayne & Calloway, 1989, 1990; O'Conner et al., 1989) to assess dementia in the elderly. Brayne and Calloway (1990) reported that different CAMCOG cutting scores produced notable variations in the prevalence of dementia when compared to the CAMCOG diagnosis. At best, these results would suggest the integration of clinical data in diagnosing dementia and caution against the overreliance on any single measure.

Cultural influences on the CAMCOG have not been adequately explored. Nearly all the research has been conducted on British populations, although Hendrie et al. (1988) found comparable results on an American sample. Apparently, a Spanish translation of the CAMDEX exists (see Lopez, Llinas, & Vidal, 1990), although I have been unable to secure a description of this research in English.

In summary, the CAMCOG appears to be a superior MSE for the evaluation of cognitive dysfunction for English-speaking patients. In cases where depression is suspected, the entire CAMDEX can be administered to improve diagnostic accuracy. Although further validation would be welcomed, the CAMCOG, as it now stands, appears to have a high level of interrater reliability, and sufficient criterion-based validity to warrant its clinical application.

Neurobehavioral Cognitive Status Examination (NCSE)

Kiernan, Mueller, Langston, and Van Dyke (1987) developed the NCSE as a cognitive MSE to assess mental abilities in five areas: language, constructions, memory, calculations, and reasoning. Recognizing the relatively low sensitivity rates of the MMSE and the CCSE, the NCSE was designed to measure specific abilities on items of graded difficulty. Including screening items, the NCSE consists of 64 items, most of which are scored as passed/failed. Unlike other MSEs, the NCSE includes a subtest called "Design Constructions" that is an analogue to the WAIS-R block designs. The NCSE was devised to screen for specific cognitive dysfunctions as well as those of mild severity, which might otherwise be overlooked by the first generation of cognitive MSEs (Schmidtt, Ranseen, & DeKosky,

1989). As noted in Table 2.2, 10 scales are computed to screen for cognitive impairment.

Kiernan et al. (1987) provided standardization data based on 60 unimpaired adults (age range = 20 – 66) and 59 geriatric volunteers (age range = 70 – 92) and found slight decrements in functioning for the elderly. Unfortunately, Kiernan et al. did not report whether differences occurred due to education, race, or gender. Moreover, these numbers appear to be quite small for the purposes of standardization.

Reliability. Kiernan et al. (1987) did not report reliability data. They stated that most of the standardization sample had nearly perfect scores, which would artificially inflate reliability estimates.[12] Obviously, tests of reliability with impaired populations (e.g., cognitively impaired and psychiatrically disordered) are needed to assess both interrater and test-retest reliabilities.

Validity. Schwamm, VanDyke, Kiernan, Merrin, and Mueller (1987) conducted the original validation study of the NCSE on 30 patients with documented central nervous system lesions. The investigators administered in a counterbalanced order the MMSE, CCSE, and NCSE. Consistent with other research, detection rates were modest for the MMSE (53.3%) and CCSE (43.3%). In stark contrast, Schwamm et al. found that 28 of the 30 patients (93.3%) were correctly identified by the NCSE. The scoring criteria on the NCSE for cognitive impairment was any low score on one or more scales. What could not be determined by this study was the matter of specificity. Using the liberal criteria of this study, what proportion of adult controls, cognitively intact elderly, and psychiatric patients would be misclassified with organic impairment? In other words, this study does not establish the discriminability of the NCSE among relevant criterion groups.

Relatively few studies have addressed the validity of the NCSE. Meek, Clark, and Solana (1989) examined test results for the Luria-Nebraska, Trail-Making Test, and NCSE on 34 inpatient substance abusers. Using the screening test of the Luria-Nebraska as a point of comparison, the NCSE had a sensitivity of 84.6% and a specificity of 47.4%. These percentages, however, are likely to be misleading, since the complete Luria-Nebraska was not administered. Implications of a study by Kewman, Vaishampayan, Zald, and Han (1991) include the possibility that medical patients may be miscategorized by the NCSE. In their study, Kewman et al. excluded patients diagnosed with neurocognitive deficits or currently receiving narcotic analgesics; they found that approximately one-third of outpatients with musculoskeletal pain were tested as impaired on the NCSE. Of course, the possibility exists that some of these patients had undiagnosed organic disorders. In both studies, the NCSE appeared to assess more patients with mild cognitive impairment than had been previously believed. Naturally, the difficulty lies in knowing how to interpret these findings. Neither study has made adequate use of appropriate measures of criterion validity (intelligence testing, standardized memory assessment, or neuropsychological test batteries).

Fields, Fulop, Sachs, Strain, and Fillit (1992; cited in McBride-Houtz, 1993) compared NSCE results to psychiatric judgment of cognitive impairment on geriatric inpatients. The NCSE appeared to "overdiagnose" cognitive impairment.

---

[12]This reasoning is not necessarily true, as restricted ranges may constrain correlations.

As observed by McBride-Houtz (1993), however, clinical judgment is hardly a gold standard against which to assess cognitive impairment.

McBride-Houtz (1993) examined the clinical usefulness of the NCSE in comparison with other MSE measures (i.e., the MMSE and CCSE) in a sample of 52 older adults with suspected cognitive impairment. Employing the General Neuropsychological Deficit Scale from the Halstead–Reitan as a criterion measure, she found that the NCSE outperformed both the MMSE and CCSE. More specifically, she found that the NCSE correlated with the overall impairment at −.67 and had a sensitivity of 82.0%. As previously noted, the availability of only two unimpaired subjects militated against establishing specificity. Interestingly, one NCSE scale, Constructions, evidenced the highest correlation with overall impairment (r = −.69).

In conclusion, the NCSE has considerable promise in its efforts to measure discrete forms of cognitive impairment. Although touted by some neuropsychologists (e.g., Tucker & Neppe, 1991), further validation would be helpful before it is routinely implemented in clinical practice. At the present time, the NCSE could certainly be employed as a screening measure for cognitive dysfunction. What appears to be relatively untested is NCSE's specificity; only one study has addressed this issue (Fields et al., 1992), and that yielded poor results. However, as a research measure, the NCSE offers considerable potential in differentiating dementia from other disorders.

Other Cognitive MSEs

The present coverage of cognitive MSEs is necessarily selective, given the array of closely related measures. Many lesser-used MSEs are reported in the literature (e.g., Barrett & Gleser, 1987; Isaacs & Walkey, 1963; Katzman et al., 1983; Whelihan, Lesher, Kleban, & Granick, 1984). In the paragraphs below, I provide a very brief summary of additional MSEs that may have particular merit in certain clinical settings.

Blessed Dementia Scale. The BDS (Blessed et al., 1968) has considerable overlap with other cognitive MSEs (Gurland et al., 1987). The BDS appears to discriminate between demented and nondemented samples (see Christensen et al., 1991) and is likely to be most useful in Great Britain because of its British content (i.e., naming monarch and prime minister).

Halifax Mental Status Scale. Fisk, Braha, Walker, and Gray (1991) devised an 11-item Canadian MSE that parallels the BDS with the exception of its Canadian content. The Halifax asks subjects to identify the capital of Canada, its prime minister, and the premier of the province. Intended for English-speaking Canadians, the Halifax scale has good test-retest reliabilities for stable patients at both 2- and 12-month intervals and appears to discriminate between demented and nondemented samples.

Mattis Dementia Rating Scale. Mattis (1976) developed an extensive MSE for the assessment of attention, initiation and perseveration, construction, conceptualization, and memory. Studies (see Nelson et al., 1986) have reported (a) good internal consistency and test-retest reliability and (b) moderate correlations with indices of organic pathology (e.g., Merskey et al., 1980). Most recently, Christensen et al. (1991) performed a meta-analysis on six studies of Mattis' scale.

They found mean effect sizes comparable to other cognitive MSEs in differentiating between demented and nondemented samples.

Cortical Function Assessment. Herst, Voss, and Waldman (1990) constructed the Cortical Function Assessment (CFA), a 10-item MSE, to (a) address cognitive abilities that are typically overlooked by brief screening measures, and (b) avoid overreliance on orientation and memory. To this end, items assess naming, writing, drawing, and stereognosis. In their initial study, the CFA shows promise with respect to internal consistency ($\alpha = .88$), test-retest reliability ($r = .95$), and correlations with other MSEs (.87 with the SPMSQ, and .92 with the MMSE).

Conclusions Regarding Cognitive MSEs

Psychologists and other mental health professionals must clearly screen clinical populations for memory and other forms of cognitive impairment. In a compelling review, Herrmann (1982) found that there was virtually no relationship between reported memory problems and actual memory impairment. More recent research (e.g., Zelinski, Gilewski, & Anthony-Berstone, 1990) has established, at best, a small association between these two facets of memory. In other words, clinicians can take little comfort in a patient's assertion that his/her memory is intact. Use of a cognitive MSE might well be considered as the first step in the investigation of potential memory dysfunction.

Studies have found cognitive MSEs as useful screens for changes in cognitive status, although these measures are likely to have a ceiling effect in treatment-outcome research. Investigations have documented the natural course of a disorder (e.g., M. F. Folstein et al., 1975; McHugh & M. F. Folstein, 1988), need for institutional placement (e.g., Fisk & Pannill, 1987; Knopman, Kitto, Deinar, & Heiring, 1988), and response to treatment regimens (e.g., Denicoff, Joffe, Lakshmanan, Robbins, & Rubinow, 1990; LaRue, Spar, & Hill, 1986; Thal, Salmon, Lasker, Bower, & Klauber, 1989). Because of their limited range, cognitive MSEs should be used only to document cognitive changes in individuals with moderate to severe dementias. In addition, patients must be screened for functional disorders which may confound these measures (e.g., see Haddad & Coffman, 1987).

Stonier (1974) offered several interesting observations that may reduce the specificity of cognitive MSEs. He found that cognitively intact patients with low MSE scores often demonstrated dramatic improvements on repeat administrations. In other words, cognitively intact patients evidenced learning on MSE items that they had previously missed. In contrast, patients with dementia typically evidenced no improvement even after four administrations. In applying these findings, psychologists may be able to improve their overall accuracy simply through the readministration of a cognitive MSE.

Clinical Applications

Comprehensive MSEs

Clinical applications of comprehensive MSEs are currently limited. Certain measures, such as the MSE Checklist and the NC-MSE, may assist psychologists in standardizing their coverage of cognitive abilities and psychopathology. The question remains, however, whether a somewhat larger investment of time for a full diagnostic interview (e.g., DIS or SADS) would not make more sense, based on the improved reliability and accuracy of diagnosis. In deciding on the utility of clinical measures, the key question is always, "Compared to what?" In contrast to an idiosyncratic interview, the MSE Checklist and NC-MSE offer modest advantages in controlling information variance and suggesting the need for further investigations.

The MSER, augmented with standardized clinical inquiries, might be useful in inpatient facilities. Extensive needs for inpatient documentation have continued unabated, fuelled by quality assurance and fears of litigation. With the computerization of some records, perhaps MSERs would allow the systematic evaluation of patients' clinical status. Moreover, comparisons could be made across line staff, with any marked discrepancies referred for thorough evaluations. From a quality assurance perspective, staff's clinical observations could be methodically reviewed, and consistent "outliers" among clinicians themselves could be identified.

The MSER may also be useful in nonclinical settings because of its emphasis of observational data. Paraprofessionals could be trained to make observations but would not need an in-depth knowledge of psychopathology. In many settings, such as correctional facilities, a substantial number of residents have significant psychopathology which may remain undetected and untreated (Teplin, 1984, 1990). The MSER might serve a useful screening function in these settings.

The MMS and its concomitant measures represent the most ambitious attempt to standardize all aspects of assessment and treatment. Its major failing resides in its very modest reliability under optimal testing conditions. As previously summarized, the MMS may serve as a model for data management in complex delivery systems. Perhaps the strongest argument for the use of the MMS is its potential as a screen for noncompliance, aggressive behavior, and suicidal ideation.

The clinical descriptions provided by these measures continue to be useful, despite the emergence of *DSM-IV*. Since these measures are not recommended for diagnostic purposes, comprehensive MSEs can still provide an adequate coverage of the patient's primary symptoms as well as a method of systematizing clinical observations.

First-Generation Cognitive MSEs

The selection of a cognitive MSE is dependent upon several factors: (a) the purpose of the assessment, (b) the use of other clinical measures, and (c) the availability of professional resources. Psychologists must decide whether to use the brief first-generation or the more comprehensive second-generation MSEs. Because of their brevity and user-friendly format, first-generation measures, particularly the MMSE, have gained wide acceptance among psychiatrists. Of the second-generation MSEs, both the CAMCOG and NCSE have distinguished themselves because of the range of clinical data available for them, and because of their diagnostic accuracy.

The first-generation MSEs are highly intercorrelated (e.g., Baldelli, Toschi, Motta, Marra, & Muratori, 1991; Herst et al., 1990; Lautenschlaeger et al., 1986;

Lesher & Whelihan, 1986). This finding is not surprising, given the considerable item overlap among the MSQ, SPMSQ, and MMSE. All three measures have good reliability, although substantially more research has been conducted with the MMSE than with either the MSQ or SPMSQ.

The MMSE is likely to be chosen, as a first-generation MSE, for several reasons (see Table 2.4). First, the MMSE appears to have slightly better clinical utility than other first-generation measures (e.g., see Christensen et al., 1991). Second, the MMSE has wider applications; it is unrestricted by age and is available in a Spanish version. Third, normative data are available for both English and Spanish versions, based on large-scale epidemiological studies. If only 5 minutes are likely to be allotted to screening for moderate to severe dementia, then the MMSE is likely to be the measure of choice.

Table 2.4
Decision Points for the Selection of Cognitive MSEs

Brevity of the screening measure
  Very brief: MSQ, MMSE, and SPMSQ
  Extended: CCSE, CAMCOG, and NCSE

Age restrictions
  Elderly only: MSQ, SPMSQ, CAMCOG
  All adults: MMSE, CCSE, and NCSE

Translations
  Spanish: MMSE and CAMCOG
  Other translations: MMSE and SPMSQ

Response styles
  Malingering: MMSE[a]

---

[a]Research examined its usefulness with feigned schizophrenia but not with dementia.

When in need of a brief screening measure, psychologists may find the cutting score (< 24) on the MMSE to be a useful first step. Many subjects who perform below this score are likely to have a moderate to severe dementia. However, many elderly patients with scores in the 24 to 27 range may also be cognitively impaired (see Jackson & Ramsdell, 1988). I would strongly recommend that psychologists pay closer attention to actual performance on individual items than to any single score. Extrapolating from Rosen and Fox (1986), any of the following should signal the need for further investigation: (a) any problems with orientation, (b) marked problems with serial-sevens (only one or two correct responses), (c) inability to spell "world" backwards, or (d) very poor recall (failure to remember more than one of the three words). Gross failures on any one of these cognitive tasks is likely to differentiate cognitively impaired patients from those with major mental illness.

The next step in the clinical evaluation of patients with poor performance on first-generation MSEs is dependent on the assessment issues. When the emphasis is on the patients' cognitive abilities, the use of intellectual and neuropsychological testing would be useful in suggesting and documenting specific impairments and indicating organic involvement (see Lezak, 1983). When differential diagnosis is paramount, referrals for neurological and neuropsychological consultations are advised.

Second-Generation Cognitive MSEs

All three second-generation MSEs deserve our attention as screening measures for cognitive impairment. The CCSE has been applied in a number of medical settings, often with satisfactory results. Several recent studies (McBride-Houtz, 1993; Schwamm et al., 1987) suggest, however, that the CCSE may have somewhat lower sensitivity than the NCSE.

The CAMCOG is designed for use with elderly populations and provides a systematic approach to assessment that includes the evaluation of functional disorders and medical conditions. The CAMCOG appears to have excellent reliability, even at the symptom level. Since the CAMCOG incorporates the MMSE, clinicians may make comparisons of MMSE scores with treatment response and outcome data. The CAMCOG provides a thorough screening of cognitive capacities and should be useful in the assessment of elderly.

The NCSE differs from other MSEs in its development of 10 specific scales. Inspection of these scales may signal potential impairment that needs further investigation. Its reliability has not been adequately assessed. However, several studies (McBride-Houtz, 1993; Schwamm et al., 1987) suggest that the NCSE has superior discriminability in distinguishing patients with mild cognitive impairment from those who are cognitively intact. Anecdotally, Mueller (1988) reported that the systematic use of the NCSE as a screening measure approximately doubled the cognitive dysfunction detected by psychiatrists in their consultations with medical and surgical patients. What is now needed is the establishment of larger normative samples and the systematic investigation of (a) interrater and test-retest reliability, and (b) specificity rates with impaired populations.

3

Diagnostic Interview Schedule (DIS)

Description, Rationale, and Development

The Diagnostic Interview Schedule (DIS) is a highly structured diagnostic interview designed to enable professional and nonprofessional interviewers to assess current and past episodes of common mental disorders (Helzer & Robins, 1988). The most recent version, the Diagnostic Interview Schedule, Version III–Revised (DIS-III-R; Robins, Helzer, Cottler, & Goldring, 1989) incorporated *DSM-III-R* diagnoses into its structure. A version for the *DSM-IV* named the DIS-IV is currently in preparation, although no timetable has been established for its validation and publication (L. N. Robins, personal communication, February 25, 1994).

The DIS-III-R consists of approximately 470 clinical ratings organized into 24 major categories. Many of the clinical ratings are composed of multiple questions, and some (particularly substance abuse items) require the completion of subcriteria. DIS-III-R items are scored with reference to both clinical relevance and possible etiology. With respect to clinical significance, three gradations are generally employed: 1 for denial of symptom; 2 for subclinical (i.e., so mild as not to require professional help or to interfere with functioning); and 3, 4, and 5 for clinically relevant symptoms. Differences in possible etiology are reflected in ratings of 3 (i.e., explained by medication, drugs, or alcohol), 4 (i.e., explained by physical illness or injury), and 5 (i.e., likely due to a psychiatric disorder). In addition, interviewers are asked to make additional ratings with regards to the onset and recency of symptoms.

Clinical inquiries are read verbatim; unlike semistructured interviews, the DIS-III-R provides no latitude for unstructured questions initiated by the interviewer. A Probe Flow Chart indicates how optional probes should be implemented to ensure accurate clinical ratings. Clinicians are provided with a detailed training manual on how to reliably code the clinical ratings of specific items (Robins, Cottler, & Keating, 1991).

The DIS differs from other diagnostic interviews in several fundamental ways. Unlike most structured interviews, the DIS attempts to identify any organic etiology of specific symptoms; that is, whether a particular symptom has a medical explanation or whether it is due to drugs or alcohol (e.g., Spengler & Wittchen, 1988). In addition, the DIS incorporates a formal assessment of cognitive impairment with the addition of the MMSE (see Chapter 2). Finally, the DIS has retained earlier diagnostic criteria for the *DSM-III*, Feighner (Feighner et al., 1972) and RDC. This feature allows researchers to make direct comparisons across diagnostic systems (see Robins et al., 1991).

The original purpose of the DIS was to assess the current episodes and lifetime prevalence of selected mental disorders (Robins, Helzer, Croughan, & Ratcliff, 1981). The DIS was designed as a research instrument for the extensive epidemiological studies conducted to ascertain the prevalence and incidence of mental disorders throughout the United States through a monumental undertaking by the Epidemiological Catchment Area Program (ECA; Regier et al., 1984). Given the breadth of the ensuing studies, with nearly 10,000 subjects from three research sites alone (Robins et al., 1984), the ECA program was compelled to use lay interviewers with modest training in clinical interviews. Because of its employment of lay interviewers, an important emphasis of the DIS is on the clarity of the structured questions and the simplicity of administration. Beyond its original intent, the DIS has been used in a variety of clinical and research settings by both clinicians and lay interviewers (Helzer & Robins, 1988).

The DIS-III-A (Robins et al., 1985) encompassed 43 *DSM-III* diagnoses. These diagnoses focus on substance abuse and dependence (i.e., alcohol, barbiturates, opioids, cocaine, amphetamines, hallucinogens, cannabis, and tobacco), schizophrenia, mood disorders, anxiety disorders, and a few others. Those disorders were selected for which there was the greatest epidemiological interest and which did not require more clinical expertise than could be expected from lay interviewers. As a result, delusional disorders, dissociative disorders, most organic disorders, most somatoform disorders, most sexual disorders, and nearly all personality disorders (APD is the exception) are not formally evaluated by the DIS.

The initial development of the DIS involved the creation of clinical inquiries that would parallel as closely as possible the *DSM-III* inclusion and exclusion criteria (for a full review of its development, see Robins, 1987; Robins & Helzer, 1991). In the generation of clinical inquiries, the authors modeled questions after those asked by experts (Helzer et al., 1985). Diagnostic interviews with actual patients were transcribed and effective phrasings were gleaned for the DIS inquiries. Moreover, optional probes were fashioned to assess severity and nonpsychiatric reasons for symptom endorsement. Revisions of the DIS inquiries involved pretesting on patient and nonpatient samples and subsequent refinement of problematic questions. These modifications resulted in Version II, on which initial comparisons were made between psychiatrists and lay interviewers (Robins et al., 1982). Additional alterations in the DIS were implemented to improve the clinical inquiries, resulting in Version III. Version III-A (Robins et al., 1985, 1988) incorporated minor changes in wording and allowed interviewers to evaluate the recency of symptoms. An important consideration in the validation of the DIS is that some studies (e.g., Helzer et al., 1985) combine more than one version, thereby confounding interpretation. Most recently, the DIS-III-R included five additional diagnoses, addressing melancholic depressive episodes, somatoform pain syndrome, and several additional substance abuse disorders.

Several computerized versions of the DIS have been developed to provide for self administrations. One argument favoring this format (see Blouin, Perez, & Blouin, 1988) is the reduction of information variance by the elimination of clinician variability in the rating of responses.[1] Several variations (see Blouin et al., 1988; Griest et al., 1984; Mathisen, Evans, & Meyers, 1987) are interactive programs that provide the necessary branching and probes in response to patients' answers. A limitation of these programs is that they do not cover all DIS diagnoses. In contrast, Wyndrowe (1987) offers a very different computerized DIS, in which a lay interviewer has access to a computer terminal and conducts the interview following the format and questions presented on the screen.

An abbreviated paper-and-pencil version of the DIS (DISSA or DIS Self-Administered; Kovess & Fournier, 1990) that covers depressive disorders, anxiety disorders, and alcoholism is also available. The justification for this very circumscribed version of the DIS is that the selected disorders are those most frequently found in nonreferred community samples. As discussed below, the DISSA may have clinical value in screening community subjects for undiagnosed mental disorders.

One notable advantage of the DIS is that it has been translated into Spanish and Chinese. Of particular interest with the Spanish versions is a cultural awareness of the heterogeneity of Hispanic patients, with systematic comparisons of Mexican-Americans, Mexicans, and Puerto Ricans (see Anduaga, Forteza, & Lira, 1991). The cross-cultural applications of the DIS will be discussed below with reference to its generalizability.

Validation of the DIS

An important facet of the DIS is its concerted attempt to establish clinical utility with nonprofessional or lay interviewers. This emphasis, inherited from its epidemiological origins, places a singular burden of the DIS's validation particularly with respect to its diagnostic reliability.

Diagnostic Reliability

The primary reliability studies have tested the reproducibility of DIS diagnoses from lay interviewers to psychiatrists (see Table 3.1). The basic paradigm has been a test-retest design with initial lay-administered DIS interviews followed at various intervals (6 weeks – 12 months) with psychiatrist-administered interviews.

The principal studies of reliability, as reported in Table 3.1 have yielded mixed results. Although Robins et al. (1981) were able to achieve a moderate level of reliability (median κ = .67) with Version II of the DIS, subsequent investigators have been much less successful in establishing test-retest reliability. In Helzer's original and follow-up studies (Helzer et al., 1985; Helzer, Spitznagel, & McEnvoy, 1987) and the research by Vandiver and Sheer (1991), the median kappa coefficients were very modest (i.e., in the .37 – .46 range). As noted in

---

[1]Of course, the counterargument is that a self-administered DIS must rely upon the patient's interpretation of questions, which may also confound information variance.

Table 3.1
General Reliability Studies of the Diagnostic Interview Schedule (DIS)

Study	Agreement
Robins, Helzer, Croughan, & Ratcliff (1981) Test-retest design was used (interval not specified) with a randomized order for lay and psychiatric interviews. The sample was 157 patients preselected on diagnosis and 60 nonpatients.	Lifetime diagnoses: $\kappa = .67$
V. Hesselbrock, Stabenau, M. Hesselbrock, Mirkin, & Meyer (1982) Interrater reliabilities were based on videotaped interviews with professional and lay interviewers/raters. The sample was 42 inpatients from an alcohol treatment unit.	Lifetime diagnoses: $M \kappa = .95$[a]
Helzer et al. (1985) Test-retest design was used with a 6-week interval; format was lay interviewers followed by psychiatrists. The sample was 370 patients preselected on 11 diagnoses.	Lifetime diagnoses: $\kappa = .43$; $Y = .63$
Helzer, Spitznagel, & McEnvoy (1987) Test-retest design was used with a 12-month interval; format was lay interviewers followed by psychiatrists. The sample was 370 patients preselected on 11 diagnoses.	Lifetime diagnoses: $\kappa = .37$
Vandiver & Sheer (1991) Test-retest design was used with a 9-month interval on modified DIS (eliminated schizophrenia, mania, organic disorders, and other disorders believed to be infrequent); the same lay interviewers were used for both administrations. The sample was 486 college freshmen.	Current diagnoses: $\kappa = .46$; $Y = .69$. Lifetime diagnoses: $\kappa = .43$; $Y = .63$

Note. κ = unweighted kappas; Y = Yule's Y. Except where otherwise noted, median statistics are reported.
[a]The overall kappa is probably inflated by the prior knowledge that nearly all patients were alcoholic.

Chapter 1, some investigators favor Yule's *Y* as a coefficient of agreement that is less sensitive to skewed distributions found with uncommon diagnoses. When Yule's *Y* is employed, the reliability estimates are at a moderate level. Interestingly, Helzer et al. (1985) found that much of the disagreement involved borderline cases in which the patient marginally met or did not meet the diagnostic criteria. In other words, psychologists should have much greater confidence in their diagnostic reliability when the patient substantially exceeds the minimum inclusion criteria.

V. Hesselbrock, Stabenau, M. Hesselbrock, Mirkin, and Meyer (1982) conducted a study of DIS interrater reliability based on videotapes of 42 inpatients residing at an alcohol treatment unit. They found almost perfect agreement (*M* κ = .95), although the numbers may be somewhat inflated since only nine disorders were represented and clinicians had foreknowledge of alcoholism, which constituted 41.2% of the diagnoses. Nevertheless, interrater reliabilities evidenced higher levels of agreement than test-retest studies.[2] This discrepancy is probably explained by the fact that test-retest studies examine both information and criterion variance, while interrater reliabilities are limited to criterion variance.

One important limitation of the above studies is their coverage of possible DIS diagnoses. In assessing the reliability of the DIS, several prominent disorders have not been formally assessed. For example, eating disorders and psychosexual disorders were not examined. Therefore, the DIS has limited clinical usefulness in cases where these diagnoses are suspected.

Several circumscribed studies have examined the test-retest reliability of specific DIS disorders (see Table 3.2). For example, Wells, Burnam, Leake, and Robins (1988) found a relatively modest level of diagnostic agreement for depression with a median kappa of .57, although this level of agreement may have been reduced by the nature of the follow-up interviews (telephone vs. face-to-face). Farrer, Florio, Bruce, Leaf, and Weissman (1989) found sex differences, with depressed females having greater consistency in reporting the onset of major depression than their male counterparts. Finally, Bushnell, Wells, Hornblow, Oakley-Browne, and Joyce (1990) established a moderate level of test-retest reliability for bulimic syndromes (median Yule's *Y* = .66).

Symptom Reliability. An alternative to diagnostic reliability is the examination of reliability estimates for symptom ratings. The reproducibility of symptom ratings is indispensable in providing an accurate description of symptomatology and in measuring changes due to the course of the disorder or response to a treatment regimen. Helzer et al. (1985) found a median correlation of positive symptoms by diagnosis of .76.[3] Wells et al. (1988) found that many depressive symptoms were reliably assessed; symptoms that were particularly problematic (i.e., κ < .40) included the following: (a) moving all the time, (b) interest in sex low, (c) tired out, and (d) thoughts slow. With reference to onset and duration of

---

[2]Insufficient data are presented to compute kappas with alcoholism excluded. However, more than half the DIS diagnoses were disorders other than alcoholism; therefore, an *M* kappa of .95 could not be achieved without a very high concordance rate among nonalcoholic disorders.

[3]Please note that these correlations only partially address the issue; the researchers did not report the correlations for each symptom, but merely the total number of inclusion criteria endorsed.

Table 3.2
Reliability Studies on Specific Diagnoses with the Diagnostic Interview Schedule (DIS)

Study	Agreement
Wells, Burnham, Leake, & Robins (1988) Test-retest design was used with a 3-month interval; format was standard interview followed by telephone interview. The sample was 230 community subjects prescreened to ensure that approximately 50% had depressive symptoms.	Depression: $\kappa = .57$. Depressive symptoms: $\kappa = .49$
Farrer, Florio, Bruce, Leaf, & Weissman (1989) Test-retest design was used with 12-month interval in the majority of cases; the sample was 335 patients with major depression.	Onset of Depression: $ICC = .48$ (males); $ICC = .81$ (females)
Bushnell, Wells, Hornblow, Oakley-Browne, & Joyce (1990) Test-retest design was used with maximum of a 4-week interval; format was lay interviewers followed by clinician. The sample was 259 community subjects preselected for possible depression, alcoholism, or bulimia.	Bulimia: $Y = .66$

Note. κ = unweighted kappas; ICC = intraclass coefficients. Except where otherwise noted, median statistics are reported.

critical symptoms (e.g., delusions/hallucinations, depression, and phobias), Wittchen et al. (1989) found surprisingly high levels of agreement, with most intraclass coefficients exceeding .70. While these studies are very promising, additional research is needed that directly addresses the interrater reliability of individual symptoms.

Reliability of Self-Administered Versions. Two studies have examined the test-retest reliability of self-administered forms of the DIS (see Table 3.3). Blouin et al. (1988) administered a computerized DIS on two occasions with a 1-week interval. Although they achieved kappa coefficients comparable to those for a standard DIS interviews (see Helzer et al., 1985; Vandiver & Sheer, 1991), what conclusions should be drawn from this research is unclear. In other words, because we do not have any direct comparisons between the computerized DIS and the standard DIS, we do not know to what degree, if any, validation of the DIS can confidently be applied to the computerized DIS.

Kovess and Fournier (1990) tested a paper-and-pencil version of the DIS in comparison to standard administrations. They found that reliability estimates for both psychiatrists and lay interviewers were similar to those found with repeated standard administrations. Several caveats must be borne in mind: (a) preselection of patients with targeted disorders may inflate estimates of agreement on the paper-and-pencil version, and (b) the self-administered version is limited to six disorders. Despite these caveats, the paper-and-pencil version may have circumscribed clinical utility.

Reliability of Spanish Versions. The three available studies would suggest that Spanish versions of the DIS have adequate reliability (see Table 3.3). Anduaga et al. (1991) conducted a small study of 15 psychiatric patients whose DIS interviews were videotaped. The tapes were independently rated by five lay interviewers, who achieved high levels of agreement (ICC = .89). The design of this study is unusual, since it does not compare lay interviewers to clinicians. Typically in DIS reliability studies, investigators attempt to demonstrate that nonprofessionals have a satisfactory level of agreement with mental health professionals.

Canino, Bird, Shrout, Rubio-Stipec, Bravo, Martinez, Sesman, Guzman, Guevara, and Costas (1987) administered a Spanish version of the DIS twice in a single day to a mixed sample of psychiatric patients and community subjects. They established a moderate level of agreement between clinicians and lay interviewers (median κ = .59) which compares favorably to English versions of the DIS.

Burnam, Karno, Hough, Escobar, and Forsythe (1983) conducted the most elegant study of the DIS Spanish version. They examined test-retest reliabilities for 61 monolingual and 90 bilingual Hispanic outpatients. Moderate reliabilities were established for the Spanish-English as well as the Spanish-Spanish administrations. Their findings also suggest moderate comparability between Spanish and English versions. Unlike most other reliability studies, the Burnham et al. effort did not preselect patients across DIS disorders. If they had been more adequately represented, some uncommon disorders might have had higher kappas.

In summary, Spanish versions of the DIS compare favorably to the standard English version. A particular advantage of the DIS over other diagnostic interviews is the care devoted to establishing the reliability of these Spanish versions. While other versions of the DIS, such as the Chinese version (see Hwu, Yeh, & Chang, 1986), have been examined for their concordance with psychiatric diagnoses, no formal estimates of their reliability are available.

Criterion-Related Validity

The bulk of DIS validational studies employ, as an external criterion, the clinical decision-making of experienced psychiatrists, who base their diagnoses on traditional interviews. This method of validation is sometimes referred to as "bootstrapping" (Robins et al., 1981) to describe a procedure using one imprecise method to improve the classificatory accuracy of another.[4] Psychologists should bear in mind the fundamental limitations of *DSM-III-R* diagnoses, as outlined in Chapter 1, in their critical review of the DIS's validity.

Original Studies. Robins et al. (1981) modeled the validation of the DIS after their earlier efforts on the Renard Diagnostic Interview (RDI; Helzer, Robins, Croughan, & Welner, 1981). By employing four recently trained psychiatrists as the gold standard, Robins and her colleagues examined the sensitivity and specificity (see Table 1.6 for a review of these terms) of the DIS across

---

[4]Bootstrapping operations are sometimes referred to as "procedural validity"; this latter term may create the false impression of a sophisticated methodology.

Table 3.3
Reliability Studies on Alternate Versions of the Diagnostic Interview Schedule (DIS)

Study	Agreement
Blouin, Perez, & Blouin (1988) Computerized version was administered twice in a test-retest design at a 1-week interval; the sample was 80 patients and 20 community subjects.	Current diagnosis: $\kappa = .49$
Kovess & Fournier (1990) Self-administered version of the DIS that is limited to mood and anxiety disorders and alcoholism was used. Test-retest design had maximum interval of 2 months; format was self-administered version followed by interview version. The sample was 237 community subjects preselected for the possible diagnoses.	Self-administered and psychiatrist: $\kappa = .45$; self-administered and lay interviewer: $\kappa = .40$
Burnam, Karno, Hough, Escobar, & Forsythe (1983) Test-retest design was used with 1-week interval by lay interviewers; monolingual subjects were administered Spanish version twice while bilingual subjects were administered both the Spanish and English versions. The sample was 151 Hispanic outpatients.	Lifetime diagnoses: Spanish to Spanish: $\kappa = .54$; Spanish to English: $\kappa = .48$
Canino, Bird, Shrout, Rubio-Stipec, Bravo, Martinez, Sesman, Guzman, Guevara, & Costas (1987b) Spanish version of the DIS was administered twice on the same day; format was random, with lay interviewers compared to psychiatrists. The sample was 60 community subjects and 129 outpatients preselected to cover representative diagnoses.	Current diagnosis: $\kappa = .59$
Anduaga, Forteza, & Lira (1991) Spanish version of the DIS was used in a videotaped study of interrater reliability; 5 lay interviewers rated a sample of 15 psychiatric patients.	Current diagnosis: M ICC $= .89$

Note. κ = unweighted kappas; ICC = intraclass coefficients. Except where otherwise noted, median statistics are reported.

diagnoses. They found a moderate level of sensitivity (range = 56 – 100%, median = 75%) with apparently higher specificity.[5] Based on their clinical interviews, the psychiatrists doubted the validity of DIS diagnoses in only a very small proportion of cases (2.7%).

The original investigators conducted subsequent studies of DIS validity which are reported in Helzer et al. (1985, 1987). Helzer et al. (1985) employed three psychiatrists to conduct most of their clinical interviews. As before, the design is contaminated by the fact that these interviewers also completed the DIS and were unavoidably influenced by its results. Not unexpectedly, when the same psychiatrist completed both the DIS and the interview, the level of agreement was nearly perfect. Somewhat less contaminated was the comparison of the lay interviewers' DIS results with the psychiatric interviews. Under these conditions, the median sensitivity was 44% (range = 20 – 72%) and the median specificity was 95% (range = 90 – 99%). The best-case interpretation would ignore the fact that these psychiatrists were influenced by their own DIS administrations (i.e., since they asked the same questions as lay interviewers, rates of agreement should be higher). Even then, the DIS diagnosis is missing the majority of the *DSM-III* disorders. At best, psychologists can feel relatively sure that when a DIS diagnosis is made, it is likely to be accurate, but they cannot assume that the absence of a particular DIS diagnosis is necessarily evidence of the absence of the corresponding *DSM-III* disorder.

Helzer et al. (1987) conducted a follow-up study to the Helzer et al. (1985) study. They found only a few significant differences between DIS and interview-based disorders in predicting subsequent diagnoses and psychiatric treatment. Somewhat optimistically, they concluded that both had satisfactory predictive validity. Across diagnoses, the average proportion of subjects receiving the same DIS diagnosis a year later was 26.3% when diagnosed by lay DIS, but not by the psychiatrist and 67.6% when diagnosed by both the lay DIS and the psychiatrist. Since diagnostic disagreements were largely composed of marginal cases, these results are hardly surprising. On the other hand, they do not appear to demonstrate discriminant validity, since other disorders were also commonplace.[6]

Studies by Other Investigators. Anthony and his colleagues (Anthony et al., 1985) conducted an elegant study of DIS construct validity. As a gold standard, they employed four research psychiatrists who independently administered an augmented version of the Present State Examination (PSE; Wing, Cooper, & Sartorius, 1974) that included *DSM-III* diagnoses. With the PSE, standardized ratings are made; however, the psychiatrists were free to make their own clinical inquiries and observations. The DIS interviews were administered to 810 community subjects by 77 lay interviewers who had completed an 8-day ECA training program.

---

[5]Caution must be taken in interpreting the results of Robins et al. (1981), as the same psychiatrists administered both the DIS and the clinical interview.

[6]Actually, the results neither prove nor disprove discriminant validity, as these other disorders may also have been present at the time of the original testing. Across diagnoses, the most surprising finding was the relative instability of the DIS APD disorder. Because this is a chronic personality disorder, I was startled that 8 of 25 patients "lost" their APD diagnosis in a 12-month period.

Anthony et al. (1985; also see M. F. Folstein et al., 1985) found very low rates of agreement on current episodes between DIS and PSE-augmented diagnoses. For the eight most common diagnoses the kappas ranged from –.02 to .35 (median = .14). Sensitivity ranged from 0% to 56% with a median of 17.5%; in sharp contrast, specificity was nearly 100% (ranging from 83 – 100%, median = 99%). Anthony et al. (1985) gently questioned the overreliance of the DIS on self-report data as well as its incomplete coverage of *DSM-III* criteria.

Erdman et al. (1987) compared DIS diagnoses for 220 psychiatric patients to their chart (typically discharge) diagnoses. Erdman et al. (1987) found disappointing levels of agreement. For current disorders, the kappas ranged from –02 to .37 (median = .12); for lifetime diagnoses, the kappas ranged from –.03 to .39 (median = .15). These results are remarkably similar to those of Anthony et al. (1985).

A second and related approach to criterion-related validity is to compare the DIS to other standardized diagnostic measures. For example, several studies have compared lifetime diagnosis on the DIS to the SADS Lifetime Version (SADS-L), while others have provided comparisons to self-administered scales.

Comparisons With the SADS-L. V. Hesselbrock et al. (1982) compared the DIS and SADS-L for 42 psychiatric patients recently admitted to an inpatient alcohol treatment unit. The lifetime diagnoses for the four common disorders (depression, alcoholism, drug abuse, and APD) had moderately high kappas, ranging from .72 to 1.00, with a median of .76. Even if we exclude the perfect agreement for alcoholism (all raters knew that patients were in an alcohol treatment unit), these results still suggest a moderate degree of convergent validity.

Hasin and Grant (1987a, 1987b, 1987c) conducted a study of 120 substance abuse patients (mostly alcoholics) that compared the DIS *DSM-III* and the SADS-L RDC diagnoses. Not surprisingly, the highest kappa coefficients were for alcohol (.60) and drug (.72) abuse. Other disorders were poorly represented in the sample, with kappas ranging from .05 to .41. These very poor results apparently reflect differences in the *DSM-III* and RDC inclusion criteria. When *DSM-III* inclusion criteria are applied to both measures, the kappa coefficients are much higher (range = .52 – 1.00, median = .85). In other words, the two measures evidence a high level of convergent validity with respect to the collected clinical data (i.e., information variance) but poor agreement when different diagnostic systems are imposed (i.e., criterion variance). Interestingly, when the DIS and SADS-L are both interpreted with *DSM-III* inclusion criteria, moderately high kappa coefficients are found for specific substance abuse disorders[7] (Hasin & Grant, 1987a).

Comparisons With Other Measures. Spengler and Wittchen (1988) examined the convergent validity of DIS coverage of psychotic symptoms with two other standardized clinical interviews: the Inpatient Multidimensional Psychiatric Scale (IMPS) and the Assessment and Documentation of Psychopathology

---

[7]For two-thirds of the substance disorders, the kappas were good (> .70). Two notable exceptions were abuse of amphetamines (.00) and narcotics (–.01), for which agreement did not exceed chance expectations.

(AMDP). In a follow-up study of 291 inpatients in Munich, all subjects were administered the DIS (Version II), the IMPS, and the AMDP. With respect to lifetime diagnoses, the DIS psychotic symptoms evidenced a high concordance rate (> 80%) with the AMDP, although the kappas ranged from .16 to .77 (median = .47). The corresponding Yule's *Y*s were substantially higher, ranging from .36 to .73 (median = .63). Less agreement was found between the DIS and the IMPS with kappas ranging from .16 to .51 (median = .31) and Yule's *Y*s of .36 to .65 (median = .42). With respect to current diagnosis, the DIS may underestimate the presence of delusions (κ with AMDP = .44) but not hallucinations (κ with AMDP = .65). This study highlights the difficulty of retrospectively evaluating psychotic symptoms (also see Pulver & Carpenter, 1983), given the differences found among all three methods (DIS, IMPS, and AMDP).

Several studies have attempted to examine the diagnostic agreement of the DIS with psychometric scales. Bonato, Cyr, Kalpin, Prendergast, and Sanhueza (1988) found poor agreement between DIS diagnoses and the MCMI. In light of the available literature, they attributed these disappointing results to inadequacies in the MCMI validation, as opposed to limitations in the DIS. Watson, Clark, and Carey (1988) found low to moderate correlations between measures of positive and negative affect and the DIS items associated with anxiety and depressive disorders. This obvious lack of psychometric studies with the DIS probably reflects the traditional deemphasis of psychological testing as a method of assessing formal diagnoses.

Validity of Specific Disorders

A number of investigators have addressed specific mental disorders and the diagnostic accuracy of the DIS. Typically, these studies have employed clinical interviews as the external criterion. These studies will be summarized by clinical syndromes.

Substance Abuse Disorders. In addition to the SADS-L studies previously reported, several investigators have examined the criterion-related validity of the DIS with substance abuse disorders. Griffin, Weiss, Mirin, Wilson, and Bouchard-Voelk (1987) compared DIS data for 124 consecutive admissions to an inpatient drug dependence unit with independent discharge diagnoses that were reviewed by a research psychiatrist. For substance abuse and dependence, the κs were moderate for alcohol (.57) and high for drugs (.89). Other specific disorders were poorly represented in the study, which resulted in low kappas (-.01 - .40) despite high rates of agreement (67 - 95%).

Ford, Hillard, Giesler, Lassen, and Thomas (1989) examined 75 substance abuse patients with dual diagnoses and compared lay-administered DIS evaluations with preliminary and discharge diagnoses. Although the kappas were generally low, the lack of agreement between the two clinical interviews raises questions on the interpretability of the results.

A team from the Addiction Research Foundation (Gavin, Ross, & Skinner, 1989; Ross, Gavin, & Skinner, 1990) examined 501 patients sent to their facility for evaluation and/or treatment. The majority of patients (56%) qualified for DIS alcohol abuse/dependence without other substance abuse; smaller percentages had drug disorders alone (18%) or combined alcohol and drug abuse disorders

(18%). For alcohol abuse/dependence, DIS disorders manifested moderate correlations of .65 with the Michigan Alcoholism Screening Test (MAST; Vinokur, & Van Rooijen, 1975) and .58 with the Alcohol Dependence Scale (Skinner & Horn, 1984). By the same token, DIS substance abuse disorders evidenced a moderately high correlation of .75 with the Drug Abuse Screening Test (DAST; Skinner, 1982). Convergent findings (see Fleming & Barry, 1991) have confirmed a moderate correspondence between DIS diagnosed alcoholism and the Short Michigan Alcoholism Screening Test (SMAST; Selzer et al., 1975).

Deykin, Buka, and Zeena (1992) examined risk factors and familial variables in depressed and nondepressed adolescent substance abusers. They were able to establish differences between adolescents whose depression preceded substance abuse and those for whom it did not. For depression episodes first, the risk factors were associated with physical abuse, gender (female), and parental problems. For substance abuse first, alcoholism in family members, drug use in siblings, and academic nonperformance were risk factors.

In summary, studies based on the SADS-L as well as clinical diagnosis suggest a moderately high convergent validity of substance abuse disorders on the DIS. This finding suggests, particularly with respect to information variance, a moderate level of correspondence in ascertaining clinical data relevant to substance abuse, both for diagnosis and rating scales.

Antisocial Personality Disorder. Two studies have examined directly the validity of the DIS APD diagnosis. Perry, Lavori, Cooper, Hoke, and O'Connell (1987) followed 70 nonpsychotic patients and community subjects over 3-month intervals for a median follow-up of 1 year. In addition to the administration of the DIS, subjects were evaluated by independent clinical interviews and follow-up administrations of the Antisocial Symptoms Scale of the Psychiatric Status Schedule (PSS; Spitzer, Endicott, Fleiss, & Cohen, 1970). In combining these criteria, the DIS evidenced a sensitivity of 96% and a specificity of 76% (κ = .65). However, the DIS appeared to overdiagnose APD in comparison to the other two methods.

Cooney, Kadden, and Litt (1990) compared DIS APD diagnoses with the PCL, the MMPI-Pd scale, and the CPI-So scale for 118 inpatients recruited for an alcoholism aftercare program. Point-biserial correlations of DIS APD diagnosis with other measures were modest: PCL (.14), MMPI-Pd scale (.28), and CPI-So scale (.43). This study offers no substantial evidence of criterion-related validity for DIS APD diagnosis.

The two APD studies vary substantially in their methodology and results. Perry et al. (1987) employed interview-based measures and found a relatively high level of agreement that included 1-year follow-up data. On the other hand, Cooney et al. (1990) used a structured interview (PCL) and two psychometric scales (MMPI-Pd and CPI-So) with disappointing results. Most surprising was the lack of agreement between DIS and PCL, since earlier research suggested a closer association (see Hare, 1985a).[8]

---

[8]A marked discrepancy was also found in the interrater reliabilities of the PCL, for which the raters in Cooney et al. (1990) found no agreement (i.e., ICC = –.12).

Borderline Personality Disorder. Swartz and his colleagues (Swartz, Blazer, George, & Winfield, 1990; Swartz et al., 1989) conducted two studies of the DIS and its diagnostic utility with borderline personality disorders. They employed as a gold standard the Diagnostic Interview of Borderline Patients (DIB; Gunderson, 1982; Kolb & Gunderson, 1980) and devised the DIS borderline index that was based on 24 DIS symptoms associated with borderline personality disorder. In an initial study (Swartz et al., 1989), the DIS borderline index had a sensitivity of 85.7% and specificity of 86.2%; these results have yet to be cross-validated.

Other Disorders. Katon et al. (1991) studied somatization disorder as diagnosed by the DIS and examined 119 patients with unexplained somatic symptoms on the SCL-90 (Symptom Checklist-90), self-reported medical history, and a questionnaire completed by primary physicians. Katon et al. (1991) established significant differences on these measures between patients with high scores and low scores. Complicating the diagnostic picture, patients with high numbers of unexplained symptoms were very often diagnosed with moderate to severe medical problems (74.7%) and/or mental health problems (81.5%).

Zimmerman and Coryell (1988) examined the concurrent validity of the DIS major depressive disorder and depression assessed by the Inventory to Diagnose Depression (IDD; Zimmerman & Coryell, 1987). Subjects for the study ($N = 613$) were first-degree relatives of inpatients with major depression. Zimmerman and Coryell (1988) found a high concordance rate when the two measures were administered at a very brief interval (i.e., less than 2 days) with a kappa of .80 (Yule's Y = .87), sensitivity of 100%, and specificity of 99.1%. The level of agreement drops substantially when the interval period is increased; the overall kappa for the study was .47 (Yule's Y = .78) with sensitivity of 47.1% and specificity of 98.6%. The authors concluded that limitations of self-report measures such as the IDD, as well as the variable clinical status of subjects, may account for the lower levels of agreement over time.

Validity of DIS Alternate Versions

Self-Administered Versions. The primary emphasis for both computerized and paper-and-pencil versions of the DIS has been to establish their levels of agreement with standard DIS administrations. For example, Kovess and Fournier (1990) found a moderate level of agreement between physicians' checklist of *DSM-III* symptoms and the DISSA (median κ = .51). Wyndowe (1987) administered diagnostic interviews and a computerized version of the DIS to 41 psychiatric patients. He found a very poor rate of agreement both on primary diagnosis (42.9% concordance, no κ reported) and overall diagnosis.

Robins and Marcus (1987) developed the DIS Screening Interview (DISSI) for use with 11 common disorders. Through the use of a hierarchical format, questions related to a particular diagnosis are skipped when a certain level of endorsement is not reached on earlier questions. Robins and Marcus cross-validated the DISSI on three additional data sets (N of approximately 12,000). They reported sensitivity of 75% or more on 11 diagnoses (exceptions were somatization, 67.0% and cognitive impairment, 44.3%) and specificity rates of 80% or more (with the exception of cognitive impairment, 76.2%).

Bucholz et al. (1991) tested the clinical utility of a self-administered DISSI in comparison to an interviewer-administered DISSI and the traditional DIS in a study of 151 psychiatric inpatients and outpatients. Using the traditional DIS as the standard, they found that the self-administered DISSI had generally satisfactory sensitivity and specificity (median of each = .79). Comparable results were found for the interviewer-administered DISSI, with the exception of APD, which was substantially less sensitive than the self-administered version. Levels of diagnostic agreement with the DIS varied widely, with kappas ranging from .34 to .87 (median = .52) for the self-administered version and .10 to .74 (median = .56) for the interviewer-administered version.

Erdman et al. (1992) compared the traditional DIS to a complete computer-administered DIS (i.e., C-DIS) and an interviewer-administered DIS, based on the computer prompts (i.e., P-DIS). This study, while using the same patient samples, differed from the Bucholz et al. study in its administration of the full DIS under these three conditions. Their results were comparable to earlier research (Griest et al., 1987) with moderate levels of diagnostic agreement (median κ =.59) between the self-administered (C-DIS) and traditional DIS interviews. The newly developed computer-prompted interview (P-DIS) appeared to offer no real advantage over the self-administered C-DIS and had a comparable level of diagnostic agreement (median κ = .61) with the traditional DIS.

The Erdman et al. study examined two additional dimensions of computer-administered diagnostic interviews: reading comprehension and response bias. After excluding from the study subjects with very low reading levels (i.e., raw scores of less than 10 on the reading subtest of Wide Range Achievement Test [WRAT; Jastak, Bijou, & Jastak, 1978]), they found no differences in symptoms and diagnoses across reading levels. They found that symptom endorsement was affected by response style, with correlations between number of symptoms and a short form of the Marlowe-Crowne social desirability scale (Greenwald & Satow, 1978) of –.30 for the traditional format and –.39 for the self-administered version. Employing the Q1 scale (Johnson, Williams, Klingler, & Gianetti, 1988) as a screening measure for unreliable or exaggerated response style, they found positive correlations of .38 for the traditional and .65 for the self-administered version. This latter finding would suggest either (a) a greater propensity to feign on the self-administered version, or (b) greater confusion among more ill psychiatric patients when they are responsible for reading and rating items on their own.

In conclusion, the computerized versions often have only modest levels of agreement with the traditional DIS. However, when the DIS is employed as a screening measure rather than a substitute, the DISSI may be an effective screen for psychopathology. Indeed, the work by Robins and Marcus (1987) and Bucholz et al. (1991) would argue strongly for this application. These computerized versions are commercially available (e.g., see Marcus, Robins, & Bucholz, 1991).

Foreign Language Versions. Studies have examined the criterion-related validity of both the Chinese (see Hwu, Yeh, & Chang, 1986) and Spanish versions (see Anduaga et al., 1991; Burnam et al., 1983; Canino, Bird, Shrout, Rubio-Stipec, Bravo, Martinez, Sesman, Guzman, Guevara, & Costas, 1987) of the DIS as compared to clinical diagnosis. To avoid redundancy, these studies will be discussed within the section on generalizability.

Generalizability and Cross-Cultural Research

Several of the original validation studies examined the generalizability of their results across the ECA research sites. For example, Robins et al. (1984) found reasonably comparable prevalence rates across three ECA sites. However, the diagnosis did differ for nine disorders, including alcohol abuse, schizophrenia, depression, and certain anxiety disorders. Since there are no compelling reasons to believe that the actual prevalence of mental disorders should vary from city to city, these results question the generalizability of particular disorders across sites. The differences in lifetime prevalences range from 28.8% in New Haven to 38.0% in Baltimore; these results suggest that a substantial proportion of diagnosed disorders may reflect local variations in DIS administrations.[9] Eaton, et al. (1989) found relatively less variation among ECA sites for current diagnoses. The notable exception was phobic disorders which evidenced marked variations in 1-year prevalences: two sites were high (16.9% at Baltimore and 15.5% at Durham, NC) and two were low (6.3% at St. Louis and 7.5% at Los Angeles). Based on Eaton et al. (1989), clinicians should exercise great care in rendering a DIS phobic disorder.

Stout, Steege, Blazer, and George (1986) found substantial differences in prevalence rates for lifetime psychiatric disorders in their comparison of patients referred to a premenstrual syndrome clinic with female community subjects from the ECA Durham site. However, these differences likely reflect differences in clinical presentation, with higher prevalence of dysthymia, anxiety, and substance abuse in the referred sample.

Cross-cultural dimensions of diagnosis play an important, although somewhat ambiguous, role in the generalizability of assessment measures. These dimensions include differences in cultural understanding, language and the nuances of understanding, and the interviewer-interviewee relationship (see Westermeyer, 1987). For example, Stefannson, Lindal, Bjornsson, and Guomundsdottir (1991) have argued that DIS diagnosis of alcohol abuse/dependence is inapplicable to Icelandic persons because of cultural differences. From a cross-cultural perspective, we will examine the clinical utility of the Chinese and Spanish versions of the DIS.

Chinese DIS

Hwu and his colleagues are responsible for the Chinese translation of the DIS (DIS-CM) and the subsequent modification of items for greater relevance in Chinese culture.[10] Hwu et al. (1986) compared clinical diagnoses to the DIS-CM for 100 psychiatric patients and 187 community subjects. They found a moderate level of agreement between the two methods, with kappas ranging from .18 to .96 (median = .54). They also found that the DIS-CM overdiagnosed several disorders in the community sample and underdiagnosed mania in the clinical sample.

---

[9]If we assume the true prevalence to be the average of the three research sites (M = 32.6%), then approximately 11% of the diagnoses would not generalize across settings.

[10]I was unable to obtain a copy of the first study (Hwu, Yeh, C. T. Chen, C. C. Chen, & T. Y. Chen, 1983) that described the development of the Chinese DIS.

Hwu, E. K. Yeh, Chang, and Y. L. Yeh (1986) examined the lifetime preva-lences of mental disorders in China as compared to U.S. data and found what they considered to be moderate to serious underestimates in the Chinese popula-tion of schizophrenia, and mood and anxiety disorders. As noted by the investi-gators, such conclusions may be confounded by cross-cultural differences which were not examined. In a follow-up study, Hwu, E. K. Yeh, and Chang (1989) found substantial differences in lifetime prevalence rates that appeared to be related both to gender and setting (urban, town, or rural). The investigators con-cluded that these variations may reflect true as well as cultural differences. Although the prevalence rates were lower than those generally found in the U.S., they noted the considerable variations in prevalence rates observed in dif-ferent countries. Moreover, research would suggest fluctuations in the preva-lence rates of certain disorders, particularly alcohol abuse, in the last decade (Hwu, E. K. Yeh, & Chang, 1988).

Studies of the DIS-CM may have limited relevance to Chinese-American popu-lations, since validity studies are based in Taiwan. In comparison to other measures, however, the DIS-CM has received the most validation for Chinese populations.

Spanish DIS

Karno, Burnam, Escobar, Hough, and Eaton (1983) translated the DIS into Spanish with an initial emphasis on the evaluation of large Mexican-American population in southern California. As reported in the diagnostic reliability sec-tion, Burnam et al. (1983) established moderate test-retest reliabilities in com-parisons of English-Spanish and Spanish-Spanish administrations. These researchers also examined sensitivity and specificity rates across 19 diagnoses. They found far-ranging values for sensitivity (from 0 – 92%, median = .50) and excellent specificity (from 69 – 99%, median = 88.5%). Several disorders had extremely low sensitivity rates (schizophreniform, manic episode, panic disorder, obsessive-compulsive disorder, somatization disorder, and organic brain syndrome).

Anduaga et al. (1991) made minor modifications in a Spanish version of the DIS for use in Mexico. This version appeared to have good interrater reliability (ICC = .89). When compared to clinical diagnoses, it demonstrated low sensi-tivity (8 – 63%, median = 39%) but high specificity (78 – 99%, median = 93%). These specificity rates are substantially lower than those found by Burnam et al. (1983) with Mexican-American samples or by Canino, Bird, Shrout, Rubio-Stipec, Bravo, Martinez, Sesman, Guzman, Guevara, & Costas (1987) with Puerto Rican samples.

Canino, Bird, Shrout, Rubio-Stipec, Bravo, Martinez, Sesman, Guzman, Guevara, & Costas (1987) carried out a separate translation of the DIS for use with Puerto Rican samples. Two translators were employed independently so that any disparities in comprehension and usage could be resolved. In addition, the DIS Mini-Mental State Examination was found to be culturally bound and was therefore substantially modified (Bird et al., 1987). The resulting DIS was admin-istered twice in Spanish, once by a psychiatrist and once by a lay interviewer, yielding a median kappa of .59 (see Table 3.3). When the DIS results by lay interviewers were compared to clinical diagnoses,[11] the sensitivity fluctuated markedly (.27 – .93, median = .65). In contrast, the specificity remained high (median = .91; range = .70 – .97). These data suggest very low correspondence for dysthymia, alcohol abuse, and somatization disorders.

Canino, Bird, Shrout, Rubio-Stipec, Bravo, Martinez, Sesman, Guzman, and Guevara (1987) examined the prevalence rates of specific psychiatric disorders in Puerto Rico. In a large-scale epidemiological study of 1,513 community subjects, these investigators found prevalence rates comparable to those established elsewhere in the United States (e.g., lifetime prevalence of any mental disorder was 28.1%).

Rubio-Stipec, Shrout, Bird, Canino, and Bravo (1989) performed an elegant factor analysis that compared a Puerto Rican sample (i.e., Canino, Bird, Shrout, Rubio-Stipec, Bravo, Martinez, Sesman, Guzman, Guevara, & Costas, 1987) with Mexican-American (Burnam et al., 1983) and White samples from Los Angeles (Burnam, Hough, Karno, Escobar, & Telles, 1987). They examined five clusters of symptoms associated with alcoholism, psychotic disorders, mood disorders, phobias, and somatization disorders. Of these, four factors (all but somatization) yielded very high congruence coefficients for both the Mexican-American and White samples. Scales based on these factors evidenced good internal consistencies (αs = .58 – .90, median = .82). The results of Rubio-Stipec et al. (1989) suggest, with the exception of somatization disorder, cross-cultural stability for second-order scales of the DIS.

Several important conclusions can be drawn from this review of DIS Spanish versions:

1. Spanish versions achieve reliability estimates that are comparable to the DIS standard version.

2. The clinical utility of Spanish versions varies with culture and nationality. Despite minor modifications, the Mexican-American version has substantially poorer sensitivity rates in Mexico. Likewise, clinicians who evaluate second and third generation Puerto Ricans residing in the United States must choose between the Puerto Rican version, with culturally specific items but no validation on American samples, and the Mexican-American version, which lacks cultural sensitivity and has differences in language usage.

3. Like many studies with the standard DIS, the major problem with Spanish versions is their rather low rates of sensitivity. Anduaga et al. (1991) provides a useful summary of sensitivity and specificity rates for Mexican-American and Puerto Rican versions.

4. Despite the previously mentioned problems with the Spanish versions of the DIS, their validational studies far surpass those for other structured interviews.

---

[11]Since these psychiatrists also administered the DIS, these estimates of agreement may be inflated.

Clinical Applications

Beyond its obvious value in epidemiological research, the principal advantage of the DIS is that paraprofessionals can be competently trained in its administration. With increased strains on the public care of the mentally ill, paraprofessionals frequently assume the primary role in assessment and nonmedical treatments. Psychologists can train and supervise paraprofessionals with the DIS and thereby substantially improve the diagnostic assessments offered in many public agencies. Ideally, a diagnostic triage should be implemented in which patients who meet or nearly meet the diagnostic criteria for mental disorders are referred to a psychologist or other trained diagnostician.

The recent publication of the *DSM-IV* must be considered in the use of the DIS. An important observation is that the DIS-IV is being developed to ensure optimal comparability with the *DSM-IV*; this version will require additional validation, particularly with diagnoses which were modified. Among the disorders covered by the DIS, the greatest number of changes occurred with anxiety disorders in their diagnostic criteria and in the addition of panic attack and acute stress disorder. Interestingly, the increased attention to substance-induced disorders (e.g., psychotic, mood, anxiety, and sleep disorders) capitalizes on a potential strength of the DIS in its attempts to establish etiologic features of individual symptoms.

Screening

The need to screen patients systematically for undetected mental illness extends beyond community mental health centers. For example, Jones, Badger, Ficken, Leeper, and Anderson (1988) found that primary care physicians routinely missed psychiatric diagnoses that were detected by the DIS. Indeed, these physicians missed (a) most mood (73.9%) and anxiety (80.0%) disorders, and (b) all organic and psychosexual disorders. Clinicians have experimented with screening measures, which employ the DIS for a more complete assessment, as part of the service delivery to large health maintenance organizations (HMOs; see Berwick et al., 1991).

Screening underserved populations with the DIS can also extend beyond the traditional patients presenting with physical or mental complaints. For example, Teplin (1990) evaluated with the DIS 542 detainees in a large urban jail. Of those with severe mental illness, approximately two-thirds (62.5%) had gone undetected when processed through the jail's primary and secondary intakes that screen for mental illness. Use of a standardized screening measure (Teplin & Swartz, 1989) and the DIS would greatly enhance the detection and subsequent interventions for persons held in custodial settings.

Use of the DIS and DIS-derived screening measures for the identification of undetected disorders requires careful attention in the training and implementation phases. Particularly in the utilization of paraprofessionals, psychologists must periodically assess staff members' competence in DIS administrations. As a note of concern, most research studies on the DIS examine interrater reliability shortly after training and do not assess whether levels of diagnostic agreement attenuate over time.

I would also encourage that subthreshold cases be recommended for complete evaluations. Helzer et al. (1985) found that most diagnostic disagreements occurred in marginal cases (i.e., those just below or just above the threshold). Screening evaluations would likely improve their sensitivity if subthreshold cases (one or two inclusion criteria below the designated threshold) were also comprehensively assessed.

Use of self-administered DIS versions have a very circumscribed clinical role for several reasons. First, the validation of these versions, as previously summarized, is quite restricted. Given the limits in diagnostic validity of the standard DIS, self-administered versions that have only a modest correspondence with the standard version compound the problems of reliability and validity. Second, the self-administered versions provide only partial coverage of the DIS diagnosis.

The use of the computer-administered DISSI would appear to be advantageous in screening large numbers of patients for possible mental disorders. A second and very different application of self-administered versions is *postscreening assessments*. In postscreening assessments, measures are employed as a double-check against missed diagnoses. In this regard, even measures with very modest sensitivity rates may be clinically useful.[12] Given the data on the DISSI that suggest generally good sensitivity and specificity, its use in this regard is strongly recommended.

Spanish and Chinese Versions

The DIS distinguishes itself from other structured interviews in its careful validation with Hispanic populations. Research on the Spanish versions suggests that its interrater reliability and concurrent validity are comparable to those found with the standardized version. As previously noted, no versions are available for Puerto Rican patients who were born and reside in the United States.

Clinical applications of the Chinese version are more circumscribed, since the studies have occurred exclusively in Taiwan. In the absence of other alternatives, however, psychologists may wish to employ the Chinese DIS in the standardized assessment of mental disorders. In such cases, psychologists must work closely with Chinese mental health professionals or paraprofessionals in order to understand important cultural differences in the presentation of symptomatology. In agencies serving large Chinese-American populations, psychologists might consider the possibility of training a Chinese-speaking paraprofessional in the administration of the DIS. In this regard the DIS has a singular advantage, as it was designed for use by nonprofessionals.

In summary, the three main advantages of the DIS are (a) administration by paraprofessionals, (b) use in screening large samples for undetected mental disorders, and (c) availability of Spanish and Chinese versions. For the convenience of the reader, these advantages are summarized in Table 3.4.

---

[12]Low sensitivity rates reduce the usefulness of screening measures, as "negative findings" may preclude the routine evaluation of existing disorders. This limitation does not apply to postscreening applications, in which the uncovering of any missed diagnosis is a decided advantage.

Table 3.4
Advantages of the DIS in Diagnostic Evaluations

1. The DIS can be administered by paraprofessionals with only modest levels of training.

2. More than other interview measures, the DIS has been translated and validated in Spanish.

3. The DIS, although having only moderate levels of sensitivity (roughly 50% across studies[a]), may be useful in clinical situations in which large numbers of individuals need to be screened for mental illness. In other words, the DIS may be valuable in the evaluation of undetected mental illness.

4. The DIS has self-administered versions (computerized and paper-and-pencil) which may also be used for prescreening and postscreening.[b]

---

[a]Since the DIS was compared to the less-than-ideal psychiatric interviews (i.e., a bootstrapping operation), the "true" sensitivity is unknown. [b]Self-administered versions have a circumscribed role because (a) they cover a limited number of diagnoses, and (b) they only approximate DIS diagnoses.

Limitations of the DIS in Clinical Practice

The DIS cannot be employed as the sole interview measure for making multiaxial diagnoses. Its coverage focuses primarily on Axis I disorders, with an emphasis on substance abuse, mood, and anxiety disorders. With reference to psychotic disorders, the DIS concentrates on schizophrenic and schizophreniform disorders, although a review of symptomatology may facilitate other diagnoses, such as delusional disorders. Somatoform and dissociative disorders are not covered. In addition, the DIS was not designed to evaluate Axis II disorders, with the exception of APD, and provides only indirect evidence for Axes IV and V.[13]

Empirical studies strongly suggest that all clinical measures can be faked (Rogers, 1984, 1987). As noted in Chapter 1, the DIS may be vulnerable to malingering and defensiveness because of (a) its high degree of face validity, (b) its clustering of symptoms by diagnosis, and (c) its structuring of questions unidirectionally so that endorsements almost always reflect impairment. In other words, patients either over- or underreporting symptoms should have little trouble in modifying their responses in a believable manner. I have found no studies that examine clinicians' ability to detect dissimulation on the basis of the DIS. Therefore, psychologists are cautioned to employ other measures such as the SIRS or the MMPI when some form of feigning is suspected. However, the DIS can be a useful ancillary measure in these cases, since it provides a systematic method for evaluating the consistency of a patient's self reporting.

Two other limitations of the DIS encompass issues of severity and etiology. In examining the course of a disorder or measuring response to treatment, systematic ratings of symptom severity become important. Because of its design, the DIS may have limited usefulness in this regard; symptoms are simply rated clinical or subclinical. On the other hand, the DIS asks interviewers to make complex judgments regarding the etiology of specific symptoms in terms of

---

[13]Typically, Axes IV and V are composite ratings derived from the overall assessment and, therefore, not assessed separately (Williams, 1985).

substance abuse or other medical explanations. The fact that some etiological distinctions are impossible to make, even after very sophisticated laboratory procedures and psychological testing, would suggest that this aspect of the DIS may be overly elaborate and unduly refined. For example, how can we truly distinguish whether paranoid symptoms arise from chronic use of psychoactive substances in a chronic drug abuser or from other more "functional" explanations? Asking clinicians to make multiple judgments (presence as well as etiology) unnecessarily complicates the assessment. On the other hand, the *DSM-IV* pays closer attention to substance-induced disorders. These distinctions, while formidable in their complexity, may assist in the diagnosis of substance-induced disorders.

The potential limitations of the DIS are summarized in Table 3.5. Psychologists must evaluate the clinical usefulness of the DIS with its strengths and limitations, not as an abstract exercise, but with specific reference to their populations, clinical settings, and referral questions.

Table 3.5
Limitations of the Standard DIS in Clinical Evaluations

1. Diagnostic coverage

   DIS, Version III-A, covers a total of 43 *DSM-III* mental disorders. Its strengths are in assessing substance abuse, mood disorders, and anxiety disorders. In addition, the DIS provides the Mini-Mental State Examination as a screen for dementia. Coverage of psychotic disorders is uneven (e.g., no delusional disorders); dissociative disorders, somatoform disorders, and personality disorders (except APD) are not included. In relation to other general diagnostic interviews, the DIS forms a middle ground between the narrow focus of the SADS and the breadth of the SCID.

2. Response styles

   The sole study by Erdman et al. (1992) would suggest that the DIS is vulnerable to both under- and overreporting. In suspect cases, psychologists may wish to employ the self-administered version as a measure of consistency or employ other measures designed to assess social desirability, defensiveness, or malingering.

3. Severity of the disorder

   The DIS typically provides two gradations in the evaluation of specific symptoms: subclinical and clinical. For symptoms in the clinical range, the DIS does not offer ratings of severity.

4. Etiological questions

   Unlike other measures, the DIS asks interviewers to make often complex judgments regarding the etiology of specific symptoms. Specifically, interviewers are asked to decide whether symptoms have a medical explanation or are the result of alcohol or other drug abuse.

4

Schedule of Affective Disorders and Schizophrenia (SADS)

Overview

Description

The Schedule of Affective Disorders and Schizophrenia (SADS; Spitzer & Endicott, 1978a) is an extensive semistructured diagnostic interview that was designed primarily for the assessment of mood and psychotic disorders. The SADS is divided into Part I for current episode and Part II (otherwise known as the SADS-Lifetime version or SADS-L) for prior episodes. In Part I, individual symptoms are rated for the worst period of the current episode and for the current time period (i.e., last week); through comparative ratings, clinicians are able to assess the severity of the disorder and minimize day-to-day fluctuations in clinical status (Endicott & Spitzer, 1978). Finally, for the assessment of key symptomatology, Spitzer and Endicott (1978b) devised the SADS-Change Version or SADS-C, which consists of 45 symptoms selected from the SADS-Part I.

An important feature of Part I is its emphasis on the degree of impairment. Most affective symptoms and behavioral observations are rated on 6 gradations (0 = no information; 1 = not at all; 2 = slight, an occasional symptom of low intensity; 3 = mild, a common symptom of low intensity; 4 = moderate, a frequent symptom or symptoms of low to medium intensity; 5 = severe, a very frequent symptom or symptoms of at least medium intensity; and 6 = extreme, unremitting symptoms of high intensity). Psychotic symptoms are typically rated on 3 gradations (0 = no information, 1 = absent, 2 = suspected or likely, and 3 = definite). Particularly with the 6-point gradations, each is anchored with a description and some also provide representative examples.

SADS-Part II or SADS-L (for simplicity, we will refer to this as the SADS-L) is organized into specific syndromes with screening criteria, individual symptoms, criteria regarding impairment, and associated features. For the specific symptoms, the scoring is dichotomous (0 = no information, 1 = no, 2 = yes), since most patients lack precision in describing symptoms from prior episodes.

The format of the SADS is semistructured, with three levels of clinical inquiries. As summarized in Table 1.4, clinicians are required to ask standard questions of each patient. In contrast, optional probes (i.e., questions enclosed in parentheses) and unstructured questions are employed selectively in order to clarify incomplete or ambiguous responses. In addition, the SADS has branching questions which serve a screening function; the nonendorsement of branching questions typically allows clinicians to skip sections of the SADS. Depending on the circumstances and the quality of elicited information, psychologists may choose to continue to administer sections of the SADS, despite a lack of endorsement of these branching questions.

The SADS was developed prior to the final revisions and implementation of the *DSM-III*. As described in the following Development section, the SADS was constructed in conjunction with the RDC. Fortunately, there is substantial convergence between the *DSM-III/DSM-III-R/DSM-IV* and RDC criteria for many Axis I disorders. However, clinicians must be knowledgeable of the two systems so that they may supplement the SADS with additional questions required to make *DSM-IV* diagnoses.

An important feature of the SADS is its in-depth examination of specific disorders. Unlike other commonly employed diagnostic measures, the SADS provides highly detailed information regarding the intensity and duration of specific symptomatology. As noted above, the SADS also provides comparison within the current episode (worst period vs. current time) and across episodes. The trade-off for this comprehensiveness is the relatively narrow spectrum of disorders covered by the SADS. The SADS allows for the diagnosis of 23 disorders and provides subcategories of schizophrenia, schizoaffective disorder, and major depression.

The SADS also integrates into its structure estimates of the patient's level of functioning. The GAS was incorporated as an overall measure of psychological impairment. In addition, several items were inserted to evaluate the patient's highest level of psychological adjustment and social functioning during the last 5 years. These latter ratings are designed to estimate (a) premorbid functioning in patients with recent onsets, and (b) highest level of functioning in chronic patients. In addition, the SADS includes a brief synopsis of potential precipitators as well as current and prior treatment.

Rationale

Studies in the early 1970s painted a rather gloomy picture for the underdiagnosis of mental disorders. A series of studies by Welner and his colleagues (Liss, Welner, & Robins, 1972; Welner, Liss, & Robins, 1972, 1973) suggested that many patients went undiagnosed and that the implementation of a structured interview and use of standardized diagnostic criteria would substantially reduce both missed diagnoses and misdiagnoses. Studies from the U.S.–U.K. diagnostic project (Cooper et al., 1972) suggested that inaccurate diagnoses across research sites could be greatly decreased through the use of structured interviews. Finally, Spitzer and Fleiss (1974) found that problems with diagnoses were magnified by very poor agreement among experienced diagnosticians across six major reliability studies.

During the 1970s, Spitzer and Endicott (1975a) experimented with several psychiatric rating forms and interviewing materials. These measures included the Psychiatric Status Schedule (PSS; Spitzer, Endicott, Fleiss, & Cohen, 1970), the Current and Past Psychopathology Scales (CAPPS; Endicott & Spitzer, 1972), the

Problem Appraisal Scales (PAS; Herz, Spitzer, Gibbon, Greenspan, & Reibel, 1974), and the Mental Status Evaluation Record (MSER; Spitzer & Endicott, 1970; Endicott, Spitzer, & Fleiss, 1975; Spitzer, Endicott, Cohen, & Fleiss, 1974; also see Chapter 2). Because of their concern with controlling criterion variance, Spitzer and Endicott (1968, 1969), and Spitzer et al. (1974) attempted to establish computer models as a method of standardizing diagnostic decision-making. These investigators concluded that limits in computer diagnosis reflected the constraints in diagnostic standards. They proposed (a) the development of the RDC for the improvement of diagnostic criteria, and (b) the creation of the SADS as a comprehensive interview for the control of information variance.

Development of the RDC and the SADS

Feighner et al. (1972) expressed dissatisfaction with the *DSM-II* diagnosis and developed their own research criteria. These criteria, widely known as the Feighner criteria, achieved a high level of diagnostic concordance for 15 disorders (see Helzer et al., 1977; Matarazzo, 1983). Spitzer et al. (1978) elaborated on these criteria and brought the total number of diagnostic categories to 23. In addition, diagnostic subtyping was developed for many of the disorders. The reliability of the RDC when employed with traditional interviews appeared high, with a median kappa of .86 (Spitzer et al., 1978). Endicott and Spitzer (1979) tested the RDC and its ability to differentiate schizoaffective and major depressive disorders.

Zwick (1983) provided a helpful critique of the RDC and its use with schizophrenic, schizoaffective, and depressive disorders. She noted that these criteria, while superior to their predecessors, warranted further refinement and validation. For example, Zwick observed that the RDC minimum period for schizophrenic symptoms (i.e., 2 weeks) is probably too brief, citing research by Helzer, Brockington, and Kendell (1981).

Comparatively little is published about the actual development of the SADS. The SADS evolved through three editions; the second edition became available in 1975 (Spitzer & Endicott, 1975b) and the third in 1978 (Spitzer & Endicott, 1978a). A primary goal of the SADS was to assist in the differential diagnosis between mood and psychotic disorders for the NIMH collaborative study on the psychobiology of depression.

The SADS was designed to be used in conjunction with the RDC (Endicott & Spitzer, 1978). The SADS items were organized into eight summary scales: depressed mood and ideation, endogenous features, depressive-associated features, suicidal ideation and behavior, anxiety, manic syndrome, delusions/hallucinations, and formal thought disorder. Very slight modifications were made in the SADS during 1979.[1]

Fyer, Endicott, Manuzza, and Klein (1985) attempted a further modification of the SADS-L to include anxiety disorders from the *DSM-III* and the *DSM-III-R*. This new version is referred to as the SADS-LA. The SADS-LA has been tested by several investigators (i.e., Leboyer et al., 1991; Manuzza, Fyer, Klein, & Endicott, 1986) whose research is summarized under the reliability and validity sections of this chapter.

---

[1]This more recent version of the SADS is designated as the third edition, 1978-1979.

Green and Price (1986) experimented with abbreviated versions of the SADS that relied upon truncated "packets" of SADS questions based on initial clinical presentation. Comparisons were made across 72 psychiatric inpatients screened for preselected diagnoses. By concentrating on only five diagnoses, Green and Price achieved moderately comparable results with kappas greater than .70.

Herzog, Keller, Sacks, Yeh, and Lavori (1992) modified the SADS-L to include eating disorders and named this version the EAT-SADS-L. Because its reliability and validity have not been reported, the use of the EAT-SADS-L should be limited to clinical research.

Validation of the SADS

More than other diagnostic interviews, the SADS has benefited from careful attention to the various elements of reliability (interrater, test-retest, and internal consistency). In the following subsections I summarize the relevant research with respect to reliability and criterion-related validity.

Diagnostic Reliability

NIMH Investigators. Researchers from the NIMH collaborative study on the psychobiology of depression conducted four studies of the SADS's reliability (i.e., Andreasen et al., 1981; Endicott & Spitzer, 1978; Keller et al., 1981). These studies were focused at three levels: symptoms (i.e, the reproducibility of individual items), summary scales, and diagnoses. In addition, research has focused on either the current episode (SADS, Part I) or lifetime diagnosis (SADS-L).

Endicott and Spitzer (1978) performed the original reliability research on the SADS (see Table 4.1). Interrater reliability by pairs of clinicians was tested on 150 newly admitted psychiatric patients who presented with mood symptoms. The reliability estimates were very high for both the summary scales (median intraclass coefficients or ICCs = .96; Endicott & Spitzer, 1978, p. 842) and RDC diagnoses (median κ = .91; Spitzer et al., 1978, p. 779) remained high for both current (median κ = .91) and lifetime (median κ = .93) diagnoses. The alpha coefficients for the summary scales was generally high (median = .80), with the exceptions of anxiety (.58) and formal thought disorder (.47). Although not specifically reported, the intraclass coefficients for the SADS, Part I were generally high for individual symptoms, with 83% of scaled items achieving kappas greater than .70.[2]

Endicott and Spitzer (1978), as part of the original validation, also conducted a test-retest reliability study on newly admitted patients interviewed by two independent clinicians at intervals of generally 1 to 3 days. The reliability estimates were generally high for summary scales (median ICC = .83) and RDC diagnoses (median κ = .72). Alcoholism was poorly represented in the study (i.e., two patients) and could not be adequately assessed.

---

[2]Almost all 6- or 7-point items appear on Part I. For the test-retest reliability, the intraclass coefficients were also generally high, with 73% of items achieving .70 or higher.

Table 4.1

General Reliability Studies of the Schedule of Affective Disorders and Schizophrenia (SADS)

Study	Agreement
Endicott & Spitzer (1978) Interrater reliabilities were determined for 150 psychiatric inpatients from four hospitals who presented with some mood symptoms; test-retest reliabilities were obtained for 60 inpatients with a typical interval of 1 to 3 days.[b]	SADS summary scales: Interrater ICC = .96; test-retest ICC = .83. RDC diagnosis[a]: Interrater κ = .91; test-retest κ = .73
Andreasen et al. (1981) Test-retest design was used with 50 nonpatients assessed by three independent clinicians. For convenience, we have labeled retests with virtually no interval (several hours) as "A" and those with a 6-month interval as "B."	Lifetime symptoms: Test-retest A: ICC = .87; test-retest B: ICC = .72[c]
Keller et al. (1981) Test-retest design was used with 25 patients with mood or schizophrenic episodes; they were evaluated independently by two clinicians on the same day.[c]	Diagnosis: ICC = .69. Summary scales: ICC = .83. Symptoms: ICC = .63
Rounsaville, Cacciola, Weissman, & Kleber (1981) Combined interrater and test-retest designs were used in a study of opiate addicts (outpatients and untreated addicts); 40 patients were jointly interviewed by clinicians and research assistants. For convenience, we have labeled retests of 20 subjects after a short interval (1 – 10 days) as "A" and of 117 subjects after a 6-month interval as "B."	Diagnosis: Inter-rater κ = .88. Test-retest A:κ = .49. Test-retest B: κ = .32
Strober, Green, & Carlson (1981) Interrater reliability was determined for 95 adolescent inpatients through joint interviews by two clinicians.	Diagnosis: κ = .75
Andreasen et al. (1982) Interrater reliabilities were assessed through eight videotapes chosen for their diagnostic complexity; videotapes were rated independently by 36 SADS-trained clinicians.	Key SADS symptoms: ICC = .76. RDC diagnosis: ICC = .75
McDonald-Scott & Endicott (1984) Interrater reliability was studied for 50 patients who participated in a longitudinal study; interviewers were mental health professionals.	SADS-C symptoms: ICC = .88. SADS-C summary scales: ICC = .93

Table 4.1   (continued)
General Reliability Studies of the Schedule of Affective Disorders and
Schizophrenia (SADS)

Study	Agreement
Rapp, Parisi, Walsh, & Wallace (1988) Interrater reliability was assessed by two clinicians on 15 elderly medical inpatients.	Current diagnosis: κ = .94
Spiker & Ehler (1984) Test-retest design was used (interval not specified) with 62 inpatients on a clinical research unit. The first evaluation by the treating psychiatrist was followed by a second evaluation with a research psychiatrist.[d]	Current diagnosis: κ = .57. Lifetime diagnosis: κ = .77
Leboyer et al. (1991) Updated SADS-L (SADS-LA; Mannuzza et al., 1986) was modified for the study of anxiety disorders and translated into French and German; interrater reliability combined with test-retest design (3-month interval) was used; consecutive samples included 35 psychiatric patients and 20 relatives.	*DSM-III-R* current diagnosis: κs of .89 – 1.00. *DSM-III-R* lifetime diagnosis: κ = .52[e]

Note. κ = unweighted kappas; ICC = intraclass coefficients. Except where otherwise noted, median statistics are reported. [a]Data from Spitzer et al. (1978); includes both current and lifetime diagnoses. [b]Although not fully reported, the ICCs for individual SADS items remained high (median ICCs > .70) for both interrater and test-retest reliabilities. [c]If subtypes of major depression are also considered, the median kappa drops to .55. [d]The investigators also report the Random Error Coefficient of Agreement (RE; Maxwell, 1977) for infrequent diagnoses; the RE was substantially higher (median RE = .88 for interrater and .87 for test-retest reliabilities). [e]If the modified anxiety section is excluded, the median kappa increases to .71.

Andreasen et al. (1981) conducted test-retest reliabilities on both the same day and at 6-month intervals for individual symptoms from the SADS summary scales (see Table 4.1). Based on this rigorous test, the intraclass coefficients for 50 nonpatients were very high for the same day (median ICC = .87) and continued high over the 6-month period (median ICC = .72). Over the 6-month interval, unreliability was observed in reporting the number of prior depressive episodes, hypomanic symptoms, and generalized anxiety. As part of the same research effort, Keller et al. (1981) examined the test-retest reliabilities on 25 patients tested twice in the same day. As reported in Table 4.1, intraclass coefficients were moderately high for individual symptoms and RDC diagnoses and high for SADS summary scales.

Andreasen et al. (1982), as part of the NIMH collaborative study, investigated the interrater reliability of videotaped SADS administrations across five research sites. She and her colleagues chose eight videotapes representing difficult diagnostic cases. These videotapes were independently rated and evaluated by 36 SADS-trained clinicians. On a symptom level, clinicians had a good level of agreement (median ICC = .76 on 57 key symptoms), with some difficulty in achieving a consensus on observational ratings (e.g., elements of formal thought disorder). Diagnostically, a moderate level of reliability was achieved (median ICC = .75) with diagnostic disagreements over RDC subtyping of depressive disorders. As a stringent test of interrater reliability, the SADS performed well, particularly at the symptom level. Supplementary analyses revealed no significant differences because of training (psychiatrist, psychologist, or social worker) and level of experience.

McDonald-Scott and Endicott (1984) examined the interrater reliability of the SADS-C on 50 patients who participated in the NIMH study on the psychobiology of depression. This study sought to address whether prior knowledge of patients' histories would confound the SADS's reliability. Various pairs of clinicians were employed to evaluate these patients, with the actual interviewer being blind to the patient's history while the observer was knowledgeable regarding the patient's background. Results established a high degree of reliability for both symptoms (median ICC = .88) and summary scales (median ICC = .93) and strongly suggested that prior knowledge does not confound reliability.

Other Investigators. Rounsaville, Cacciola, Weissman, and Kleber (1981) conducted a combined interrater and test-retest reliability study of the SADS-L with opiate addicts. They established high interrater reliabilities (κ = .72 – 1.00, median = .88) on 40 subjects. However, an attempt by the same investigators to establish test-retest reliability on a small sample (N = 20) was relatively unsuccessful. Although "frequent" ($\geq$ 3) disorders, such as major depression and alcoholism, had satisfactory kappas, others were very poor. At the 6-month interval, kappas are generally low for anxiety disorders and minor depression, with a disappointing overall kappa of .32. Whether this reliability estimate partly reflects the fluctuating clinical status of opiate addicts is not known.

Strober, Green, and Carlson (1981) conducted an interrater reliability study of the SADS with adolescent inpatients. They augmented the SADS with items related to adolescent disorders. When SADS-derived diagnoses are considered, the kappa coefficients of disorders that are sufficiently represented ($n \geq 5$) range from .64 to .94 with a median of .75. Although the results are certainly acceptable, their interpretation is partly confounded by the addition of an unspecified number of non-SADS items.

Leckman, Sholomsaks, Thompson, Belanger, and Weissman (1982) examined interscorer reliability on 469 cases previously collected as part of an epidemiological study, using the SADS-L to assess lifetime prevalence of RDC disorders. The SADS-L protocols were reevaluated by two clinicians, resulting in a moderate level of interscorer consistency (median κ = .73). These results have only limited clinical relevance because (a) interrater reliability was not assessed, and (b) certain modifications were made in the SADS-L protocols.

Spiker and Ehler (1984) yielded somewhat lower kappas in their test-retest study of 62 inpatients over an unspecified interval. The median kappa was .57 across seven diagnoses. Particularly low was the diagnosis of schizoaffective disorder, depressed type (κ = .24). Lifetime diagnosis was somewhat improved (median κ = .63), with the problematic disorder being labile personality. Without detracting from these findings, it should be noted that these low reliabilities occur with disorders that are not typically diagnosed with the *DSM-III-R*.

The 1991 Leboyer et al. reliability study differed from earlier studies in several respects. First, the study used two language translations (German and French). Second, the study examined the usefulness of the SADS-LA, which includes an augmented section on anxiety disorders. Third, the study evaluated the diagnostic reliability for *DSM-III* and *DSM-III-R* disorders rather than RDC diagnoses. Leboyer et al. (1991) found excellent agreement ($\kappa \geq .89$ for *DSM-III-R* disorders) on estimates of interrater reliability. Test-retest reliability at 3-month intervals evidenced considerable variability: kappas for *DSM-III* disorders ranged from .07 to .92 (median = .64), while kappas for *DSM-III-R* disorders ranged from .27 to .78 (median = .52). In general, anxiety and schizoaffective disorders were the most problematic.

Reliability of Specific Disorders. As reported in Table 4.2, two of three studies (Mazure & Gershon, 1979; Merikangus, 1981) that focused on SADS lifetime reliability with mood-disordered patients found good agreement ($\kappa > .70$) in a test-retest design at 6-month intervals. For example, Mazure and Gershon (1979) found diagnostic agreement on 40 of 48 cases with a kappa of .79. Importantly, clinical documentation suggested that two of the eight discrepant cases resulted from further deterioration in the patients' status, warranting the modification of diagnosis from minor to major depression. Although not described in detail, Hurt, Friedman, Clarkin, Corn, and Aronoff (1982) reported very high reliability coefficients (> .90) in an inpatient study of mood-disordered patients. In contrast to other research, Bromet, Bunn, Connell, Dew, and Schulberg (1986) found poor agreement (median $\kappa = .34$) on 131 community subjects reinterviewed at an 18-month interval. Several methodological problems are apparent in the Bromet et al. study which limits its interpretability. First, these researchers did not readminister the complete SADS-L, but only the depression subsections. What biasing effect this may have had on the reporting of symptoms is unknown. Second, the study was conducted in the context of an environmental disaster (Three Mile Island). How well these data generalize to nontraumatized communities is also not known.

Investigators have examined the SADS's reliability for various disorders. For example, Rosen et al. (1984) found a moderately high interrater reliability (ICC = .77) for 54 male schizophrenic patients. Similarly, Hasin and Grant (1987a) found excellent interrater agreement ($\kappa = .91$) in a small sample of psychiatric patients from a substance abuse unit.

Manuzza et al. (1989) examined the test-retest reliability of the SADS-LA for anxiety disorders alone. They found a moderate level of agreement across diagnostic systems (see Table 4.2). When the interval between administrations was brief (< 7 days), the level of agreement was generally high (median $\kappa = .88$). Of the six anxiety disorders, substantial problems with test-retest reliability was found for simple phobias and generalized anxiety disorder. Fyer et al. (1989) examined the reliability of individual symptoms in the Mannuzza et al. study and found considerable variations in kappa coefficients by disorder: panic attacks (range = .25 – .90; median = .46), generalized anxiety (range = .08 – .54; median = .35), obsessions and compulsions (range = .60 – .73; median = .66), social phobia

Table 4.2
Reliability Studies with the Schedule of Affective Disorders and Schizophrenia (SADS) for Specific Disorders

Study	Agreement
Mazure & Gershon (1979) Test-retest design at a 6-month interval was used; the study evaluated 49 subjects in a mixed sample of mood-disordered patients, their first-degree relatives, and medical-patient controls.	Lifetime diagnosis: κ = .79
Merikangas (1981)[a] Test-retest design was used on the SADS-L with a 6-month interval; 50 spouses of inpatients with major depression were evaluated.	Lifetime diagnosis: κ = .77
Rosen et al. (1984) Interrater reliability was studied with 54 male schizophrenic inpatients; interviewers were three psychiatrists/psychologists teams.	Current diagnosis: ICC = .77
Bromet , Bunn, Connell, Dew, & Schulberg (1986) Test-retest design had an 18-month interval; the study employed 131 female community subjects from semirural areas. A restructured SADS-L was used on the first administration and only SADS-L depression sections on second administration.[b]	Lifetime diagnosis: κ = .34
Hasin & Grant (1987) Interrater reliability was studied with 11 inpatients of a substance abuse unit.	Lifetime diagnosis: κ = .91
Manuzza et al. (1989) Test-retest design had a variable interval (1 – 60 days); 104 patients with a current or prior anxiety disorder were studied.	Lifetime diagnosis: RDC κ = .76; *DSM-III* κ = .82; *DSM-III-R* κ = .68[c]
Kendler, Gruenberg, & Kinney (1994) Interrater reliability was evaluated for 40 patients within the schizophrenic spectrum.	Diagnosis: κ = .91

Note. κ = unweighted kappas; ICC = intraclass coefficients. Except where otherwise noted, median statistics are reported.
[a]Unpublished dissertation that was cited in Bromet et al. (1986). [b]The kappa coefficient is slightly higher if probable depressions are also considered (i.e., median κ = .41) or the same interviewers were used for both administrations (i.e., median κ = .44). During the 18-month interval, nearly half of those diagnosed as depressed on the second administration had experienced a major depressive episode; this emergence of depression following a serious nuclear accident (Three Mile Island) may have lowered the reliability estimates. [c]Fyer et al. (1989) reported the kappas for individual anxiety symptoms.

(range = .49 – .66; median = .60), and simple phobias (range = .20 – .79; median = .59). Of these symptoms, those associated with phobias (simple and social) proved the most effective.

Other Perspectives. An integral component of the SADS is its overall rating of impairment through the GAS. Endicott et al. (1976) evaluated the GAS's inter-rater reliability in a series of four studies with adult samples. In two studies, a total of 79 psychiatric patients were interviewed by research staff, resulting in ICCs of .76 and .91. Two additional studies involved the review of clinical materials; these studies yielded moderate levels of agreement (ICCs of .69 for patient records and .85 for case vignettes).

Simon, Endicott, and Nie (1987) studied the consistency of self-reporting, often referred to as "temporal stability," in a test-retest design with 762 inpatients (admission and discharge SADS) and 193 outpatients (after a 2-month interval). They employed clinical staff whose reliability had been assessed in previous NIMH studies. The study differed from more formal evaluations of test-retest reliability in that the same clinical staff conducted both the initial and follow-up SADS evaluations; this lack of blindness to earlier diagnoses has likely inflated the level of diagnostic consistency. Simon et al. (1987) found nearly perfect agreement for lifetime RDC diagnoses, with a range of .80 to 1.00 and a median of .99. High agreement was also found for subtypes of major depression. One major advantage of this study over research with small samples was that specific diagnoses had sufficient representation. Because of its lack of blindness, the study reflects more on diagnostic consistency than on interrater reliability.

Conclusions. The SADS has performed impressively with respect to inter-rater and test-retest reliabilities. On a symptom level, the SADS has had moderately high ICCs in studies of interrater (Endicott & Spitzer, 1978) and test-retest (Andreasen et al., 1981; Keller et al., 1981) reliabilities. With respect to summary scales, two studies have found high reliabilities (i.e., ICCs > .80; Endicott & Spitzer, 1978; Keller et al., 1981). More variation was found on diagnosis, although studies generally found good agreement for both interrater and test-retest reliabilities. Investigators not associated with the NIMH collaborative studies had somewhat lower reliability estimates; this was particularly true in test-retest designs with lengthy intervals (e.g., Rounsaville et al., 1981). For example, Spiker and Ehler (1984) found only a moderate level of agreement on current diagnosis (median κ = .57).

The SADS consistently outperforms other general diagnostic interviews. Moreover, the reliability of its individual symptoms is unparalleled in structured interviewing. Perhaps the only drawbacks of the SADS with respect to diagnostic reliability are its emphasis on RDC classification and its more limited spectrum of mental disorders.

Criterion-Related Validity

Validational studies of the SADS are closely tied to RDC diagnosis. The first efforts at establishing validity were therefore linked to Syndeham's criteria of diagnostic validity, with an emphasis on exclusion criteria (differential diagnosis) and outcome criteria. The early outcome studies are summarized by Feighner et al. (1972) and Spitzer et al. (1978) as they relate to RDC criteria. Since that time, several studies have attempted to refine the inclusion/exclusion criteria for depression. Endicott and Spitzer (1979) examined closely the differences between (a) psychotic depression and schizoaffective disorders, and (b) endogenous and nonendogenous major depression. With respect to the latter, they concluded that 2-year outcome data did not support the commonly held notion that endogenous depression had poorer outcomes; indeed, the opposite may be true (also see Gallagher & Thompson, 1983). Klerman, Endicott, Spitzer, and Hirschfeld (1979) employed the SADS to explore neurotic depression and determined that this diagnostic entity did not have sufficiently distinct inclusion and exclusion criteria.

Loebel et al. (1992) followed 70 first-episode schizophrenic inpatients, who were evaluated with the SADS and had monthly follow-ups with the SADS-C for a period up to 3 years. They found that a gradual onset without treatment and premorbid adolescent adjustment predicted patients' remissions, while the severity of symptoms and age of onset did not. Untreated psychotic symptoms associated with schizophrenia appeared to have important implications to future treatment success.

Large numbers of studies have explored the genetic and family correlates of mental disorders with the SADS and the SADS-L.[3] For example, Maziade et al. (1992) reviewed the major genetic-linkage studies for bipolar disorders and found that most of those studies which used structured interviews (76.7%) involved the SADS or the SADS-L. While the findings of these studies are mixed, the authors have found the SADS to be useful in this type of etiological research.

Kendler, Gruenberg, and Kinney (1994) utilized the SADS-L to examine genetic patterns of schizophrenic adoptees. They found a clear genetic pattern for schizophrenia and schizophrenia spectrum disorders that differentiated this constellation from other psychiatric disorders. These data are highly relevant to establishing the etiological basis of schizophrenia.

Kessler, Cleary, and Burke (1985) conducted a 6-month follow-up study of 166 primary care patients, based on repeat administrations of the SADS-L. Their research suggests that the GAS was sensitive to change in both remitted and new cases of mental illness. Interestingly, a substantial proportion of mood and anxiety disorders remitted, although most new cases went unrecognized and therefore untreated by primary care physicians. Predictably, personality disorders evidenced a chronic course with very few remissions or new cases.[4] Over shorter periods of time (i.e., 2 months), the SADS-RDC diagnoses appear to demonstrate remarkable diagnostic consistency (Simon et al., 1987); only hypomanic disorder evidenced substantial variability (i.e., changes in 24.4% of the cases).

A handful of studies have examined outcome criteria for specific disorders. For example, research has considered whether schizophrenics with more positive (e.g., hallucinations and delusions) SADS symptoms have a better prognosis

---

[3]Interestingly, Chapman, Mannuzza, Klein, and Fyer (1994) found that care must be exercised in how familial histories are collected, since patients and relatives often perceive mental disorders within the family very differently.

[4]The sole exception was labile personality disorder; its inclusion criteria may be confounded by maladaption to chronic physical illness.

than those with predominantly negative (e.g., flattened affect and decreased motivation) symptoms. Studies have yielded mixed results towards confirming (e.g., Andreasen & Olsen, 1982) and disconfirming (e.g., Rosen et al., 1984) this hypothesis. Several studies have also examined the treatment-responsiveness of SADS-diagnosed manic syndromes. Secunda et al. (1985) examined the SADS and the GAS in conjunction with several observational methods. They found that the SADS manic symptoms discriminated manic episode and bipolar disorder from other diagnoses. In addition, the SADS-C manic scale combined with rating scales successfully predicted treatment outcome. Similarly, Freeman, Clothier, Pazzaglia, Sesem, and Swann (1992) found the SADS-C and GAS useful in measuring treatment response in manic patients. Moreover, the results converged with findings from the Brief Psychiatric Rating Scale (BPRS; Overall & Gorham, 1962).

Coryell et al. (1994) conducted a multisite NIMH study with the SADS concerning episodes of major depression. They found a remarkable consistency across centers on the course of episodes. Regardless of the number of episodes or referral sources, the course of most episodes was well-defined, with recovery for 60% of the cases in 6 months and 80% in 12 months.

Hokanson, Rubert, Welker, Hollander, and Hedeen (1989) employed three successive administrations of the SADS-L, the Interpersonal Checklist (LaForge & Suczek, 1955), the Self-Esteem Inventory (Filippo & Lewinsohn, 1971), and social activity logs in a study of depressed college freshmen. They compared depressed subjects ($n = 37$) and those who became depressed ($n = 27$) to normals ($n = 43$) and those with other disorders ($n = 17$). They found significant differences in concomitant characteristics of depression to be low social contact, anhedonia, and increased stress. Differences for new cases of depression were less clear but appeared to be related to general indices of psychopathology.

Rounsaville et al. (1981) studied the diagnostic stability of 117 opiate users across a 6-month period and demonstrated the predicted consistency for substance abuse disorders (i.e., 100%). Other common disorders evidenced moderately high consistency from the initial assessment to the follow-up: major depression (77.4%), alcoholism (88.2%), and antisocial personality disorder (76.9%). Understandably, less frequent disorders exhibited greater variability. Additional follow-up by the same research group (Kosten, Rounsaville, & Kleber, 1986) suggested complicated interactions between life stresses, depression, treatment, and the outcome of opioid dependence.

The original and subsequent research on the course and outcome of the SADS-derived diagnoses is generally positive. A small group of studies have explored the convergent validity of the SADS-RDC diagnosis, while the bulk of SADS validity studies address its concurrent validity. These two forms of validity will be addressed individually.

Convergent Validity. Dean, Surtees, and Sahsidharan (1983) combined the PSE (Wing, Cooper, & Sartorius, 1974; Wing, Nixon, Mann, & Leff, 1977) with the SADS in order to compare diagnostic systems. In a study of 576 female community subjects, generally good agreement was found for RDC major depression the ICD-8 diagnoses, with relatively poor agreement on the other two common diagnoses: minor depression and generalized anxiety disorder. Despite the large initial sample, the results are somewhat tempered by the relatively small number of diagnoses (*n* = 80) and narrow representation of mental disorders.

Boyd, Weissman, Thompson, and Myers (1983) performed SADS interviews on 510 community subjects and examined diagnostic criteria for alcoholism based on, among others, the RDC, *DSM-III*, and ICD-9. Despite some variation, the concordance between *DSM-III* alcohol abuse and RDC alcoholism was 78.8%; between ICD-9 alcohol dependence and RDC, 64.7%. In both cases, the RDC classification was more encompassing. In other words, RDC almost never missed either *DSM-III* alcohol abuse (3.7% missed) or ICD-9 alcohol dependence (8.3% missed). Moreover, the SADS was found useful in collecting data for other diagnostic systems.

Hill, Gallagher, Thompson, and Ishida (1988) explored the suicidal ideation and behavior for elderly patients with SADS-RDC diagnoses of major depression. They found that three scales contributed to the prediction of suicidality as measured by the SADS: the Hopelessness Scale (Beck, Weissman, Lester, & Trexler, 1974), the Beck Depression Inventory (BDI; Beck, Ward, Mendelson, Mock, & Erbaugh, 1961), and health ratings. Although it was not the direct focus of their work, Hill et al. (1988) found predicted interrelationships among hopelessness, depression, and suicidal ideation.

L. J. Chapman et al. (1984) administered a slightly modified SADS-L that included additional items related to schizotypal and prepsychotic symptoms. When compared to measures of social adjustment and impulsive nonconformity, L. J. Chapman et al. (1984) found predicted differences on these scales with typically nonconforming disorders (APD and substance abuse) as well as with schizotypal disorders. Following this line of research, Eckblad and L. J. Chapman (1986) provided similar evidence for hypomanic disorder on the basis of self-report inventories.

Concurrent Validity. In the original validity study, Endicott and Spitzer (1978) correlated the SADS summary scales with the Katz Adjustment Scales, completed by subjects and relatives, and the Symptom Checklist-90 (SCL-90; Derogatis, 1977). The mean correlations of the SADS summary scales with the Katz were .42 for relatives and .40 for subjects; similarly, the mean correlation with the SCL-90 was .47. Although relatively modest, such validity coefficients are typical in the presence of multiple sources of data (Cronbach, 1970).

Hesselbrock et al. (1982), as described in Chapter 3, examined the diagnostic concordance for the SADS-L and the DIS. They found moderately high kappas (.72 – 1.00, median = .76) for four common diagnoses. Diagnostic agreement was lower on infrequent diagnosis, which resulted in an overall concordance of 93/133 or 69.9%.

Endicott et al. (1976) examined the concurrent validity of GAS in comparison to ratings on the MSER. They found that GAS ratings at the time of admission and 6 months later correlated with the MSER at .44 and .62, respectively. In addition, a higher percentage of patients with GAS ratings under 40 (i.e., 48.3% in 9 months) were rehospitalized, in comparison to those patients with moderate GAS ratings of 40 to 61 (29.4%) and high GAS ratings above 62 (27.8%) .

A body of research has examined the concurrent validity of depression as diagnosed on the SADS. Several studies have examined agreement between the

SADS and SADS-C and the Hamilton Depression Rating Scale (HDRS; Hamilton, 1960). Endicott, Cohen, Nee, Fleiss, and Sarantakos (1981) compared 48 inpatients on both measures; they found that the HDRS correlated at .84 with depression syndrome, .80 with endogenous features, .60 with anxiety, and −.69 with GAS. Although the correlation with anxiety is unfortunately high, the other validity coefficients offer strong support for the SADS-C validity with depression. Subsequently, Hurt et al. (1982) compared SADS diagnostic interviews to interviews based on the HDRS. They found a moderately high negative correlation ($r = -.71$) between the HDRS and the GAS, which is consistent with the Endicott et al. (1981) study.

Bromet et al. (1986) found that low scores on the SCL-90 depression scale and few reported depressive symptoms on the SADS were associated with low incidence of subsequent depression. They did not formally assess the level of association between the two measures. Myers and Weissman (1980) assessed the diagnostic agreement between the self-report measure, the Center of Epidemiologic Studies Depression scale (CES-D; Radloff, 1977), and SADS-RDC diagnosis. With use on 482 community subjects, agreement was found for 14 of 22 (63.6%) depressed persons and 432 of 460 (93.9%) nondepressed persons. Again, no correlations between the measures were reported.

Rapp and his colleagues (Rapp, Parisi, & Walsh, 1988; Rapp, Parisi, Walsh, & Wallace, 1988) examined SADS-RDC diagnoses for an elderly sample of 150 medical inpatients. They found highly significant differences between SADS-RDC depression, other disorders, and controls, in the predicted direction, for the BDI, the Self-Report Depression Scale (Zung, 1965), and the GDS (Yesage et al., 1983). As expected, depression was often associated with very poor physical health.

Rogers, Harris, and Wasyliw (1983) compared SADS-C and SCL-90 administrations across two time periods with a small sample of forensic patients. As a stringent test of concurrent validity, they compared individual symptoms for 23 comparable variables. Overall, they found moderate to moderately high correlations (i.e., M rs = .54 for the first, and .68 for the second administration). These findings compare favorably to the initial validity studies with the SCL-90/SADS-C (i.e., M r = .48; Derogatis, 1977). However, Rogers et al. expressed concern regarding the variability of individual reliability estimates across administrations.

In contrast to the previous studies, Johnson, Magaro, and Stern (1986) examined the discriminant validity of the SADS-C in comparison to the BDI and HDRS. They compared scores on these measures on community controls, depressed patients, and paranoid and nonparanoid schizophrenics. They established that depressed patients had higher scores than other groups on all measures, including the SADS-C depression scale.[5] In addition, the SADS-C depression scale correlated highly with the BDI (.81) and the HDRS (.96). Finally, they found predicted correlations between the GAS and the BDI (−.50) and HDRS (−.45) as estimates regarding the severity of depression. This study by

---

[5]Because the SADS-C is an abbreviated version of the SADS, items for the SADS summary scales associated with depression were compiled into a single depression subscale. Also of interest, schizophrenic patients scored higher than other groups on the schizophrenia subscale, which was derived from psychotic items of the SADS-C.

Johnson et al. (1986) is methodologically superior to other concurrent validity studies in its use of diagnostically different clinical samples; these avoid the restricted range of other studies and allow a testing of discriminant validity.

Hasin and Grant (1987a, 1987b, 1987c; see Chapter 3) compared the DIS diagnosis with the SADS-L on depression and other disorders. In general, they found very poor agreement for several diagnoses in a study of 120 drug abusers. With respect to depression, the kappa was negligible (.13). Not surprisingly, the two measures showed moderately high levels of agreement for substance abuse. Why this study is at variance with other research is difficult to explicate. Possibly, the unreliability often found with substance abusers is partially responsible.

Alternate Versions. Green and Price (1986) experimented with shortened versions of the SADS that comprised RDC "packets." Since the questions included in these packets are substantially different from those found in the SADS, their equivalency with the SADS must be fully tested. In testing 33 patients on both the RDC packets and the SADS-RDC, a high level of concordance was achieved (90.9%; κ = .94). However, only the diagnoses of depression and alcoholism were adequately represented. Therefore, I cannot recommend the use of the RDC packets at this time, even for screening purposes.

Leboyer et al. (1991) tested the reliability of the SADS-LA for French and German translations. Apparently, these translations represented a consensus approach among mental health professionals from both countries, although no independent translations or back-translations to English were performed. Results for current diagnosis were high (κs = .89 – 1.00). Unfortunately, the data combined interrater and test-retest reliability.

Response Styles and SADS Validity. The validity of any diagnostic interview depends partly on its ability to detect feigned disorders. In other words, if malingered disorders are not discovered, then diagnostic accuracy must necessarily suffer. No studies have directly addressed the ability of the SADS to withstand systematic attempts at malingering. However, Rogers (1988) performed a normative study[6] of the SADS with 104 forensic patients. He proposed several potential strategies that would suggest highly atypical response patterns: (a) a pattern of rare symptoms endorsed by 5% or less of the forensic sample, (b) pairs of symptoms which either are contradictory or occur together infrequently, and (c) endorsement of many symptoms with extreme severity. Inspection of these strategies may alert psychologists to the potential of feigning.

Rogers (1988) also suggests nonempirical guidelines for evaluating the consistency of patients' self-reports and the integration of collateral SADS interviews (also see Rogers & Cunnien, 1986). In addition, the emphasis of SADS-L on the onset and course of mental disorders places a special burden on feigners in attempting to make the malingered disorders believable in describing current and past episodes.

Summary. Studies of the RDC, as summarized by Feighner et al. (1972) and Spitzer et al. (1978), document the concerted efforts to establish consistent outcome criteria for RDC diagnosis. Relatively few studies have attempted to

---

[6]Greene (1988) promulgated this normative approach to malingering, in which highly atypical responses in a socially deviant pattern are seen as indirect evidence of feigning.

examine the convergent validity of SADS-RDC diagnosis and other classification systems, such as the *DSM-III* and *DSM-III-R*. One exception was research by Boyd et al. (1983) who found a moderately high concordance on alcohol abuse of approximately 80%. Concurrent validity studies generally support the use of the SADS, especially in the assessment of mood disorders and overall impairment (GAS). The study by Johnson et al. (1986) is particularly noteworthy in establishing the discriminability of SADS-C scales for depressed and schizophrenic patients.

The primary limitation of the SADS appears to be its clinical applicability to substance abusers. Available research raises questions on the diagnostic stability of the SADS with drug abusers (Rounsaville et al., 1981) as well as the inconsistency of clinical data across the SADS-L and DIS (Hasin & Grant, 1987c). A second constraint is the lack of cross-validated research on translated versions of the SADS.

Generalizability and Cross-Cultural Research

Studies of very experienced clinicians (Andreasen et al., 1981; Keller et al., 1981) suggest that the SADS validity is generalizable across research sites and inpatient and outpatient populations. Researchers from the NIMH collaborative studies on the psychobiology of depression conducted interviews at five centers (Boston, Chicago, Iowa City, New York, and St. Louis) which yielded highly consistent results. In addition, Andreasen et al. (1982) found very good reliabilities across research sites for videotaped SADSs.

Few studies have examined the prevalence rates of SADS–RDC diagnoses for different community samples. For example, Weissman and Myers (1980) conducted a longitudinal study of 511 subjects who were systematically evaluated in 1967, 1969, and 1975; SADS was administered during the 1975 assessment period only. As found in previous research, the lifetime prevalence of depression occurred almost twice as frequently in females than in males. Minorities had a lower, but statistically nonsignificant, prevalence of major depression.

Unlike the DIS, the SADS has paid relatively little attention to cultural diversity in establishing its validity. Several larger studies do not report ethnic status (Andreasen et al., 1981; Kessler et al., 1985) or alternatively, limit their sample either exclusively (Simon et al., 1987) or almost exclusively (Boyd et al., 1983; Bromet et al., 1986) to Whites.

Vernon and Roberts (1982) conducted a large-scale study of current and lifetime diagnoses based on community samples of 219 Whites, 187 African-Americans, and 122 Mexican-Americans. These investigators found comparable prevalence rates for most mental disorders. The notable exceptions were several mood disorders, which were approximately twice as prevalent in African-Americans and Mexican-Americans as in the White samples. Overall, the study would suggest generalizability across minority groups.

Research is generally lacking on translated versions of the SADS, as noted in the previously described validity studies. In addition, no data are available on its use with Hispanic populations other than English-speaking Mexican-Americans;

psychologists may wish to rely on the DIS for these patients. Certainly, more work is needed with respect to ethnic diversity and minority status and their potential influences on SADS evaluations.

Clinical Applications

Kessler et al. (1985) underscored the need for systematic assessment of primary care patients through the use of SADS or other structured interviews. When compared to the SADS-L, Kessler et al. found that nonpsychiatric physicians who performed the role of primary care providers recognized only 20% of chronic mental disorders that were present for at least 6 months. Moreover, these same physicians missed nearly every new case of mental disorders; they recognized a mere 3% of new cases over the same 6-month period. With the introduction of the SADS, the diagnosis and subsequent treatment is likely to improve vastly.

Psychologists and other mental health professionals have often been reluctant to devote the necessary resources for the organized and periodic evaluation of problematic patients. One exception is research by Rogers and Wettstein (1985), who readministered the SADS-C at 3- to 4-month intervals over an 18 month period to potentially dangerous outpatients.[7] They found significant differences on the initial SADS-C for successful and rehospitalized patients; readmitted patients had (a) much lower GAS scores, (b) many more symptoms in the clinical range, and (c) increased severity on specific symptoms. When the last assessment was examined prior to hospitalization, these differences were maintained. While their results are likely to be specific to their patient population, the Rogers and Wettstein study illustrates the usefulness of the SADS-C in the systematic monitoring of treatment changes, including both improvement and decompensation.

The SADS and SADS-C are well suited for documenting changes in clinical status for patients with major mental illness. Among the general diagnostic measures, the SADS offers more comprehensive coverage than its alternatives for mood and psychotic disorders. For studies that assess either the course of these disorders or treatment response, the SADS would appear to be the measure of choice. Not only does it provide severity ratings; it also incorporates associated clinical features which may be important markers regarding chronicity and response to specific treatments.

The SADS is also useful in medical settings (Cavanaugh & Wettstein, 1989; Weddington, Segraves, & Simon, 1986). Rapp and his coinvestigators (Rapp, Parisi, & Walsh, 1988; Rapp, Parisi, Walsh, & Wallace, 1988) found that the SADS was an effective diagnostic measure for medical patients. Their research suggested a relative lack of attention to mental disorders by medical staff: none of 27 depressed patients had been accurately diagnosed by treating physicians. Of grave concern is that fact that patients without depression were more likely than those with depression to be prescribed antidepressants. The inclusion of a structured interview such as the SADS would likely improve both diagnosis and clinical intervention.

---

[7]All patients had been found not guilty by reason of insanity on very serious charges and were evaluated as "high risk" when entering the outpatient treatment program.

The hallmark of the SADS is its impressive interrater reliabilities for current episodes. In clinical settings where highly reliable diagnoses are critical for mood and psychotic disorders, psychologists would do well to consider the SADS, based on the reproducibility of its results for individual symptoms, summary scales, and diagnosis. The SADS could also be integrated with sections of the SCID to produce a more comprehensive diagnostic framework for disorders, particularly personality disorders.

Of the general diagnostic measures, the SADS should also be considered in evaluations where the veracity of self-reporting is at question. Although this has not been tested in an experimental design, Rogers (1988) performed a normative study and established guidelines for when feigning should be considered. By the same token, Rogers (1988) also provided threshold criteria for when psychologists should consider defensiveness or the underreporting of symptoms. For example, he suggested that the endorsement of four or fewer symptoms for the current episode was very unusual (< 1% of patients) and should signal the need for a thorough assessment of underreporting.

Rogers and his colleagues (Rogers, 1986; Rogers & Cavanaugh, 1981; Rogers & Cunnien, 1986; Rogers, Thatcher, & Cavanaugh, 1984) have made a strong argument for the use of the SADS in forensic evaluations. Because of its impressive interrater reliability and adequate test-retest reliability over lifetime diagnoses, the SADS lends itself to the assessment of impairment at specific time periods. For example, insanity evaluations require an assessment of symptomatology/impairment at a discrete time period, namely the time of the offense. In two related studies, Rogers (Rogers, Cavanaugh, & Dolmetsch, 1981; Rogers et al., 1984) was able to establish significant differences in SADS summary scales and the GAS for patients clinically determined to be sane and insane. The SADS provided clear evidence of pervasive psychotic symptomatology in those evaluated as insane. Likewise, the SADS may be adapted to civil forensic cases, such as personal injury. Under these circumstances, the SADS current episode (i.e., Part I) can be administered for three discrete time periods: just prior to the injury, soon after the injury (e.g., 3 – 6 months), and for the present time. This expanded version of the SADS provides a structure for understanding the acute and long-term effects of the injury. In addition, clinicians can assess whether the reported progress (a) is consistent with other clinical data and (b) fits a typical pattern of treatment response. Thus, the SADS lends itself to a variety of forensic evaluations.

The advent of the *DSM-IV* has little direct impact on the clinical usefulness of the SADS. As noted in the introduction to this chapter, the SADS was organized by RDC rather than *DSM* criteria and addresses a constellation of primarily psychotic and mood disorders. The SADS was designed to collect comprehensive data on these disorders. Towards this end, the individual SADS items cover nearly all the symptoms for schizophrenic and mood disorders found in the *DSM-IV*. With respect to longitudinal diagnosis in Part II, the greatest change is found in APD which has been successively modified in each version of *DSM* (see Chapter 1). For the diagnosis of APD, psychologists will need to augment the SADS with extensive questioning about *DSM-IV* inclusion criteria.

Major modifications of *DSM-IV* anxiety disorders are likely to affect the diagnosis of anxiety disorders with both the SADS and the SADS-LA. Psychologists may wish to use the anxiety questions of the SADS to screen for potential anxiety disorders, since the clinical inquiries address most anxiety symptoms. Prior to rendering a *DSM-IV* anxiety disorder diagnosis, supplementary questioning will be required.

In summary, the SADS is adaptable to a wide range of clinical settings where reliable and precise measurement is imperative. Because of its versatility, I would argue for the inclusion of the SADS in the clinical training of psychologists, with the level of preparation on par with that of more traditional psychometric approaches. For purposes of clarity, Table 4.3 includes a summary of the SADS's primary advantages in clinical assessments.

The SADS also has several limitations in clinical practice. Among these is its requirement of more intensive training than most diagnostic interviews. Towards this objective, the Biometric Research at the New York State Psychiatric Institute has videotapes and other training materials available. Many research programs have implemented week-long training programs in the administration and scoring of the SADS. Other drawbacks (see Table 4.4) include its focus on mood and schizophrenic disorders to the relative exclusion of other Axis I disorders, and its use of RDC diagnostic criteria.

Table 4.3
Advantages of the SADS in Diagnostic Evaluations

1. Interrater reliability

   The SADS, more than any other diagnostic measure, has outstanding interrater reliabilities for current episodes that extends from individual symptoms to summary scales and diagnoses. In addition, the SADS compares favorably to other measures on lifetime diagnoses.

2. Symptom severity

   The SADS provides severity ratings for many symptoms experienced during the current episode; these ratings allow psychologists to accurately estimate the salience of particular symptoms as well as treatment response.

3. Associated symptoms

   The SADS provides comprehensive coverage of symptomatology associated with mood and psychotic disorders. In addition to inclusion criteria, the SADS attempts to assess associated features and clinical characteristics of particular disorders. For example, the SADS items addressing major depression include an additional 20 clinical ratings beyond those needed to make the diagnosis.

4. Suspected feigning

   The SADS has some clinical guidelines for when to suspect feigning. While preliminary in nature, they are substantially better than those available for other general diagnostic interviews.

5. Convergent validity

   Convergent validity studies tend to confirm the validity of the SADS-RDC diagnoses.

Table 4.4
Limitations of the SADS in Clinical Evaluations

1. Narrow band of diagnosis

   Although the SADS is designed to cover 23 mental disorders, the majority of its diagnoses are mood disorders and their subtypes. For a comprehensive review of Axis I disorders, psychologists must supplement the SADS with additional clinical interviews.

2. RDC-based diagnosis

   One complication with the use of the SADS is that the clinical inquiries are focused on RDC diagnostic criteria, rather than *DSM-III-R* or *DSM-IV*. Although the diagnostic systems are often very close, psychologists must be aware of the differences and augment the SADS with additional clinical inquiries.

3. Sophisticated training requirement

   As a semistructured diagnostic interview, the SADS requires that the psychologist be well versed in diagnosis and have a working knowledge of the SADS's administration and scoring. (Training materials are readily available.)

4. Absence of translated versions

   Unlike the DIS, for example, relatively little attention has been paid to validation of non-English versions of the SADS.

5

Structured Clinical Interview for *DSM-III-R* Disorders (SCID) and Other Structured Interviews for Axis I Disorders

Structured interviews for Axis I disorders, beyond the DIS, the SADS, and the PSE, lack the large-scale studies that incorporate normative (epidemiological) and longitudinal research. These additional structured interviews often correspond with the assessment models of the DIS and SADS. For example, the RDI (Helzer et al., 1981) was the predecessor of the DIS, while the Composite International Diagnostic Interview (CIDI; World Health Organization, 1987) is largely an outgrowth of the DIS. Likewise, the CASH (Andreasen et al., 1992) draws heavily on earlier research with the SADS. In contradistinction, the SCID (Spitzer, Williams, & Gibbon, 1987a, 1987b) was specifically devised to parallel the *DSM-III-R* with respect to inclusion criteria and decision rules.

My decision to include the SCID in this composite chapter on Axis I disorders reflects on the notable absence of extensive validational research. Despite the auspicious beginning of the SCID as a systematic method of assessing *DSM-III-R* diagnoses, major studies of its reliability and discriminant validity have generally not been forthcoming. Perhaps the encompassing nature of the SCID, with its extraordinary coverage of diagnoses, militates against the collaborative research that has been the hallmark of the SADS and the DIS.

I have also chosen to include the PSE in this summary chapter despite its extensive validation. My rationale for this decision is that the PSE, although developed as part of the U.S.–U.K. Diagnostic Project (see Cooper et al., 1972), represents a "crystallization of Anglo-European clinical methods and concepts, much influenced by the phenomenological approach of Jaspers and Schnieder" (Luria & Guziec, 1981, p. 250). As such, it is unlikely to be employed by North American psychologists in clinical practice and applied research.

Major modifications in the *DSM-IV* have centered on anxiety disorders. For each of the Axis I structured interviews, psychologists must take into account the addition of panic attack and acute stress disorder as new diagnoses. In addition, the inclusion criteria have been modified for nearly all of the existing anxiety disorders. Psychologists may wish to continue to use the current structured interviews and augment their questioning when significant symptoms of anxiety are present. Most other major Axis I changes occurred in disorders not typically covered by general structured interviews (e.g., somatoform and dissociative disorders).

This chapter focuses extensively on the development and validation of the SCID and the PSE. This discussion and analysis will be followed by brief reviews of other Axis I structured interviews.

Structured Clinical Interview for *DSM-III-R* (SCID)

Description and Rationale

Spitzer, Williams, Gibbon, and First (in press) described the early development of the SCID from its initial conceptualization in 1983 to its first draft in 1985. With funding from NIMH, an extensive field trial was carried out in the mid-1980s (see Williams et al., in press). The most recent version is available through the investigators (Spitzer, Williams, & Gibbon, 1987a, 1987b) at a nominal cost or, with slight modifications and at substantial cost, from the American Psychiatric Press (Spitzer, Williams, Gibbon, & First, 1990b).[1]

The SCID for Axis I disorders is actually a constellation of three closely related measures: (a) the SCID-P (Patient version with complete coverage of psychotic symptoms) is intended for general clinical use; (b) the SCID-P with Psychotic Screen (Patient version with a highly abbreviated coverage of psychotic symptoms) is used in some outpatient settings in which psychotic disorders are unusual; and (c) the SCID-NP (Non-Patient version with a different introduction but coverage similar to SCID-P with Psychotic Screen) is aimed at non-clinical populations. In addition to these versions, the SCID-II (Spitzer et al., 1987b) is an entirely separate component, designed to assess personality disorders (see Chapter 9). Spitzer et al. (in press) also described several research versions of the SCID that include specialized questions for panic disorders (see Williams, Spitzer, & Gibbon, 1992) and treatment of schizophrenia (Schooler, Keith, Severe, & Matthews, 1989).

The SCID-P is comprised of an Overview Section (sociodemographic data, current problems and symptoms, treatment history, and chart of significant life events), Summary Score Sheet (lifetime and current diagnoses, plus Global Assessment Functioning Scale or GAF), and nine modules for disorders/ syndromes. The organization of mood and psychotic disorders involves two steps: (a) clinical ratings of symptomatology, and (b) integration of symptoms for diagnosis and differential diagnosis. In comparison, the remainder of the SCID is organized in modules that combine symptoms and diagnosis.

The most complex and challenging module of the SCID-P is Psychoactive Substance Use Disorders. Psychologists and other mental health professionals are

---

[1]Instruments developed under NIMH funds (e.g., the SADS) typically cannot be sold for a profit.

asked to identify significant substance abuse in eight drug classes: (a) sedatives-hypnotics-anxiolytics, (b) cannabis, (c) stimulants, (d) opioids, (e) cocaine, (f) hallucinogens/PCP, (g) other, and (h) polydrug use (i.e., at least three of the above categories). Each reported drug class is then rated on as many as 15 symptoms.

Table 5.1
Organization of the Structured Clinical Interview for
DSM-III-R (SCID-P)

Disorder/syndrome	Number of symptoms/ratings
Mood syndromes	
Major Depressive	33
Manic	33
Dysthymia	18
Psychotic and associated symptoms	
Delusions	19
Hallucinations	11
Clinical Observations	12
Differential diagnosis of psychotic disorders	
Brief Reactive Psychosis	5
Schizophrenia	11
Schizophreniform	6
Schizoaffective	3
Delusional	7
Mood disorders	14
Psychoactive substance abuse disorders	
Alcohol	18
Non-Alcohol	130
Anxiety disorders	
Panic	25
Agoraphobia	13
Social Phobia	16
Simple Phobia	16
Obsessive-Compulsive	14
Generalized	25
Somatoform disorders	
Somatization	39
Somatoform Pain	5
Undifferentiated	7
Hypochondriasis	6
Eating disorders	
Anorexia Nervosa	9
Bulimia Nervosa	10
Adjustment disorder	8

The organization of the SCID-P is hierarchical, with explicit decision trees for when to discontinue administration of each module. The advantage of this organization is that the interviewer minimizes unnecessary expenditure of time on symptoms which are unlikely to qualify for a particular disorder. The disadvantages of this approach are that diagnoses may be occasionally overlooked and critical ratings of psychopathology are frequently absent.

The scoring system for individual symptoms is based on a 3-point rating: 1 for absent/false, 2 for subthreshold (i.e., the criterion is nearly met), and 3 for threshold/true (i.e., the criterion is met or exceeded). Nearly all symptoms are rated for the current episode. Moreover, clinicians are asked to make several additional distinctions. For mood disorders, ratings of both current and past episodes are required. For psychotic symptoms and mood syndromes, judgments regarding etiology (organic/not organic) are mandated. Interviewers are encouraged to use all sources of clinical data in making their ratings.

Clinical inquiries are organized into Standard Questions, Branching Questions, Optional Probes, and Unstructured Questions. The majority of questions are composed of standard questions, presented in regular type in the left columns of the SCID-P, that are routinely asked of each patient. In addition, branching questions are occasionally used. These are presented with prefatory instructions which are capitalized, such as "IF YES," "IF UNCLEAR," and "IF NOT ALREADY KNOWN." Finally, optional probes are presented in parentheses and should be used to clarify clinical ratings of diagnostic criteria. One important feature of the SCID-P is the attention paid to the patient's own description of symptoms. Certain clinical inquiries, particularly those addressing mood states, will specify "OWN EQUIVALENT" as explicit permission to use the patient's own words to describe symptomatology. The SCID-P and other versions are "semi-structured" in that the interviewer must augment the SCID inquiries with his/her own clinical inquiries in cases of inadequate or ambiguous information.

The primary purpose of the SCID is to provide comprehensive coverage of most *DSM-III-R* Axis I disorders. As noted by Spitzer et al. (in press), the SCID-P is not exhaustive; seven major diagnostic categories are not addressed (i.e., developmental disorders, organic mental disorders, dissociative disorders, sexual disorders, sleep disorders, factitious disorders, and impulse control disorders). In addition, less common mood, anxiety, and somatoform disorders are also not covered. Nevertheless, the SCID-P provides the broadest coverage among diagnostic interviews for Axis I disorders. The SCID-P distinguishes itself from other diagnostic interviews, with the exception of the DIS, in its formal coverage of *DSM-III-R* diagnostic criteria.

The trade-off for diagnostic interviews, described in Chapter 1, is breadth versus depth. Because of its breadth, the SCID-P evaluates the majority of diagnostic criteria by single inquiries, since more extensive questioning would unduly lengthen the interview process. Even so, some clinicians are selective in their administration of SCID-P modules, which may introduce additional information variance into the diagnosis.

Reliability Studies of the SCID

Williams et al. (in press) described the primary reliability study conducted with SCID-P in a test-retest design. A total of five clinical sites (total N = 390) and two nonclinical sites (total N = 202) were employed. The clinical sites represented a range of inpatient and outpatient settings, with prevalent diagnoses of mood, anxiety, schizophrenic, and substance abuse disorders. Interviewers with a minimum of background information and unaware of other diagnostic results performed SCID-P interviews. The interval period between SCID-P interviews ranged from 24 hours to 2 weeks. An important dimension of the reliability study was the use of interviewers from different centers in actual SCID-P interviews.

The weighted kappas for current diagnoses across clinical sites ranged from .40 to .86, with a median of .59.[2] A major cause of concern was the substantial variation among clinical sites for common disorders. For example, the range of kappas for major depression varied markedly, from .37 to .82. Even more remarkable was the extraordinary variability in agreement for alcohol abuse/dependence (.00 – .73). Weighted kappas across current diagnoses fluctuated considerably from .49 to .67. Interestingly, lifetime diagnoses were somewhat higher (median κ = .68) and fell in the moderate range.

Weighted kappa coefficients were very modest for the nonclinical samples, based in part on the low prevalence of mental disorders. For the five disorders with sufficient representation ($\geq$ 10), the range of kappa was .19 to .53 with a median of .42. Because of their correction for low-base rates, I would argue that these kappa coefficients should be given little weight in evaluating the reliability of the SCID.

Riskland, Beck, Berchick, Brown, and Steer (1987) conducted an interrater reliability study on three groups of outpatients: 24 generalized anxiety, 25 major depressive, and 26 other disorders. Sixteen psychologists participated in the study that employed videotapes for reliability checks. They found an overall concordance of 83%, with a moderate level of agreement (median κ = .72).

Alnaes and Torgersen (1988) reported a SCID study of 298 outpatients, of whom 30 were videotaped for interrater reliability. Although there appears to have been an excellent concordance (99%) on mood, anxiety, and adjustment disorders, the authors did not report kappa coefficients, except for major depression (.86). While these data are promising, we have no way of knowing which disorders were reliable and which were not.

Skre, Onstad, Torgersen, and Kringlen (1991) employed a Norwegian translation of the SCID in an audiotaped interrater reliability study as part of a larger family study of mental disorders. With the use of three raters per subject, they employed a generalized kappa. For disorders with adequate representation ($n \geq$ 5), the kappas were consistently high, with a range from .70 to .96 and a median of .88. This study underscores the potential for the SCID to produce reliable diagnoses.

Several studies have investigated the SCID's reliability with small targeted samples. For example, Goldsmith et al. (1992) examined the interrater reliability of the SCID in a self-referred sample of obese persons seeking weight reduction treatment. Apparently, the level of overall diagnostic agreement was adequate (κ = .78), although details about the disorders and range of agreement were not

---

[2]The median was calculated for 11 disorders that had sufficient representation ($\geq$ 10 patients).

forthcoming. Williams, Spitzer, and Gibbon (1992) performed a highly targeted reliability study on panic patients. Raters were members of a collaborative study on panic disorders who knew that patients would have at least some panic disorder symptoms. Since nearly all the patients (88.6%) had panic disorders, this study is not a stringent test of the SCID's reliability.

Hayward et al. (1992) examined the interrater reliability of the SCID-NP with sixth- and seventh-grade girls. Here several caveats must be borne in mind: (a) the SCID-NP is not intended for children, and (b) subjects appeared to have been administered only questions associated with panic disorders. Within the narrow scope of panic symptoms, moderate to high (.66 – 1.00) kappa coefficients were reported.

Validation of the SCID

Perhaps because of the SCID's one-to-one correspondence with the *DSM-III-R*, studies have paid relatively little attention to criterion-related validity for differential diagnosis. The two notable exceptions are panic and depressive disorders. In addition, relatively few studies have examined the convergent validity of the SCID with psychometric methods.

One investigation of differential diagnosis with the SCID was carried out by the Quebec pedigree studies (see Maziade et al., 1992). These investigators compared diagnoses by a senior psychiatrist, who reviewed audiotapes of the SCID interviews and clinical records, with a second psychiatrist who reviewed all the materials except for the audiotapes. They found good agreement between these raters and the field interviewers who conducted the SCIDs (κ = .83). Consistent with the research program, diagnoses were chiefly for mood and schizophrenic disorders.

Alnaes and Torgersen (1989a) examined differences between depression and panic disorder with three diagnostic groups: panic-only, depressed-only, and combined. Although some differences in familial variables were observed, they did not form any pronounced pattern. More interesting was the overlap among disorders, with as many as five Axis I diagnoses in addition to Axis II disorders. Worrisome in terms of diagnostic overlap, roughly two-thirds of the depressed-only and panic-only groups, and 95% of the combined group, warranted the diagnosis of a personality disorder from the anxious cluster. Similar overlaps are reported for other mood disorders (Alnaes & Torgersen, 1989b).

Several research teams have addressed the course and treatment outcome of SCID-diagnosed panic disorders. Noyes et al. (1990) examined the baseline and follow-up assessment (*M* = 36.5 months) for 89 patients with panic disorders. They found that panic disordered subjects evidenced poorer adjustment than controls on the Social Adjustment Scale (Weissman, Paykel, & Prusoff, 1972), although they tended to show improvement at follow-up in both self- and observer-rated symptoms. Primary predictors of subsequent adjustment were self-rated anxiety and level of initial impairment. Interestingly, the SCID subtypes related to phobic avoidance were also related to subsequent phobic symptoms and general adjustment. With respect to differential diagnosis, patients with severe phobic avoidance or agoraphobia were more likely than less avoidant patients to have major depression (51% vs. 20%) and personality disorders (48%

vs. 23%). Additional studies, cited below, address the comorbidity of panic and depressive disorders.

Treatment studies with SCID-diagnosed panic disorders have focused on both medication and placebo trials. Ballenger et al. (1988) conducted a multisite trial of alprazolam on panic patients and agoraphobic patients. In an 8-week trial, they found that the majority of medicated patients had a resolution of panic attacks (55%), although nearly one-third in the placebo condition (32%) also experienced a cessation of panic attacks.[3] Coryell and Noyes (1988) examined a subset of 47 placebo patients from the Ballenger et al. study. They found that the decreased frequency of panic attacks (i.e., fewer episodes and better outcomes) accounted for patients having better recoveries without treatment. Inexplicably, patients with concurrent major depression manifested a nonsignificant trend towards a greater resolution of panic symptoms than those without depression (34.4% vs. 18.2%). In a similar study, Reich (1990) found no differences in panic symptoms for placebo patients who dropped out of studies compared to those who completed the required 8 weeks.

Maier, Buller, Sonntag, and Heuser (1986) compared SCID diagnoses of panic disorders with ICD-9 classifications for 97 patients presenting with panic attacks. Despite the lack of correspondence between the two diagnostic systems (i.e., ICD-9 does not diagnose panic disorders), the results were rather disconcerting. Substantial numbers of SCID panic patients were categorized by ICD-9 under affective psychosis or neurotic depression, and only a minority (30.9%) warranted any diagnosis of anxiety disorder.

Studies have also examined precursors and biological markers of panic disorders. For example, Rosenbaum et al. (1988) found that the children of panic-disordered and agoraphobic patients exhibited greater behavioral inhibition than controls. A finding important from an etiological perspective was that children of patients with major depression manifested considerably less inhibited behavior. In addition, panic patients have evidenced cardiovascular differences which may, at times, be interpreted as panic attacks (see Gaffney, Fenton, Lane, & Lake, 1988; Shear et al.,1987). Other research has suggested a small but negligible relationship between panic disorders and thyroid function (Lesser, Rubin, Lydriard, Swinson, & Pecknold, 1987).

The comorbidity between panic-disordered and depressed patients has been a matter of diagnostic and treatment concern. Pecknold et al. (1987) found significant differences in the imipramine-binding sites between depressed and panic-disordered patients. Based on the Ballenger et al. (1988) study, Lesser et al. (1988) investigated the role of secondary depression in panic-disordered patients. They found no significant differences in number of panic attacks or severity of phobias for panic patients with or without depression. Moreover, patients treated with alpraxolam reported parallel improvements in anxiety and depressive symptoms. Other studies have documented the role of personality features associated with panic and depressive disorders and the efficacy of subsequent interventions (Reich, Noyes, Hirschfeld, Coryell & O'Gorman, 1987; Reich

---

[3]The fluctuating clinical course of panic disorders militates against developing stable outcome criteria against which to validate these diagnoses.

& Troughton, 1988a). In sum, the results appear equivocal on the differentiation of panic and depressive disorders on the bases of etiology, symptom presentation, and treatment response.

Other research has addressed diagnostic overlap with the SCID for patients with generalized anxiety disorder and psychotic disorders. For example, Strakowski et al. (1993) found variable overlap for patients experiencing their first psychotic episode. One encouraging finding was that diagnostic overlap, with the exception of substance abuse, appeared to be relatively dispersed across a range of other disorders. In addition, delusional disorders appeared to have minimal overlap with mental or medical disorders. Brawman-Mintzer et al. (1993) found considerable diagnostic overlap of generalized anxiety disorder, both with other anxiety disorders and with depression. In sum, these findings are not surprising and likely reflect the current status of diagnosis rather than any particular limitation of the SCID.

Duncan (1987) compared the SCID diagnosis for schizophrenia and bipolar disorders for 48 outpatients who were also administered the DIS and had their clinical records systematically reviewed. They found that the SCID diagnosis outperformed that of the DIS and accurately identified 77% of schizophrenic and 85% of bipolar disorders. Both measures evidence only modest agreement with the record review, which suggests either limitations in record-keeping or constraints of SCID-based diagnosis.

Studies have also addressed the validity of SCID diagnosis for other specific diagnoses. For example, Stuckenberg, Dura, and Kiecolt-Glaser (1990), through the use of receiver operating characteristics analysis, found in a study of 177 elderly community subjects that the HDRS, the BDI, and the Brief Symptom Inventory depression scale (BSI; Derogatis & Spencer, 1982) successfully predicted major depression on the SCID. The latter two scales (BDI and BSI) had sensitivities and specificities greater than .70. Copolov and his associates (Copolov et al., 1989) failed to find differences between depression and other disorders on the dexamethasone suppression test. Other research has examined schizophrenia (Schooler et al., 1989), eating disorders (Schmidt & Telch, 1990; Schwartz, Aylward, Barta, Tune, & Pearlson, 1992), alcoholism (Buydens-Branchey, Branchey, & Noumair, 1989), cocaine dependence (Weiss, Griffin, & Hufford, 1992), PTSD (Pitman, Altman, & Macklin, 1989), and HIV-infected males (Williams, Rabkin, Remien, Gorman, & Ehrhardt, 1990).

In general, the validation studies of the SCID are disappointing. Unlike studies of the SADS and the DIS, systematic investigations of the SCID and its relationship to either clinical diagnosis or other structured interviews have not been forthcoming. Although extensive studies were conducted on the SCID and panic disorder, studies of other diagnostic categories have received relatively little attention. The SCID assumes that the *DSM-III-R* and *DSM-IV* are the gold standards of diagnosis. The SCID is viewed as having "procedural validity" in accurately representing these gold standards. Despite the parallelism between SCID inquiries and *DSM-III-R* criteria, the thoroughness and adequacy of its questions deserve further investigation. Comparisons with the SADS and DIS as well as with self-report measures would be most helpful.

Clinical Applications

For current diagnosis, the SCID-P offers the widest coverage of Axis I disorders with clinical inquiries that parallel *DSM-III-R* inclusion criteria. The SCID was designed to provide clinicians with a comprehensive user-friendly assessment method that would allow the reliable and systematic evaluation of most mental disorders. The SCID has partially met this goal: it provides greater coverage of several diagnostic categories, such as somatoform and eating disorders, than found in other structured interviews. Moreover, the SCID is very comprehensive in its evaluation of substance abuse.

My reservations regarding the routine clinical use of the SCID are threefold. I will address each reservation individually.

First and foremost, the SCID has not been adequately tested with respect to its reliability. The study by Williams et al. (in press) uses a very stringent standard for reproducibility of diagnosis (i.e., a test-retest model with raters from different centers). Unfortunately, the results are only marginally acceptable, with extraordinary variation even with common disorders (e.g., depression and alcohol abuse) that typically achieve high reliability on other interview methods. The interesting question is how well other diagnostic interviews would perform under these stringent conditions. Beyond the Williams et al. (in press) study, the efforts to evaluate the SCID's reliability are limited to very circumscribed diagnoses and, therefore, lack generalizability to other clinical settings. The notable exception is the study of Skre et al. (1991) which suggests considerable promise; however, this study has limited applicability to North American populations since it involved a Norwegian translation.

The second reservation has already been mentioned in the summary paragraph on the SCID's validity. Despite the SCID's parallel structure with the *DSM-III-R*, much more research is encouraged on the relationship of the SCID to other diagnostic measures to establish convergent, if not concurrent, validity. For example, if the DIS and the SCID, both based on *DSM* criteria, evidenced high agreement on common diagnoses, psychologists and other mental health professionals would have a stronger basis for rendering their diagnostic conclusions. On the other hand, marked disparities between the two measures would demand further investigation.

The notable exception to the second reservation is the assessment of panic disorders. As previously noted, the SCID has distinguished itself in the thorough evaluation of panic and agoraphobic disorders with reference to their diagnostic criteria, correlates, and treatment outcome.

The third reservation addresses the vulnerability of the SCID to response styles. A preliminary study by Rogers, Bagby, and Prendergast (1993) suggested that the SCID-P could be faked by schizophrenic patients. With the use of the SIRS as the criterion, these investigators compared response patterns of patients strongly suspected of fabricating bogus symptoms ($n = 13$) to schizophrenics who appeared honest in their presentation of symptoms ($n = 30$). On most psychotic symptoms, the groups were indistinguishable, although dissimulating schizophrenics tended to endorse tactile hallucinations and psychotic symptoms over most of the last 5 years.

The SCID may certainly be used for current episodes in diagnosing those disorders with moderate reliability estimates across research sites. The SCID is the structured interview of choice among general diagnostic measures for non-alcoholic substance abuse, somatoform, eating, and panic disorders. With more extensive validation, the SCID has the potential to improve diagnostic validity for most common disorders. At present, however, psychologists must weigh its obvious advantages (e.g., compatibility with *DSM-III-R* and *DSM-IV* and broad coverage of mental disorders) against its current shortcomings (e.g., modest reliability and lack of emphasis on the severity of symptoms), in deciding how to implement the SCID in their professional practices.

Present State Examination (PSE)

Description and Rationale

The PSE was originally developed to standardize the assessment of psychopathology through the use of accepted clinical inquiries and operationalized definitions (Wing, Birely, Cooper, Graham, & Isaacs, 1967). With its phenomenological emphasis on clinical description, the PSE has organized signs and symptoms into 36 syndrome scores, summarized in Table 5.2. Inspection of Table 5.2 reveals a syndromal structure that is very different from other structured interviews. For example, signs/symptoms of depression may be included in each of the four general clusters and on as many as eight syndromes.

Wing and his colleagues (Wing et al., 1990) described the origins of the PSE in preliminary studies conducted in the late 1950s. After five editions, the first study of the PSE was published (Wing et al., 1967). The seventh and eighth editions were studied extensively in relationship the to U.S.-U.K. Diagnostic Project (Cooper et al., 1972) and the WHO-sponsored International Pilot Study of Schizophrenia (World Health Organization, 1979). Although the PSE was intended as a descriptive measure, more recent studies have examined its usefulness with ICD-8 and ICD-9 diagnoses.

Two substantially different versions of the PSE continue to be used in clinical settings based on the eighth (Wing et al., 1974) and ninth editions (Wing, 1976). The eighth edition provides an exhaustive coverage of psychotic and neurotic characteristics, with approximately 500 items. For most symptoms, the interviewer is provided with a standard question and is encouraged to ask additional inquiries. Although similar in content and organization, the ninth edition is a much briefer version that has eliminated items that are rarely recorded. As such, the PSE ninth edition requires ratings of only 140 symptoms and characteristics. Luria and Guziec (1981) have made a detailed comparison of the two editions and found that the eighth edition has more than twice the depressive items and four times the psychotic symptoms as the ninth edition. Moreover, these commentators observed that ninth edition, unlike the earlier edition, has amalgamated multiple symptoms into single ratings.

The justification for employing the PSE is its standardization of clinical inquires for assessing comprehensively the symptoms and characteristics of psychiatric patients. Wilmink et al. (1989), in an extensive study of 2,000 medical patients, found that Dutch general practitioners missed the majority of mental

Table 5.2
Organization of the Present State Examination (PSE)

Delusional and hallucinatory syndromes
    Nuclear syndrome
    Depressive delusions and hallucinations
    Auditory hallucinations
    Delusions of persecution
    Delusions of reference
    Grandiose and religious delusions
    Sexual and fantastic delusions
    Visual hallucinations
    Olfactory hallucinations
    Subcultural delusions and hallucinations

Behavior, speech, and other syndromes
    Catatonic syndrome
    Incoherence of speech
    Residual syndrome
    Affective flattening
    Hypomania
    Overactivity
    Motor slowness
    Nonspecific psychotic syndrome
    Agitation
    Self-neglect

Specific neurotic syndromes
    Depressed mood
    Obsessional syndrome
    General anxiety
    Situational anxiety
    Hysteria
    Special features of depression

Nonspecific neurotic syndromes
    Depersonalization
    Ideas of reference
    Tension
    Lack of energy
    Worrying
    Irritability
    Social unease
    Loss of interest and concentration
    Hypochondriasis
    Somatic symptoms of depression

disorders as assessed by the PSE. Moreover, Saghir (1971) compared the PSE to unstructured interviews, all of which were administered by experienced psychiatrists. He found that PSE interviews were much more comprehensive in their coverage of psychopathology, with nearly twice the clinical inquiries per category. Interestingly, unstructured interviews were rated with substantially more empathetic statements and interpretations than were PSE interviews with the same patients. In sum, the study suggested that the PSE may standardize clinical inquiries and reduce information variance.[4]

The scoring system for the PSE is roughly analogous to the SCID, with 3-point ratings: 0 for symptom absent, 1 for occasional or not severe, and 2 for almost continuous or severely distressing. In addition, two other ratings are possible: X for asked but unsure of the rating or no reply, and Y for not asked or inapplicable. As noted by Cooper, Copeland, Brown, Harris, and Gourlay (1977), clinicians should be conservative in making their ratings; when in doubt, the lower rating should be given. In general, these ratings are limited to the last 4 weeks, since more extended periods may constrain the PSE's reliability. In cases where extensive case records are available, previous episodes may be rated on the Syndrome Check List (see Wing, 1980).

Reliability of the PSE

The early reliability studies were conducted by Wing et al. (1967) and Kendell, Everitt, Cooper, Sartorius, and David (1968). Wing et al. (1967) reported on a series of small studies that employed the third, fourth, and fifth editions of the PSE. On 172 patients they reported "complete agreement" on diagnoses in 83.7% of the cases. On much smaller samples (20 – 53), they found high correlations, particularly for the fifth edition, for interrater and test-retest reliability. Kendell et al. (1968) on the seventh edition combined interrater and test-retest reliability in a study of 37 psychiatric admissions. With the use of three experienced psychiatrists, they found promising product-moment correlations for interrater reliability for scales (.58 – .97, median = .85). Although the test-retest reliabilities were acceptable (median r = .65), the range was extraordinary (−.05 – .78), with four scales evidencing very poor reliability (< .40): Ideas of Reference, Elevation of Mood, Depersonalization, and Perceptual Disturbance.

Luria and McHugh (1974) employed six videotaped PSEs, each of which was rated by four to six psychiatrists on the eighth edition. Using Kendell's coefficient of concordance, high levels of agreement were achieved for diagnosis (W = .80) and phenomenological sections (W = .94), although the interpretation of results is limited by the small number of cases. In a further study of the eighth edition, Cooper et al. (1977) evaluated 30 random outpatients with a mixed group of raters. Correlations for syndromes evidenced a marked range across both interrater (.34 – .96, median = .76) and test-rest (.16 – .82, median = .50) reliability. Combining the two studies, there appears to be evidence of satisfactory interrater reliability for the eighth edition but only modest test-retest reliability.

---

[4]Saghir (1971) did find considerable variability among PSE interviewers in the extensiveness of their questioning.

Wing, Nixon, Mann, & Leff (1977) conducted the major reliability study of the ninth edition. Initial interviews were conducted by four female interviewers on abbreviated PSEs and were audiotaped whenever possible. Psychiatrists conducted follow-up interviews after substantial intervals, employing the full ninth edition. The level of agreement for syndromes ranged widely for interrater (κs = .25 – .85, median = .63) and test-retest (κs = .00 – .49, median = .39). Although the authors report that psychiatrists made few additional ratings as a result of their full administration, the incomparability of the two administrations may have artificially lowered the test-retest estimates.

Two additional studies of the ninth edition have employed abbreviated PSEs. Remington, Tyrer, Newson-Smith, and Cicchetti (1979) examined the interrater reliability of a 26-item PSE on 52 anxious and depressed patients and found a moderate level of agreement (ICC = .70). Rodgers and Mann (1986) conducted a large community study on a 48-item version of the ninth edition. Interviews were performed by 56 trained female nurses on a predominantly female sample. A total PSE score was highly correlated with psychiatrists' ratings of audiotapes (r = .96), with a satisfactory agreement on individual symptoms (median weighted κ = .70). Unaccountably, reliability estimates for individual symptoms were reported only for female subjects.

Several studies have inspected the reliability of translated versions of the full PSE-9. For example, Lasage, Cyr, and Toupin (1991) examined the interrater reliability of a French translation of the ninth edition PSE. They evaluated the reliability estimates for four nursing assistants on 18 psychiatric patients and found a median kappa of .70. Assumed, but untested, in this study was the comparability of the English and French versions. Mignolli, Faccinicani, Turit, Gavioli, and Micciolo (1988) conducted a combined interrater and test-retest (interval of 4 – 9 days) reliability study on 30 psychiatric patients, obtaining excellent interrater and test-retest reliabilities (M weighted κ = .96 and .83, respectively). Goekoop et al. (1991) assessed the interrater reliability of a Dutch PSE-9 on 40 outpatients and 59 inpatients. Overall agreement was good for self-report responses (M κ = .85) but poor for the observational ratings (M κ = .39). Obviously, replications are needed with each translated version, although the Italian version appears to be very reliable.

Several additional studies are relevant to the PSE's reliability. For example, Sturt (1981) combined data from four earlier studies (total N = 1,085) and found that the total PSE (ninth edition) had high internal consistency with an alpha of .89. Wing, Henderson, and Winckle (1977), in a study of 50 nonpsychotic patient referrals, evaluated either a psychologist or a psychiatrist; they found that the psychologist rated more symptoms than his psychiatric counterpart. Since the ratings were conducted at different centers (i.e., nonrandom assignment of patients) with different patients, the study offers no firm conclusions regarding unreliability. Nonetheless, the study raises an interesting question regarding interprofessional agreement on the PSE.

PSE reliability studies do not tend to follow a standard methodology, which constrains its cross-validation (see Table 5.3). Indeed, the studies vary with respect to the PSE edition, its completeness (abbreviated or full versions), training and background of the evaluators, and the samples studied. In brief, the eighth and ninth editions appear to have adequate interrater reliability for syndromes/scales. Much less is known about the interrater reliability of individual symptoms or diagnoses. Similarly, the test-retest reliabilities have not been sufficiently tested and are highly variable even within studies. In summary, psychologists may feel comfortable in their use of the PSE (eighth and ninth editions) for the evaluation of syndromes/scales, but should remain circumspect with respect to its other applications.

Table 5.3
Reliability Studies of the Present State Examination (PSE)

Study	Agreement
Wing, Birely, Cooper, Graham, & Isaacs (1967) Interrater reliability was studied with 172 patients[a] composed of three inpatient and five outpatient samples; psychiatrists were used as interviewers and raters. Test-retest reliabilities did not specify interval.	Interrater, nonpsychotic sections: $r = .94$; interrater, psychotic sections: $r = .91$. Test-retest, nonpsychotic sections: $r = .76$; test-retest, psychotic sections: $r = .92$
Kendell, Everitt, Cooper, Sartorius, & David (1968) Combined interrater ($n = 37$) and test-retest ($n = 25$) reliability study was conducted on the seventh edition with newly admitted inpatients evaluated by different pairs of three psychiatrists; the interval for retesting was described as "a few days."	Interrater scales, $r = .85$. Test-retest items: $\kappa = .41$[b]; test-retest scales, $r = .65$
Luria & McHugh (1974) Interrater reliability was evaluated using the eighth edition. Four to six psychiatrists observed six videotapes of psychiatric inpatients.	Diagnosis, $W = .80$. Phenomenological sections, $W = .94$
Cooper, Copeland, Brown, Harris, & Gourlay (1977) Interrater and test-retest reliability study was conducted using an abbreviated eighth edition. Five raters (two without mental health backgrounds) interviewed 30 unselected outpatients; repeat administrations on 26 patients were conducted after a 1-week interval.	PSE sections, interrater $r = .76$. PSE sections, test-retest $r = .50$
Wing, Nixon, Mann, & Leff (1977) Interrater ($n = 28$) and test-retest ($n = 95$) reliability study had a community sample; psychiatrists administered the complete ninth edition while lay interviewers administered abbreviated versions. Test-retest interval was typically 1 to 5 weeks (range = 5 – 84 days).	Syndromes, interrater $\kappa = .63$. Syndromes, test-retest $\kappa = .39$

Table 5.3   (continued)
Reliability Studies of the Present State Examination (PSE)

Study	Agreement
Remington, Tyrer, Newsom-Smith, & Cicchetti (1979) Interrater reliability study focused on 26 items of the ninth edition. Five interviewers of varied backgrounds observed videotapes (20 cases) or had separate interviews on the same day (32 cases); patient group was limited to anxiety and depressive disorders.	26 symptoms, ICC = .70
Rodgers & Mann (1986) Interrater reliability study with an abbreviated ninth edition was conducted on a community sample (*N* = 526). Interviewers were 56 female nurses; audiotapes were rated by psychiatrists.	Total PSE score, *r* = .96. 48 symptoms (women only), κ = .71[c]

Note. W = Kendall coefficient of concordance; *r* = product-moment correlations; κ = unweighted kappas; ICC = intraclass coefficients. Except where otherwise noted, median statistics are reported.
[a]Actual numbers used in the calculations are much smaller, ranging from 20 to 53. [b]This calculation is a *M* statistic based on two raters and 25 patients. [c]Actually, the authors report an "index of association," which apparently is highly correlated (*r* = .98) with kappa.

Validation of the PSE

The PSE, because of its phenomenological perspective, has devoted relatively little attention to its relationship to diagnosis. Luria (1979) examined the mean differences for PSE syndromes for four diagnostic groups (total *N* = 35) and found preliminary differences in the expected directions. Wing, Mann, Leff, and Nixon (1978) evaluated 62 nonpsychotic patients and 123 female subjects with depressive or anxiety states on the basis of psychiatric interviews and abbreviated ninth edition PSEs. The two methods were highly convergent on whether individuals had a mental disorder (*r* = .89); the data are less clear, however, regarding the concordance for specific diagnoses.[5] Bebbington, Sturt, and Kumakura (1983) reviewed the concordance rates among the PSE, *DSM-III*, and hospital diagnoses for 146 depressed patients. They found an agreement of 76.5% for *DSM-III* and 84.8% for hospital diagnoses. Huxley, Korer, and Tolley (1987) compared PSEs to social worker diagnoses, with moderate agreement on depression (66.0%) and modest agreement on paranoid schizophrenia (50.0%). Maurer, Biehl, Kuhner, and Loffler (1989) administered the PSE ninth edition, which was augmented by *DSM-III* systems, to 30 acute schizophrenic and 51 discharged depressive patients. They found an 82% concordance rate for depression and stable diagnoses across three admissions, and approximately 60%

---

[5]The study was limited primarily to depressive disorders with less representation of anxiety disorders. Although differences in PSE ratings are reported by disorder, the level of diagnostic agreement is not.

concordance for schizophrenia. Unlike other Axis I diagnostic interviews, the PSE does not report extensive validation studies on a broad range of mental disorders.

Watt, Katz, and Shepherd (1983) conducted a diagnostic outcome study of the PSE with 121 schizophrenic patients who were divided into treatment and nontreatment conditions and reevaluated after 1 and 5 years. The study documented differences in outcome, with substantial numbers either having a single episode (16%) or multiple episodes with little residual impairment (32%). Unfortunately, these investigators did not examine symptom or syndromal differences that might predict the course of the disorder.

Other outcome studies have examined the PSE in the context of mood and anxiety disorders. For example, Robinson, Starr, and Price (1984) documented depression secondary to stroke in 103 elderly medical patients. Although they found immediate and delayed onset of depression, no comparison groups were available to test the significance of the findings in an older medical sample. Catalan, Gath, Bond, and Martin (1984) administered the PSE to 84 psychiatric patients at a 7-month follow-up. Predictably, they found that the more severely impaired patients and those treated with medication tended to manifest greater impairment than others at follow-up. The Catalan et al. study provides data on the usefulness of the PSE in documenting chronic disorders.

PSE studies have placed a major emphasis on concurrent validity with the General Health Questionnaire (GHQ; Goldberg, 1978) and other self-report measures. In an early study, Henderson, Duncan-Jones, Byrne, Scott, and Adcock (1979) established an overall correlation between the PSE and the GHQ of .76. More recently, Banks (1983), in a study of 200 community adolescents using the 28-item version of the GHQ, had an optimum sensitivity of 100% and specificity of 84.5%. Interpretation of the study is limited by the very few numbers of mentally disordered youth (n = 7). Ormel, Koeter, Van Den Brink, and Giel (1989) conducted a longitudinal study on 175 psychiatric outpatients with three administrations of the PSE ninth edition and the 28-item GHQ. The two measures evidenced moderate relationships across the three time periods with correlations of .55, .54, and .71, respectively. Moreover, an analysis of covariance suggested that changes in patient status were observed across administrations on both measures. Wilmink and Snijders (1989) employed a 30-item GHQ to predict PSE results in sample of 292 primary care patients. They found a sensitivity of 91% and a specificity of 62%. Finally, Wilmink and Snijders compared the GHQ to the PSE with 1,994 Dutch medical patients; they found that the GHQ has a sensitivity of 42% and a specificity of 85%. In summary, the PSE provides moderate evidence of concurrent validity for the presence or absence of any mental disorder, but not for particular mental disorders.

Peveler and Fairburn (1990) compared the SCL-90-R to an abbreviated version of the PSE in samples of 113 diabetic and 75 bulimic patients. The two measures evidenced moderate correlations for symptom totals (.59 for diabetics and .74 for bulimics) and indices of overall impairment (.64 for diabetics and .73 for bulimics). Given the atypical samples, the convergence of the two measures is very encouraging. However, the use of a shortened 46-item PSE limits the study's generalizability.

Sturt (1981), in the previously mentioned study, examined the relationship of social functioning to PSE syndromes and found highly significant differences. In contrast, Sturt and Wykes (1987) examined the relationship between the PSE (ninth edition) and social functioning in a sample of 66 chronic psychiatric patients. While community versus institutional placement was related to impairment in social functioning, no such relationship was found between total symptom score on the PSE and the Social Behavior Scale (Wykes & Sturt, 1986).[6] In a study of depression, Parker and Blignault (1983) found that treatment status predicted the total score on the PSE (i.e., depressed untreated subjects had lower ratings than their treated counterparts).

Studies have examined the usefulness of the PSE in epidemiological research. For instance, Bebbington, Hurry, Tennant, Sturt, and Wing (1981) studied the prevalence of mental disorders in a London borough on 800 community residents, with an overall prevalence of ICD diagnoses of 6.1% males and 14.9% females. In a follow-up study, Bebbington, Hurry, and Tennant (1988) found that PSE syndromes related to anxiety and depression evidenced predictable elevations in subjects, both patients and nonpatients, who had recently experienced adverse or threatening events. Similarly, Byrne (1984) and Mayou, Peveler, Davies, Mann, and Fairburn (1991) reported that psychiatric patients were likely to have greater problems with social adjustment, which was also reflected in their presence of psychiatric disorders, as assessed on the PSE ninth edition.

The usefulness of a structured interview can be assessed indirectly by epidemiological comparisons across samples/cultures. If dissimilar prevalence rates are established by employing a measure such as the PSE, then the generalizability of the PSE is questioned. Review of the major epidemiological studies in the last decade (e.g., Hodiamont, Peer, & Syben, 1987; Lehtinen, Lindholm, Veijola, & Vaisanen, 1990; Mavreas, Beis, Mouyias, Rigoni, & Lysktsos, 1986; Vazquez-Barquero et al., 1987) suggests comparable prevalence rates for males (range = 7.2 – 8.6%) but substantially more variation for females (range = 7.5 – 22.6%). Although cultural influences could affect the prevalence of mental illness, this more-than-twofold difference between countries with low prevalence (Netherlands & Finland) and high prevalence (Spain & Greece) is cause for concern.

A number of studies have examined the relationship of the PSE to biological markers. For example, Bachneff and Engelsmann (1983) related EEG recordings to psychiatric syndromes as measured by the eighth edition PSE. Without becoming unduly technical, they found meaningful differences on key PSE symptoms that were associated with systematic variations in computer-averaged electric potentials. As a further example, ratings on the PSE ninth edition for psychotic symptoms appear to be associated with increased dimethyltryptamine excretions, which decreased as the clinical status improved (see Murray, Oon, Rodnight, Bireley, & Smith, 1979). Moreover, the potential efficacy of the PSE to document changes due to medication trials has been noted (e.g., see Nair,

---

[6]Freeman, Cheadle, and Korer (1979) also found no differences in PSE scores for inpatient, day-treatment, and outpatient subjects.

Bloom, Debonnel, Schwartz, & Mosticyan, 1984). Finally, Smith, Carr, Morris, and Gilliland (1988) used selected items for the PSE to study differences in response on the dexamethasone suppression test. On 52 consecutive admissions, levels of cortisol concentration was related to the level of psychomotor retardation of the PSE. Studies of biological markers provide, at best, only indirect evidence of validity, since their results are often open to multiple interpretations.[7]

Family studies have found the PSE, in combination with the SADS-L and the PDE, to be useful in documenting the prevalence of mental disorders in the off-spring of schizophrenic mothers. Parnas et al. (1993) found greater prevalence of schizophrenia and schizotypal personality disorder but not schizoid personality disorder.

In summary, the PSE eighth and ninth editions were intended to system-atize the symptoms and clinical characteristics associated with Axis I disorders. Because of this intent, less emphasis has been placed on the relationship to clinical diagnosis or other diagnostic measures. The validational studies focus on "psychiatric morbidity" or the presence of a major disorder rather than the specific symptomatology associated with a specific disorder. North American mental health professionals must take care not to judge the PSE in ethnocentric terms, since the PSE was constructed from an Anglo-European perspective. As an important caution, PSE studies appear to fall into three major categories: (a) full administration of the eighth edition, (b) full administration of the ninth edition, and (c) highly abbreviated administration (i.e., typically 40 items) of the ninth edition. The generalization across these versions has not been adequately investigated.

Clinical Applications

The PSE, especially the full eighth edition, provides an unparalleled phenomenological review of relevant symptomatology and associated features. In particularly challenging treatment cases, such an exhaustive review may provide a richer and more complete view of the relevant phenomenology than what is typically found in routine *DSM-III-R* diagnoses. For example, a patient with atypical psychosis may be understood within non-*DSM* psychopathology with reference to assessment and treatment outcome.

A second important feature of the PSE is its extensive use in international studies with an emphasis on cultural and cross-cultural matters. With assistance from the World Health Organization, the PSE has been translated into 40 different languages. Studies have shown its clinical usefulness in European countries (e.g., Garyfallos et al., 1991; Hodiamont, Peer, & Syben, 1987; Hout & Griez, 1984; Lasage et al., 1991), English-speaking countries (i.e., Ni Nuallain, O'Hare, & Walsh, 1990; Romans-Clarkson, Walton, Herbison, & Mullen, 1990), and African countries (Gillis, Elk, Ben-Arie, & Teggin, 1982; Katz et al., 1988; Okasha & Ashour, 1981; Orley & Wing, 1979).

The WHO-sponsored study by Katz et al. (1988) illustrates the culturally specific dimensions of mental disorders. Samples of Indian (n = 86) and Nigerian

---

[7]Studies (e.g., C. G. Lyketsos, G. C. Lyketsos, Richardson, & Beis, 1987) have also examined the relationship of the PSE to medical conditions, although this line of research has little direct bearing on PSE validity.

(*n* = 123) schizophrenics were assessed on the PSE and ICD-9. They found differences in the subtypes of schizophrenia as well as symptomatology. For example, Indian schizophrenics possessed more systematized delusions and olfactory hallucinations. In contrast, Nigerian schizophrenics had more delusions of control, thought insertion, and visual hallucinations. Swartz, Ben-Arie, and Teggin (1985) found that certain symptoms were culturally bound, and therefore difficult to interpret meaningfully. Nevertheless, North American psychologists who evaluate substantial numbers of patients from other cultural backgrounds may find the PSE a useful adjunct to their assessments.

The limitations of the PSE to North American practice are readily apparent. While reliability studies suggest a moderate level of agreement for symptoms and syndromes, studies vary across editions and tend to focus on a limited range of diagnoses. As previously noted, the PSE has been studied in relationship to ICD-9 diagnoses, but not systematically with *DSM-III-R* disorders. In general clinical practice, most psychologists may feel more comfortable with the SADS or SCID than the PSE, because of their diagnostic applications. In epidemiological and community studies, the DIS may have greater relevance than the PSE because of its more extensive reliability and validity studies.

Other Structured Interviews for Axis I Disorders

Renard Diagnostic Interview (RDI)

The RDI (Helzer, Robins, Croughan, & Welner, 1981) was developed by a psychiatric team at the University of Washington, commonly referred to as the "St. Louis group," for administration in large-scale studies by nonphysicians with a minimum of clinical training. The St. Louis group had been instrumental in establishing the Feighner criteria (see Chapter 4) for improving the reliability of diagnostic criteria. In addition, these researchers began to experiment with structured interviews for improving diagnostic reliability. Their first efforts (Helzer et al., 1977) suggested that a moderately high level of diagnostic agreement could be achieved by trained psychiatrists. Given this early success, Helzer et al. proceeded with the development of the RDI.

Description of the RDI. Helzer, Robins, Croughan, & Welner (1981) do not provide a comprehensive description of the RDI. Nonetheless, the RDI, as the forerunner of the DIS, appears to have a parallel structure. Clinical inquiries are scored on five ratings: 1 for not present, 2 for present but not meeting minimal criteria for severity, 3 for present but always the result of drugs/alcohol, 4 for present but due only to a physical illness or injury, and 5 for present and not explainable by medication, substance abuse, or physical complications. The RDI is organized with standard and branching questions. Because of its intended use by nonprofessional interviewers, the format is highly structured with explicit decision rules.

The RDI, unlike the DIS, is focused solely on the Feighner criteria, which permits a circumscribed range of diagnoses. Diagnosis can be accomplished either by the interviewer or through a computer scoring program. Since the RDI is nonhierarchical, no primary diagnosis is rendered and an unlimited number of co-occurring disorders are allowed.

Validation of the RDI. Helzer, Robins, et al. (1981) administered the RDI to randomly selected inpatients during their first 2 days of admission. The basic design required the administration of a standard diagnostic interview as well as RDI on two occasions. Altogether, 120 inpatients completed at least two of the three assessments. Five psychiatrists conducted the standard diagnostic interviews. An addition, four psychiatrists and four nonphysicians were responsible for administrations of the RDI. Interviewers were blind to other assessment results and were not permitted to review clinical records.

Estimates of reliability were based on 99 patients in a test-retest design at intervals ranging from 1 to 3 days. For the four common diagnoses (alcoholism, depression, mania, and phobic neurosis), the median kappa was .56 (range = .53 – .77). Interestingly, the lay interviewers appeared to slightly outperform their psychiatric counterparts (i.e., in examining different pairs, the *M* kappas for psychiatrist-psychiatrist was .52 as compared with lay interviewer-lay interviewer of .62 and lay interviewer-psychiatrist of .65).

Validity was examined through a bootstrapping operation that compared RDI diagnoses to standard diagnoses. For the four common diagnoses previously listed, the overall sensitivity was 79% and the specificity was 87%. Although the RDI is described by Helzer et al. as a valid measure, I am particularly concerned with the narrowness of diagnostic coverage (four disorders) and the lack of cross-validation.

Clinical Applications. The RDI is important from a historical perspective in providing the conceptual basis for more recent structured interviews, such as the DIS and the CIDI. From a clinical perspective, however, there are insufficient data to recommend its use either with patient populations or in community surveys. At present, preliminary data suggest moderate test-retest reliability and good external validity for four disorders. However, the RDI is designed for use with the largely discarded Feighner criteria, has only circumscribed applications to these criteria, and lacks any systematic cross-validation. For these reasons, the RDI is not recommended for clinical settings.

Comprehensive Assessment of Symptoms and History (CASH)

Andreasen (1987), with her colleagues, developed the CASH for evaluating signs, symptoms, and history in patients with major psychoses and mood disorders. Realizing the continuing changes in diagnostic systems, Andreasen developed the CASH to assess symptomatology and biological, psychological, and social correlates of mental disorders. By focusing on symptoms and correlates, Andreasen hoped to avoid the variability and possible arbitrariness of diagnostic standards.

The CASH was designed as one component of an assessment battery. Other components included the Scale for the Assessment of Negative Symptoms (SANS; Andreasen, 1984a), the Scale for the Assessment of Positive Symptoms (SAPS; Andreasen, 1984b), and follow-up measures to the CASH. Substantial research on the SANS and SAPS suggested their potential usefulness in predicting treatment outcome. What remains untested is the incremental validity of these components on both diagnostic and symptomatic levels.

Description of the CASH. The CASH is organized into three major sections: present state, past history, and lifetime history. For the present state, the clinician addresses psychopathology during the last month.[8] The CASH diverges from other Axis I interviews in its emphasis on social class and economic status. Psychopathology for the current episode is divided into psychotic, manic, and major depressive syndromes. Many of the clinical inquiries are reproduced without modification from the SADS. Unlike the SADS, however, the CASH provides severity ratings (i.e., 0 = not at all, 1 = questionable, 2 = mild, 3 = moderate, 4 = marked, and 5 = severe) for nearly all symptoms, including psychotic symptoms. Moreover, the CASH differs from the SADS in its extensive clinical observations. For instance, the CASH requires more extensive observations of formal thought disorder, including circumstantiality, pressured speech, distractible speech, thought blocking, perseveration, and clanging. In addition, the CASH provides a section on handedness and laterality that was adapted from Benton (1967) as well as administration of the MMSE.

The Past History section summarizes psychopathology for previous episodes of psychotic and mood disorders. Three nominal ratings (presence or absence) are made of past symptoms: (a) ever present, (b) present in the initial 2 years of the disorder, and (c) present much of the time since the onset of the disorder. The Lifetime History section addresses substance abuse disorders, prodromal symptoms of schizophrenia, and hypomanic and dysthymic symptoms. Substance abuse symptoms are scored for current and past use, while other symptoms are evaluated on whether they are premorbid, prodromal, intermorbid, or residual. Similar to the SADS, the clinician makes overall ratings of social and overall functioning which include the GAS.

Andreasen, Flaum, and Arndt (1992) reported that the CASH was devised to provide a comprehensive data base concerning clinical description and specific psychopathology. They justified the development of the CASH on the basis that the diagnosis of mental disorders have not yet identified critical components of establishing specific diagnoses: pathophysiology and etiology. While they chided other research for being unduly narrow and preoccupied with *DSM* diagnosis, they did not offer a compelling rationale for how they selected symptomatology that extends beyond the current nomenclature. Item development and refinement are not clearly described.

Validation of the CASH. Andreasen et al. (1992) provided the first published study on the CASH's validity. Because it is a descriptive model, the essential requirement of the CASH is the reliability of clinical ratings at the symptom level. To address this important issue, Andreasen et al. administered the CASH to 30 consecutive admissions with prominent psychotic and mood symptoms. Eight clinicians participated in the reliability study that included two raters (interrater reliability) followed by a readministration by a third rater (test-retest reliability) within 24 hours. Because the CASH includes approximately 1,000 individual ratings, Andreasen et al. provided only a brief distillation of findings. For interrater

---

[8]An exception to this rule occurs when the current episode is less than 6 months in duration. Under these circumstances, the clinician is instructed to rate each symptom at its worst during that 6-month period.

reliability, the ICCs were excellent with approximately 61% meeting or exceeding .75. Like most structured interviews, the test-retest reliability was significantly lower, with less than half (roughly 45%) having ICCs of .65 or higher.

Andreasen et al. (1992) also examined the diagnostic agreement, although only three disorders were adequately represented (≥ 5 cases); estimates of interrater reliability were only moderate (i.e., κs = .45, .61, and 1.00). Comparable estimates for the three disorders were found in the test-retest design (κs = .52, .72, and .90). A review of global ratings found that they tended to be moderately high for both positive symptoms (grand median ICC = .73) and negative symptoms (grand median ICC = .70); it should be noted that these global ratings combine interrater and test-retest reliabilities across current and past episodes.[9] Mood symptoms tended to have good interrater (median ICC = .83) and moderate test-retest (median ICC = .58) reliability.

In summary, the initial reliability study yielded promising results. Three cautions must, however, be considered. First, the study involved a very limited sample size, with patients preselected for prominent psychotic or mood symptoms. Second, the test-retest reliability was performed at a very short interval, typically less than 24 hours. Third, the study involved clinicians highly experienced with the CASH (minimum of 1 year) who were trained by Andreasen and other investigators.

Andreasen et al. (1992) reported that two validity studies have been completed and are forthcoming in publications. The first study provided evidence of convergent validity by comparing patients' responses on the CASH to an informant's observations of the patient that were recorded on a second CASH. Although the details are not provided, these investigators report that most items correlated at .70 or higher with a "consensus" CASH.[10]

The second validity study adopted an innovative research design to test the accuracy of patients' retrospective reporting of symptoms. Patients were tested at 6-month intervals over a 24-month period; the study examined the stability of patients' self reporting over prior periods of time. Interestingly, patients were relatively inaccurate at reporting negative symptoms. A full report of this second study is also planned.

Clinical Applications. The CASH appears to have considerable potential as a measure for reliably assessing Axis I symptomatology. At present, however, further reliability and validity studies are essential before adoption for clinical use. Two promising advantages of the CASH are its incorporation of other validated scales, including the SANS, SAPS, MMSE, and GAS, and the development of abbreviated versions for measurement of treatment outcome. With additional validation, the CASH may offer an important contribution to clinical interventions with Axis I disorders.

---

[9]It is important to observe, however, that test-retest reliability for negative symptoms during the initial 2 years of a psychotic disorder had no reliability (ICC = .00).

[10]The consensus CASH was apparently an amalgamation of all available diagnostic data following the LEAD model of validation. The obvious shortcoming of this approach is the non-independence of measures.

Polydiagnostic Interview (PODI)

Philipp and Maier (1986) developed the Polydiagnostic Interview (PODI) as a systematic method for deriving psychiatric diagnoses for psychotic and mood disorders. The "polydiagnostic" component of the PODI refers to its emphasis on multiple diagnostic systems; the PODI integrates *DSM-III* and RDC criteria and compares them to other diagnostic models found chiefly in the research literature.[11] The purpose of the PODI is the assessment of different diagnostic approaches and their clinical relevance. In addition, the PODI stresses reliable evaluation at the symptom/sign level as a way of circumventing the arbitrary conventions of any single diagnostic system.

Description. Philipp and Maier (1986) constructed the PODI for the assessment of multiple diagnostic systems. For *DSM-III* diagnoses, they adopted large portions of the SCID because of its array of diagnoses and direct parallel with *DSM*. They supplemented SCID questions with specific items from the PSE, ninth edition. The most recent version consists of more than 180 ratings and requires 2 to 3 hours to complete.

Philipp and Maier simplified complex diagnostic criteria by dividing them into subcomponents. When items were not available on either the SCID or the PSE, clinical inquiries were constructed. They also added Andreasen's Scale for the Assessment of Negative Symptoms (SANS). Finally, clinical observations were systematized and decision rules were implemented for how to proceed when discrepancies between self report and observations were noted. A computer program is employed for integrating subcomponents and applying different diagnostic criteria. As part of its development, an initial study of interrater reliability (*N* = 40) was conducted and employed in revising the PODI.

Validation of the PODI. The final version of the PODI was used in an interrater reliability study of 137 psychiatric inpatients. They reported that the majority of affective and psychotic criteria had kappas of .80 or higher, but do not provide any measure of central tendency. Agreement regarding clinical observations was apparently somewhat lower but was always above their threshold of moderate consistency ($\geq$ .50). For some unexplained reason, reliability estimates were computed only for individuals who manifested the disorder. For example, a kappa for "expansive mood" is derived solely from the 18 manic patients included in the study. A more stringent test of interrater reliability would be to compute reliability coefficients for the full sample.[12] Moreover, no information is provided on the background of the interviewers or their training with the PODI.

Philipp and Maier acknowledged the difficulties in establishing the diagnostic validity of the PODI, since comparisons with other measures are vitiated by the very fact that the PODI is an amalgamation of measures. Because of this

---

[11]These include an additional 10 research models for depression, 3 for manic disorders, 3 for schizoaffective disorders, and 8 for schizophrenic and paranoid disorders. Examples are the Vienna Research Criteria and the Schneiderian first rank symptoms (see Berner et al., 1983).

[12]In diagnostically homogeneous samples, higher levels of agreement are expected. In addition, this limiting of diagnostic groups increases dramatically the base rates for individual symptoms and, thus, inflates the kappas.

limitation, they assert that the PODI has some evidence of procedural validity in its systematic application of subcriteria and criteria to diagnosis. I find this evidence of validity to be necessary but not sufficient. Other Axis I interviews have struggled with criterion-related validity with comparisons to related interview measures (perhaps in this case the SADS?) and multiscale inventories. Although far from perfect, such research can provide valuable data on convergent and discriminant validity. Moreover, factor analytic models might provide preliminary evidence of construct validity.

Clinical Applications. The PODI is an ambitious project for the integration of diagnostic criteria from a wide range of nosological and research models. Strictly speaking, the PODI is not a structured interview but an amalgamation of previously developed measures (SCID and PSE). As such, the emphasis has been on its use as a decision model for comparing different diagnostic systems (M. Philipp, personal communication, April 14, 1993).

The PODI has not been adequately tested for clinical use. The sole reliability study is flawed by inflated reliability coefficients. No data are currently provided regarding its validity. In the absence of further research, the PODI is not recommended for clinical practice.

Composite International Diagnostic Interview (CIDI)

The Composite International Diagnostic Interview (CIDI) was developed under the auspices of the World Health Organization (1987). The CIDI is based on the DIS-Version III and augmented with questions from the PSE. The purpose of this expansion was to provide more detailed coverage of PSE items and provide a measure that would be clinically useful on an international basis.

The CIDI was designed primarily for epidemiological studies to provide estimates on the prevalence of mental disorders in different countries. Its chief advantage over the DIS and other diagnostic measures (see Semler et al., 1987) is that it allows researchers and clinicians to compare inclusion criteria from four diagnostic systems: (a) Feighner criteria, (b) research diagnostic criteria, (c) *DSM-III*, and (d) ICD-9 classes derived from the PSE. A unique feature of the CIDI are questions regarding the age of onset of most symptoms; this provision allows for information regarding the development and sequencing of symptoms with respect to specific disorders. Symptoms are recorded for their presence as well as their recency.

As an overview to the CIDI, Robins et al. (1988) recognized both the value of the DIS in generating *DSM-III* diagnoses as well as its involvement in the European tradition which was best exemplified in the PSE. In integrating the two measures, they incorporated 63 PSE items into the DIS structure. Field trials attempted to address its feasibility in different cultures.

Validation of the CIDI. Studies have focused primarily on the reliability of the CIDI and its concordance with diagnosis. Semler et al. (1987) employed a German translation of the CIDI which was administered to a diagnostically diverse sample of 60 psychiatric inpatients. In a test-retest design (M interval of 1.7 days), the four interviewers achieved moderate reliability for lifetime diagnoses with a median kappa of .63 (range = .41 to .84). Subclassifications of anxiety and mood disorders yielded modest kappas. When different time frameworks were employed (i.e., 4 weeks, 6 months, 12 months, and lifetime), different patterns emerged. Very brief time periods did not effectively assess episodic disorders (e.g., manic episodes) or substance abuse disorders. Despite high concordance rates, the rarity of these disorders during this brief period militated against satisfactory reliabilities. These investigators recommend further validation with larger samples.

Wittchen et al. (1989) performed a further analysis of the Semler et al. study. They calculated the onset of symptoms and found a moderate level of agreement (73.5% across interviews, median ICC = .78 for 17 CIDI items). In addition, CIDI results were compared to clinical diagnosis (ICD-8) and the age of onset of specific syndromes. They found a moderate level of agreement, with a median ICC of .74.

Farmer, Katz, McGuffin, and Bebbington (1987) compared the CIDI diagnoses with the PSE for a sample of 30 psychiatric patients with symptoms of depression, psychosis and eating disorders. Agreement between the PSE and CIDI–PSE equivalent items was discouragingly low. For 44 comparisons in which equivalent items were rated, the range of kappas was .00 to .86, with a median of .28. One problem with this analysis was the poor representation of certain PSE symptoms, which prevented an adequate testing of reliability. Greater agreement was achieved for the CIDI on PSE syndromes (median r = .52) and total PSE score (r = .64). The investigators agreed with Semler et al. (1987) that the CIDI and PSE evidence poor comparability.

Recent efforts with the CIDI have produced prevalence rates and risk factors for mental disorders in large-scale epidemiological research (e.g., Kessler et al., 1994; Sartorius et al., 1993; Wittchen, Zhao, Kessler, & Eaton, 1994). These studies offer little direct evidence of diagnostic validity.

Clinical Applications. The CIDI is an ambitious WHO project for the validation of a diagnostic measure that would amalgamate the DIS and PSE into a composite assessment generalizable across diverse cultures. Unfortunately, the validation to date has fallen far short of its aspirations. Little is known about CIDI reliability either within the same or across different cultures. Attempts to compare its results to the PSE, despite considerable overlap, have produced only modest results. Psychologists would do best to use either the DIS or the PSE in epidemiological or clinical applications because of the CIDI's psychometric limitations. I would, therefore, recommend that the CIDI not be employed in clinical practice.

Other Structured Interviews

A variety of structured interviews have been employed on a limited basis, either as the foundation of diagnostic research or as a circumscribed attempt to improve clinical practice. I have summarized a representative sampling of these interviews in the following paragraphs.

Interview Guide for DSM-IV Psychiatric Disorders. Zimmerman (1994) developed the Interview Guide as an easily accessible reference for Axis I and II disorders. The Interview Guide includes *DSM-IV* criteria with sample questions. Unlike other semistructured interviews, the Interview Guide does not offer any formalized ratings. Intended as a pocket reference, the Interview Guide has not been validated.

Psychiatric Diagnostic Interview (PDI). Othmer, Penick, and Powell (1981) constructed the Psychiatric Diagnostic Interview (PDI) as a structured interview that could be reliably administered by paraprofessionals. The PDI consists of 12 basic syndromes for current and lifetime diagnoses which were based originally on RDC criteria but were later supplemented with *DSM-III* items. Viatori (1985) described the organization of the PDI with each syndrome arranged into Cardinal (central criteria), Social Significance (impact on social, vocational, and family functioning), Auxiliary (associated symptoms), and Time Profile (onset and duration). The interrater and test-retest reliability of the PDI appear to be satisfactory (Othmer et al., 1981). As evidence of concurrent validity, Weller et al. (1985) compared the PDI with the DIS for 86 inpatients. They found good agreement between the two measures, with an overall kappa of .72. The PDI has been successfully applied to research on forensic patients (e.g., Walters, Mann, Miller, Hemphill, & Chlumsky, 1988) and alcoholism (e.g., Larson & Heppner, 1989).

Iowa Structured Psychiatric Interview (ISPI). Tsuang (1974) developed the Iowa Structured Psychiatric Interview (ISPI) for use in epidemiological research on schizophrenic, depressive, and bipolar disorders. In addition to these disorders, the ISPI screens for anxiety disorders and substance abuse history. Reported symptoms and behavioral observations are scored on dichotomous ratings (presence or absence). One notable difference between the ISPI and other diagnostic interviews is its emphasis on social and family history.

Royal Park Multidiagnostic Instrument for Psychosis (RPMIP). McGorry, Kaplan, Dossetor, Copolov, and Singh (1988) constructed the Royal Park Multidiagnostic Instrument for Psychosis (RPMIP) as a semistructured diagnostic interview that was designed to assess functional psychoses from several diagnostic systems. According to Jackson et al. (1991), the RPMIP has demonstrable reliability with *DSM-III* psychotic disorders. Given these promising results, the RPMIP deserves further investigation.

6

Axis I Interviews
for Children and Adolescents

Traditionally, the assessment of psychopathology in children and adolescence was achieved by individualized behavioral observation and indirect means, such as play therapy, with considerable skepticism for self-reporting (B. Herjanic, M. Herjanic, Brown, & Wheatt, 1975). As summarized by Achenbach (1985), the last two decades have yielded a proliferation of instruments for direct measurement, including standardized rating scales and structured interviews. These developments parallel the emergence of the *DSM-III* and adult diagnostic measures. Following a brief overview of child diagnostic interviews,[1] I will focus primarily on four diagnostic interviews: (a) the Schedule of Affective Disorders and Schizophrenia for School-Age Children (Kiddie-SADS or K-SADS; Chambers et al., 1985), (b) the Child Assessment Schedule (CAS; Hodges, Kline, Stern, Cytryn, & McKnew, 1982), (c) the Diagnostic Interview for Children and Adolescents (DICA; Herjanic & Reich, 1982), and (d) the Diagnostic Interview Schedule for Children (DISC; Costello, Edelbrock, Dulcan, Kalas, & Klaric, 1984).

Rutter and Graham (1968) constructed the Isle of Wight Inventory, which combined unstructured and structured components. For much of the interview the questions are unstructured, with the precise wording left to the interviewer's discretion. The interviewer also asks the child to complete standardized tasks which are incorporated into systematic ratings of psychopathology on 21 categories. As a forerunner of structured interviews, the Isle of Wight Inventory also included a parent interview, with questions extending beyond symptomatology to child-family relationships and marital/family issues.

B. Herjanic et al. (1975) set the stage for child diagnostic interviews by systematically assessing the reliability of self-reporting by children aged 6 to 16. With 50 outpatient children, these researchers assessed the completeness and accuracy of self-reports in comparison to parent reports on the same structured interview. Although reported as simple concordance rates, B. Herjanic et al. found good agreement of factual information and symptoms (> 80%) and moderate agreement of descriptions of behavior (75%) and mental status (69%). These investigators also found good interrater reliability and concluded that structured interviews were likely to assume a significant role in child assessment.

---

[1]For simplicity, I will use the term "child" to encompass children and adolescents, unless otherwise specified.

Reliable assessment of children involves the corroboration of self-reporting with standardized observations and collateral interviews by parents, teachers, and mental health professionals. Towards this end, Achenbach, McConaughy, and Howell (1987) performed a meta-analysis of 119 studies of children from various settings (e.g., clinics, regular and special classrooms, and facilities for delinquents). They found that informants who had a similar relationship with the child (e.g., both parents or two different teachers) evidenced a moderate level of agreement among themselves (rs = .54 – .64, median = .58). In contrast, different sets of informants (e.g., parent vs. teacher) yielded only modest levels of agreement (rs = .24 – .42, median = .27). Comparable levels of agreement were found when child ratings were compared to informants (rs = .20 – .27, median =.25). As might be expected, higher correlations were found for externalized (e.g., hyperactivity and delinquency) than internalized (e.g., social withdrawal and anxiety) problems.

What is the significance of the Achenbach et al. study to child assessment? As noted by the authors, clinical data from any single source is unlikely to capture the complex array of psychological problems experienced by many children. For psychologists practicing with children and adolescents, the systematic integration of multiple data sources appears essential to the assessment process.

We will now turn our attention to the four major diagnostic interviews for children. As noted by Gutterman, O'Brian, and Young (1987), these interviews share much in common: generally comparable age groups (from 6-18 to 8-17), parallel interviews (parent/child), and computer algorithms. In addition, these interviews rely upon the *DSM* taxonomy for their gold standard, which may artificially limit their "true" validity (see Edelbrock & Costello, 1990). Significant differences occur in organization, ratings of severity, and training of interviewers (see Hodges, 1993). For each measure, I provide a similar framework to facilitate cross-comparisons. The section on each diagnostic interview is organized into three components: description, validation, and clinical applications. The chapter concludes with a synopsis of additional structured interviews for children.

A common issue for these four structured interviews is the substantive changes that occurred in the diagnostic standards of *DSM-IV*. Significant changes were implemented for pervasive developmental disorders with modifications of autistic disorder and the introduction of Rett's and Asperger's disorders. Communication disorders have sustained important alterations in diagnostic criteria. These disorders are not covered by the major structured interviews for children.

Changes in *DSM-IV* which affect structured interviews have included modifications of anxiety disorders, with the subsuming of overanxious disorder as part of generalized anxiety disorder, and simplification of the criteria for separation anxiety disorder. As noted with adult interviews, many of the criteria for anxiety disorders have also been modified. In addition, other childhood disorders have experienced minor alterations. As a general guideline, psychologists will need to familiarize themselves thoroughly with the *DSM-IV* and the considerable changes in *DSM-IV* criteria. As a practical manner, child interviews will provide most of the data base necessary to make the necessary diagnoses. Perhaps the most troublesome changes are those implemented for minimum duration (e.g.,

3 months for elimination disorders and 1 month for selective mutism and separation anxiety disorder). Psychologists will need to make the necessary modifications for duration and frequency to ensure the clinical utility of structured interviews. Moreover, *DSM-IV*-compatible versions are anticipated for several of these interviews in the near future.

The Schedule of Affective Disorders and Schizophrenia for School-Age Children (K-SADS)

Description

The Schedule of Affective Disorders and Schizophrenia for School-Age Children (K-SADS) was originally developed in 1977 by Drs. Puig-Antich and Chambers as part of an effort to study prepubertal depression and its similarities to adult depression. When these investigators moved to Columbia University, they devised parallel items to the SADS so that direct comparisons could be made between adult and child symptomatology (W. J. Chambers, personal communication, July 2, 1993).

The original version (Puig-Antich & Chambers, 1978) was designed for sequential administrations with first the parent(s) and then the child. Clinical data from both sources are combined into summary ratings. When marked discrepancies occur, the child is presented with the parent's perspective in an effort to resolve the inconsistency. Like the SADS, ratings are made for the worst period of the last episode as well as for the last week.

The interview process begins with an unstructured interview in which the purpose of the assessment is explained and presenting problems are explored. Clinical inquiries are provided to survey potential symptoms and troubles experienced by the child. The organization of questions closely parallels the SADS itself. For example, the majority of questions on mood disorders use identical wordings and scoring criteria as the SADS. Additional questions are employed, however, to assess symptoms from the child's perspective. Similarly to the SADS, nonpsychotic symptoms are typically rated on a 6-point scale of severity: 1, not at all; 2, slight–subthreshold; 3, mild; 4, moderate; 5, severe; and 6, extreme.

The K-SADS includes several components not found in the SADS. For instance, the K-SADS has an expanded section on anxiety disorders in which separation anxiety plays a prominent role. The APD section of the SADS is transformed into an extended section on conduct symptoms. Each RDC criterion for conduct disorder is examined by multiple questions, typically four to six, and additional symptoms are addressed (gang activities, bullying, and homicidal acts).

Psychotic symptoms, while uncommon in children, are addressed extensively. Interestingly, the coverage of psychotic symptoms is occasionally more thorough than in the original SADS, such as clinical inquiries concerning command and religious hallucinations. Hallucinations are systematically differentiated from illusions, eidetic imagery, elaborated phantasies, and imaginary companions. In contrast to hallucinations, the delusions and formal thought disorder sections closely parallel the SADS.

The goals of the K-SADS, as articulated by W. J. Chambers (personal communication, July 2, 1993), are fourfold. First, the K-SADS provides a direct symptom-by-symptom interview with parent and child data. Second, the K-SADS presents clear definitions of symptoms and behavior. Third, the K-SADS offers a semiquantitative rating of intensity/severity of symptoms and behavior. Fourth, the K-SADS is intended for use by trained clinicians to produce clinical judgments, integrating sources of data and implementing sophisticated estimates of symptom severity.

Several modifications have made to the original K-SADS. The K-SADS was expanded to the K-SADS-E (Epidemiologic Version; Orvaschel, Puigh-Antich, Chambers, Tabrizi, & Johnson, 1982) which included the following diagnostic categories: attention deficit disorder, alcohol abuse and dependence, drug abuse and dependence, and suicidal behavior. Most recently, Ambrosini, Metz, Prabucki, and Lee (1989) worked on the latest version (January, 1988) of the K-SADS, namely the K-SADS-III-R. As the name suggests, the K-SADS-III-R was designed to assess *DSM-III-R* disorders and provides clinical data on 31 different diagnoses: 10 mood, 5 anxiety, 5 psychotic, 4 behavioral, 2 eating, and 5 other disorders. The K-SADS-III-R was subsequently updated in July 1992 (Ambrosini, 1992) with the incorporation of 17 items from the Hamilton Depression Rating Scale. The psychometric properties of the K-SADS-III-R will be described in subsequent sections. According to Ambrosini (personal communication, August 11, 1993), the K-SADS-III-R is unlikely to undergo any substantial revisions with the advent of *DSM-IV*, since most childhood disorders that are included in the K-SADS-III-R have not been significantly altered.[2]

Reliability

Pilot work on the K-SADS suggested that the diagnostic interview had considerable promise for the assessment of child psychopathology. For example, Puig-Antich, Blau, Marx, Greenhill, and Chambers (1978) worked on the construction of a predecessor to the K-SADS but did not establish its reliability. Strober, Green, and Carlson (1981) broadened the adult SADS to include several disorders with children and adolescents and achieved an overall concordance with a kappa of .74. These studies formed the basis for more formal research on the K-SADS and its reliability.

Orvaschel et al. (1982) conducted a small but interesting study on 17 mood-disordered children who were outpatients at the New York Psychiatric Institute. She and her colleagues tested the usefulness of the K-SADS-E in the retrospective assessment of diagnosis and key symptoms. They found that symptoms reported retrospectively were almost invariably endorsed during the initial K-SADS. Some discrepancies did occur because symptoms reported earlier were overlooked. Although a high kappa was reported for the retrospective diagnosis, interpretation of this statistic must be tempered by very limited range of diagnosis. On the small list of specific symptoms, the K-SADS-E and the K-SADS evidenced moderate consistency between child and parent versions (median κ = .64 and .63, respectively).

---

[2]According to Ambrosini (personal communication, August 11, 1993), a K-SADS-IV was developed in 1986 by Puig-Antich, but does not appear to be widely used. The K-SADS-IV is unrelated to the *DSM-IV*.

Chambers et al. (1985) performed the first major study of K-SADS reliability (see Table 6.1). Outpatient children and adolescents, who were not in an emergency, were approached about their willingness to participate in the study. The study required separate K-SADS interviews with parents and children, with a repeat evaluation within 72 hours. For 52 children, estimates of test-retest reliability and interinformant agreement were derived. As summarized in Table 6.1, good reliability was found for the summary scales (median $r = 72$), although the diagnostic agreement was rather modest (median $\kappa = .54$). Moreover, the reliability for individual symptoms associated with five disorders appeared particularly encouraging, with a median kappa of .58. Finally, interinformant agreement was moderate, with median ICC of .58. Overall, the Chambers et al. study suggested that the K-SADS has substantial merit for the consistent assessment of child psychopathology.

Table 6.1
Reliability Studies for the Schedule of Affective Disorders and Schizophrenia for School-Age Children (K-SADS)

Study	Agreement
Orvaschel, Puigh-Antich, Chambers, Tabrizi, & Johnson (1982) Test-retest reliability was determined for 17 mood-disordered outpatients (ages 6 – 11) based on the K-SADS with retesting (interval, $M = 12$ months) on the K-SADS-E; cross-informant consistency was assessed by separate parental interviews.	Diagnosis, $\kappa = .86$. Parent-child consistency on symptoms (K-SADS), ICC = .64[a]. Parent-child consistency on symptoms (K-SADS-E), ICC = .63[b]
Chambers et al. (1985) Test-retest reliability was studied (interval of < 3 days) for 52 outpatient children and adolescents, ages 6 to 17, with six interviewers (five were psychiatrists); cross-informant consistency was assessed by separate parental interviews.	Individual symptoms, ICC = .58[c]. Summary scales, $r = .72$. Diagnosis, $\kappa = .54$[d]. Parent-child consistency on symptoms, ICC = .58
Hammen (1988) Interrater reliability study examined 35 children participating in a family stress study; the children were evaluated by clinical psychology graduate students.	Diagnosis, $\kappa = .84$
Ambrosini, Metz, Prabucki, & Lee (1989) Interrater reliability study of 25 outpatients, ages 6 – 17, employed the K-SADS-III-R with two interviewer/raters; separate interviewers were used for outpatients and their parents.	Diagnosis based on child interview, $\kappa = .76$. Diagnosis based on adult interview, $\kappa = .89$. Summary scales, ICC > .90[e]. Individual symptoms, ICC > .80[e]

Table 6.1   (continued)
Reliability Studies for the Schedule of Affective Disorders and Schizophrenia for School-Age Children (K-SADS)

Study	Agreement
Apter, Orvaschel, Laseq, Moses, & Tyano (1989) Combined interrater (*n* = 70) and test-retest (*n* = 70, 1-week interval) design used two highly trained interviewers with a Hebrew translation on consecutive admissions to an adolescent inpatient unit; cross-informant consistency (*n* = 40) was assessed by separate parental interviews.	Interrater diagnosis, κ = .78. Test-retest diagnosis, κ = .78. Interrater summary scales, ICC = .93. Test-retest summary scales, ICC = .84. Child-parent agreement, diagnosis, κ = .42. Child-parent agreement, summary scales, ICC = .57

Note. κ = unweighted kappas; ICC = intraclass coefficients; *r* = product-moment correlations. Except where otherwise noted, median statistics are reported.
[a]This median statistic reflects only 21 variables, most related to depression. [b]This kappa reflects the ability of the K-SADS-E to retrospectively assess symptoms reported originally on the K-SADS on the 21 selected variables. [c]This median statistic reflects only 43 variables included on the summary scales. [d]Based on five disorders, three of which are depressive disorders. [e]Incomplete data do not allow the computation of median statistics which are higher than the estimates provided.

Subsequent research has corroborated the K-SADS's reliability. For example, Hammen (1988) established an interrater reliability on 35 children recruited for a study of family stress with excellent diagnostic agreement (κ = .84). With the use of two highly trained interviewers, Apter, Orvaschel, Laseg, Moses, and Tyano (1989) examined the reliability (interrater, test-retest, and interinformant) for a Hebrew translation of the K-SADS-E, the slightly expanded epidemiologic version. On an inpatient adolescent (*M* = 16.3 years) sample, good levels of agreement were found for diagnosis (κ = .78 for both interrater and test-retest) and high levels for summary scales (median ICCs = .93 for interrater and .84 for test-retest). Interinformant agreement was generally modest (κ = .42 for diagnosis and ICC = .57 for summary scales).

Ambrosini et al. (1989) examined the interrater reliability of the most recent version, the K-SADS-III-R, on a group of 25 patients that excluded psychotic and mentally retarded. The format for the study was videotapes, which were independently evaluated by a second rater. For the seven syndromes with adequate representation (≥ 5), median κs for the present episode were good for the child interviews (.76) and excellent for the parent interviews (.89). In addition, the majority of summary scales and individual symptoms appeared to have excellent reliability, although insufficient data were presented to calculate these estimates.

Weissman, Warner, and Frendich (1990) examined the diagnostic reliability of the K-SADS-E (test data, not clinical interviews) in addition to other clinical data in establishing diagnoses for 38 children. At best, these kappas are evidence of interscorer agreement; reliabilities for three disorders ranged from kappas of .69 to .93 and were moderately associated with the Global Assessment Scale for Children (GAS-C; Shaffer et al., 1983).

In summary, the K-SADS has good reliability that compares favorably with that of other child diagnostic interviews.[3] Without exception, estimates of inter-rater reliability have been in the moderate to high range. Similarly, test-retest reliability appears to be generally adequate. Interinformant agreement appears to be problematic with all interview measures; in the case of the K-SADS, the estimates (> .40) appear better than most. Since the research encompasses the K-SADS, K-SADS-E, and the K-SADS-III-R, additional cross-validation would be most useful. With that caveat in mind, the K-SADS offers clinically useful data at three levels of analysis: individual symptoms, summary scales, and diagnosis.

Validity

Chambers et al. (1985) devoted most of their efforts to the reliability of the K-SADS, paying comparatively little attention to its validity. Although the K-SADS summary scales evidence moderate internal consistency, the relationship of these scales to external criteria was not explored. Ryan et al. (1987) examined patterns of symptomatology for 95 prepubertal children and 92 adolescents with a diagnosis of major depression with differences in affective symptoms between the two groups. Childhood depression was marked more by anxiety, somatic complaints, and hallucinations, while adolescent depression was characterized more by anhedonia, hopelessness, serious suicide attempts, weight changes, and hypersomnia. Diagnostic overlap was observed for conduct, anxiety, and substance abuse disorders. Principal components analysis identified five factors that contribute to our understanding of childhood and adolescent depression: endogenous symptoms, negative-cognitions, anxiety, appetite/weight changes, and conduct problems. These findings offer a mixed picture for the diagnostic validity of major depression as assessed by the K-SADS. Longitudinal research is needed to evaluate whether differences that occur between childhood and adolescent depression represent developmental changes or the course of the disorder. As noted in Chapter 1, diagnostic overlap is always a complicating dimension in attempting to establish inclusion criteria that consistently differentiate one disorder from others.

Apter, Bleich, Plutchik, Mendelsohn, and Tyrano (1988) examined the SADS summary scales in relationship to clinical diagnoses[4] for 140 consecutive adolescent patients in Tel-Aviv hospital. Comparisons across the three most common disorders (schizophrenia, major depression, and conduct disorder) revealed highly significant differences in the predicted directions for depression and schizophrenia. While lower on most scales, adolescents with conduct disorders evidenced a higher frequency of suicidal thoughts and behavior.

Several studies have assessed concurrent validity by comparing K-SADS with diagnoses based on other interview-based measures. The three primary studies in this regard have examined the K-SADS in relationship to the DISC (see

---

[3]The only exception found was a small study of interinformant concordance by Ivens and Rehm (1988) who report negligible agreement. Unfortunately, they report kappas for only a small number of depressive symptoms; this finding has little relevance to the K-SADS as a whole.

[4]Apter et al. (1988) reported that clinical diagnosis was achieved through a consensus of the treatment and research teams. Although it is not explicitly stated, I am assuming that the treatment team did not have access to K-SADS data. Otherwise, the results are hopelessly contaminated.

Cohen, O'Conner, Lewis, Veliz, & Malachowski, 1987), the CAS (Hodges, McKnew, Burbach, & Roebuck, 1987), and the DICA (Carlson, Kashani, Thomas, Vaidya, & Daniel, 1987). I will examine each of these studies individually.

Cohen et al. (1987) administered the DISC to 101 children, aged 9 to 12, as part of an epidemiological study. K-SADS interviews occurred at an interval of 3 to 4 months after the DISC. The two diagnostic measures appeared virtually unrelated, although the very small number of definite diagnoses militated against significant findings. When comparing possible diagnoses, the range of kappa coefficients was between .08 and .27.[5] Of course, the interpretation of these results is confounded by the extended interval between the two measures. We have no way of knowing whether the lack of observed association reflects clinical changes in the research population. As noted by Cohen et al., long intervals between tests, use of nonclinical populations, and mixing of lay and professional interviewers are likely to lead (individually and collectively) to poor levels of agreement.

Hodges et al. (1987) employed the K-SADS-E and the CAS to 29 children referred for outpatient services. They found that both measures yielded substantially more diagnoses for parent-based than on child-based interviews. For four diagnostic groupings (attention deficit, conduct, anxiety, and affective), they found very modest kappas for child interviews alone (i.e., median = .44, range = .36 – .52), with higher coefficients for parent alone (i.e., median = .60, range = .51 – .75) and child/parent consensus (i.e., median = .61, range = .59 – .65). Although relying on a very small sample, the results suggest a moderate convergence of the two measures.

Carlson et al. (1987) administered the K-SADS and the DICA to the parents of 30 inpatient children whose mean age was 10.1 years. As a departure from concurrent validity studies, the children were administered only one of the two interview measures. Results of the two measures were compared to clinical diagnoses rendered by two child psychiatrists who were blind to K-SADS and DICA. For the six more common disorders, the K-SADS evidenced a modest convergence with clinical diagnoses (median κ = .50, range = .16 – .69) which was roughly comparable to the DICA (median κ = .40, range = .15 – .75). With the clinical diagnosis as a gold standard, the K-SADS appeared to underdiagnose oppositional disorder, while the DICA overdiagnosed overanxious and separation anxiety disorders. Unfortunately, direct comparisons were not made between the K-SADS and the DICA.

Other studies have compared the K-SADS to Stony Brook Child Psychiatric Checklist (SBC; Gadow & Sprafkin, 1987), Child Behavior Checklist (CBCL; Achenbach & Edelbrock, 1979, 1983), and the Adolescent Mood Scale (AMS; Costello, Benjamin, Angold, & Silver, 1991). Costello et al. (1991) examined mood variability on the AMS in 30, mostly depressed, adolescent inpatients. They found few differences on the basis of K-SADS diagnoses. Grayson and Carlson (1991) administered the K-SADS-E and the SBC to 63 inpatient children (M age = 9.5). Kappa coefficients provided very low to moderate estimates of association

---

[5]When possible SADS diagnoses were compared to "probable" DISC diagnoses the coefficients increased, yet remained very modest (< .40). Readers should note that the questions and criteria for oppositional disorder were created by the investigators and were not a component of the K-SADS.

(median κ = .53, range = .16 – 76). In contrast, Apter et al. (1988) found virtually no relationship between social competence as measured by the CBCL and the GAS-C; unfortunately they did not examine directly the results from the CBCL and the K-SADS. However, Biederman et al. (1993) employed the Kiddie-SADS-E to examine CBCL scales for 133 ADHD patients and 118 normal-control boys. They found highly significant differences in the predicted direction between (a) CBCL Attention Problems and ADHD diagnosis, (b) CBCL Delinquent Behavior and conduct disorders, and (c) CBCL Anxiety/Depression and anxiety disorders.

Studies have also examined the validity of the K-SADS through investigations of clinical correlates. Hammen (1988) conducted a 6-month follow-up study of 79 children involved in a family stress study. She found that initial diagnosis was the strongest predictor of follow-up diagnosis in depressed and nondepressed children. The stability of diagnosis compared to stress life-events and self-concept is encouraging. In the assessment family correlates, several studies have assessed risk factors for children for mentally disordered parents, utilizing either the K-SADS or K-SADS-E for children and the SADS for parents. Both Orvaschel (1988) and Hammen et al. (1987) found familial patterns for depression. Lahey et al. (1988) found a similar link for conduct disorders but not for attention-deficit disorder with hyperactivity. In addition to establishing predicted familial patterns, the studies illustrate the usefulness of the parallel K-SADS and SADS investigations.

In summary, studies have demonstrated predicted differences for the K-SADS and K-SADS-E for clinical diagnosis and familial patterns. Studies of concurrent validity have yielded mixed results. Given its methodological constraint, the negative results of the Cohen et al. (1987) study should be interpreted cautiously. In contrast, both Hodges et al. (1987) and Carlson et al. (1987) yielded moderately positive results which are comparable to the cross-measure studies with adult diagnostic interviews (e.g., SADS and DIS). At present, however, no studies have investigated the diagnostic validity of the K-SADS-III-R.

Clinical Applications

The K-SADS, like its adult counterpart, offers detailed clinical criteria for rating both the presence and severity of specific symptomatology. Clinical ratings are made separately for the parent and child for both the present episode and last week, and then combined into summary ratings. The complexity of the ratings is an advantage when carefully applied and, understandably, a disadvantage when one is faced with time constraints or less standardized administrations. A paramount question for each child psychologist is, "Am I willing to administer the K-SADS following its rigorous procedures?" If the answer is no, then the K-SADS has the potential of becoming an elaborate pretense.

The K-SADS and its revisions offer clinicians a broad range of symptoms and clinical characteristics for mood and psychotic disorders which are likely to provide a relatively complete diagnostic picture of these disorders. The most recent revision, the K-SADS-III-R, has adopted the *DSM-III-R* criteria for its validity and has yet to investigate formally the newly included disorders. Therefore, clinicians are likely to be on solid ground when employing the K-SADS and K-SADS-E to assess common disorders for which the K-SADS was developed, rather than rely solely on the K-SADS-III-R for the coverage of most childhood disorders. In other words, if the K-SADS-III-R is employed, then the diagnostic interview should be supplemented by clinical interviews to ensure comprehensive coverage of the recently added disorders.

The parallel coverage of the K-SADS and SADS allows for a systematic evaluation of symptoms from childhood to adulthood. Clinically, psychologists will need to choose which measure to employ with older adolescents. For example, Kutcher, Yanchyshyn, and Cohen (1985) found the SADS to be useful in the evaluation of adolescent depression with inpatients ranging in age from 13 to 18 (*M* age = 16.5). The advantage of the K-SADS-E and K-SADS-III-R is their coverage of childhood disorders. In contrast, the advantage of the SADS is its superior reliability and validity. One possible avenue is screening adolescent patients beforehand for possible childhood disorders. If none appear present, then the SADS might be employed.

The reliability estimates for child diagnostic interviews are generally lower than those for adults. The reason for this decline is not completely understood, but probably reflects routine use of multiple sources (parent and child), the child's lesser ability for accurate and consistent self-reporting, and less clear emergence of symptoms in children and adolescents. Within this framework, the K-SADS appears to be moderately reliable. Interinformant agreement (parent and child) appears to be highly variable, with a tendency for children to underreport and parents to overreport symptoms.

In general, the K-SADS and K-SADS-E appear to be clinically useful measures that are likely to be strong candidates for child and adolescent diagnoses. With further validation, the K-SADS-III-R may bridge the breadth-versus-depth issue found with the SADS. Until then, the K-SADS has special merit in the examination of mood, schizophrenic, anxiety, and conduct disorders. For clinical settings that provide a family context to assessment and treatment, the parallel nature of the K-SADS and SADS is advantageous.

Diagnostic Interview Schedule for Children (DISC)

Description

The original version of the NIMH Diagnostic Interview Schedule for Children (DISC) was developed by Herjanic, Puig-Antich, and Conner in 1979 as part of a feasibility study on child psychiatric interviews (NIMH, 1991). Reflecting the authors' own backgrounds, the initial version drew from existing measures (e.g., the DICA and the K-SADS). Virtually no description has been published of the original version. In 1981, Costello and his colleagues were awarded a grant for the revision of the DISC, which was subsequently completed in 1984 (A. J. Costello, Edelbrock, Dulcan, Kalas, & Klaric, 1984). As noted by E. J. Costello, Edelbrock, and A. J. Costello (1985), this updated version addressed most *DSM-III* diagnoses that could be applied to children. Further revisions were made in the DISC to improve its applicability to both clinical and epidemiological settings. As a result, the DISC–Revised version or DISC-R was published in 1988 (see Shaffer et al., 1988). With further modifications, the most recent version of the DISC, the DISC-Version 2.3 (DISC-2.3) was developed in 1991 to provide diagnostic compatibility with *DSM-III-R* and the then-anticipated *DSM-IV* (NIMH, 1991).

Efforts were made to simplify the language and sentence structure of the DISC in order to improve children's comprehension and accuracy. As reported by Edelbrock, A. J. Costello, Dulcan, Kalas, and Conover (1985), questions consist of easily understood words, and sentences rarely exceed 10 words in length. In addition, complex sentences are divided into multiple questions, with an opportunity provided to respond to each subquestion. In evaluating children's responses, interviewers are instructed not to take their answers at face value. Instead, the children are asked further questions to clarify their responses and may be asked to provide examples. Despite these precautions, children and some parents are likely to misunderstand some questions regarding obsessions, compulsions, and certain psychotic symptoms (see Breslau, 1987).

The DISC and its revisions are composed of a structured interview in which both clinical inquiries and ratings of responses are highly standardized. Because of its epidemiological applications, the DISC is highly structured so as to enable nonprofessional interviewers to conduct interviews in a systematic and reliable manner. For the sake of simplicity, I will limit the description to the most recent version, the DISC-2.3.

The DISC-2.3 comprises six modules: Anxiety Disorders, Miscellaneous Disorders (i.e., eating, elimination, and tic disorders), Affective Disorders, Schizophrenia and Other Disorders, Disruptive Behavior Disorders (e.g., attention deficit disorder with hyperactivity, oppositional defiant disorder, and conduct disorder), and Alcohol and Other Substance Abuse Disorders. Each module is organized by diagnosis and subdivided into components of the disorder. For example, social phobia is composed of 8 general components assessed through 29 clinical inquiries/ratings. In addition to the six modules, an introductory section surveys sociodemographic information and history of health and mental health treatment, and includes a timeline to establish important events in the last 12 months.

The DISC-2.3 consists of two parallel versions, the DISC-Child (DISC-C) and the DISC-Parent (DISC-P). The primary difference between the two versions is the rewording of the questions from "Do you..." in the child version to "Does (he/she)..." in the parent version. Interview time for children is approximately 90 minutes and for parents, 2 hours and 30 minutes (Zahner, 1991). The method of integrating DISC-C and DISC-P data is not specified.

The scoring for the DISC is considerably simpler than for its adult counterpart, the DIS. Instead of attempting to establish clinical distinctions on the basis of etiology, the DISC provides a three-point rating system: 0 for "no," 1 for "sometimes or somewhat," and 2 for "yes." According to Weinstein, Stone, Noam, Grimes, and Schwab-Stone (1989), ratings of 1 should be considered subclinical, since their inclusion in diagnostic models leads to overdiagnosis. The DISC provides two additional ratings: 8 for "not applicable," and 9 for "don't know." For evidence of psychotic symptoms, interviewers are required to provide detailed observations that may be rated by clinicians.

Breslau (1987) examined DISC records for a community sample of 240 children and young adults. By employing an expanded scoring system that required examples and descriptions, she found that both children and their mothers frequently misinterpreted questions regarding compulsions and delusions. One of the dangers of a structured interview is that it does not allow the interviewer any latitude to investigate responses more fully. Clinicians who utilize the DISC may be sensitized to this problem and follow the standard administration of the DISC with additional probes to ensure that respondents fully understand the clinical inquiries.

Reliability

The Costello team and their colleagues (E. J. Costello et al., 1985; Edelbrock et al., 1985) conducted a very large study of DISC interrater and test-retest reliability. In the initial study, E. J. Costello et al. (1985) reported a sample of 316 psychiatrically referred children with extremely high levels of interrater reliability ($r > .99$). Unfortunately, details were not provided about the interviewers or the setting. The test-retest reliability after an interval of 1 to 2 weeks appeared to be satisfactory for total symptom scores (see Table 6.2) across child and adult versions.

Edelbrock et al. (1985), employing the same sample, provided a much more detailed description and analysis of 242 children (inpatients and outpatients) on whom test-retest data were available from both children and parents. The sample, although approximately two-thirds male, was well-balanced with respect to race (White and African-American) and socio-economic status (SES). As observed in Table 6.2, the age of the children played a dramatic role in the estimates of test-retest reliability. Preteenagers and particularly younger children (ages 6 – 9) were inconsistent in their self-reporting. In contrast, both teenagers and parents produced good test-retest reliabilities (ICCs > .70).

Anderson, Williams, McGee, and Silva (1987) employed videotapes of 60 11-year-old community subjects to test interrater and test-retest reliability. As summarized in Table 6.2, the interrater reliability appeared to be very satisfactory for both individual symptoms as well as broad diagnostic categories. Unfortunately, they report very little data on the test-retest reliability and only allude to the consistency across diagnostic categories. In general, however, the Anderson et al. (1987) study is strongly supportive of the DISC's reliability.

Lahey et al. (1990) evaluated the DISC's interrater reliability with 44 boys (ages 7 – 12) referred to outpatient treatment for disruptive behavior. They reported kappa coefficients for the four common disorders (conduct,

Table 6.2
Reliability Studies of the Diagnostic Interview Schedule for Children (DISC)

Study	Agreement
E. J. Costello, Edelbrock, & A. J. Costello (1985) Combined interrater and test-retest reliability with a 1- to 2-week interval employed separate interviews for 316 psychiatrically referred children and their parents.	Interrater, total symptom score, $r = .99$. Test-retest (child), total symptom score, $r = .75$. Test-retest (adult), total symptom score, $r = .84$

Table 6.2   (continued)
Reliability Studies of the Diagnostic Interview Schedule for Children (DISC)

Study	Agreement
Edelbrock, A. J. Costello, Dulcan, Kalas, & Conover (1985) Further analysis of Costello et al. (1985) was conducted on 242 children, ages 6-18, on whom test-retest data was available (median interval period of 9 days); each child and parent was interviewed twice, once by a clinician and once by a lay interviewer in counterbalanced order.	DISC-C *M* symptom score (ages 6-9), ICC = .43. DISC-C *M* symptom score (ages 10-13), ICC = .60. DISC-C *M* symptom score (ages 14-18), ICC = .71. DISC-P *M* symptom score (ages 6-9), ICC = .76. DISC-P *M* symptom score (ages 10-13), ICC = .73. DISC-P *M* symptom score (ages 14–18), ICC = .75
Anderson, Williams, McGee, & Silva (1987) Interrater and test-retest reliability study used sixty 11-year-old community subjects who were administered the DISC on three occasions (at approximately 4-month intervals). Protocols were blindly scored at different time intervals by two experienced clinicians.	Interrater individual symptoms, κ > .50[a]. Interrater and test-retest for broad diagnostic categories, κ = .86
Lahey et al. (1990) Interrater reliability study used 44 boys that were referred to university clinics for predominantly disruptive behavior disorders.	Individual symptoms, κ = .92. Diagnoses, κ = .91
Shaffer et al. (1993) Interrater reliability study used 10 videotaped child interviews of patients (ages 11-17) by four professional interviewers.	Diagnoses, ICC = 1.00
Schwab-Stone et al. (1993) Test-retest reliability study used 37 parent-child pairs with children primarily from an outpatient sample; test interval was 1 to 3 weeks. A total of 24 professional interviewers were employed.[b]	Diagnosis (parent only), κ = .80; diagnosis (child only), κ = .64; diagnosis (parent + child), κ = .59. Number of symptoms (parent only), ICC = .86; number of symptoms (child only), ICC = .66; number of symptoms (parent + child), ICC = .72

Note. κ = unweighted kappas; ICC = intraclass coefficients; *r* = product-moment correlations. Except where otherwise noted, median statistics are reported.
[a]Of the 70 symptoms that were endorsed in at least three cases, nearly two-thirds had kappas exceeding .50. [b]The sample size varied slightly across conditions (i.e., ≥ 37). Please note that the "number of symptoms" is a composite estimate and does not provide evidence on the reliability of individual symptoms.

oppositional-defiant, dysthymia, and attention-deficit disorder with hyperactivity) which were very high for both symptoms and diagnosis. They did not report reliabilities for less frequent disorders and symptoms, which are likely to be substantially lower.

Several studies (Schwab-Stone et al.,1993; Shaffer et al., 1993) have examined the reliability of the DISC-R as part of a consortium of NIMH-sponsored research. Shaffer et al. (1993) found nearly perfect agreement for the five diagnoses with sufficient representation. Schwab-Stone et al. (1993) achieved a moderate level of agreement for test-retest reliability across a 1- to 3-week interval. Reliabilities were consistently high for diagnosis and number of symptoms for the DISC-R when it was administered to the parent alone. In contrast, the DISC-R child-only condition was highly variable in diagnosis (.16 – .77) as well as number of symptoms (.44 – .77).

In summary, the DISC appears to have excellent reliability, particularly with older children. Both versions (DISC-C and DISC-P) have adequate test-retest reliability for symptom clusters, which compares favorably to that of other child interview formats. Although not analyzed by race, the initial study had an adequate sampling of African-Americans. Overall, the results would support the clinical use of the DISC in achieving a stable and reproducible diagnosis.

Validity

The validation of the DISC has involved its concurrent validity with traditional diagnosis and psychometric measures, most notably the CBCL. In addition, studies have investigated other features of diagnostic validity, including the discreteness of specific disorders, risk factors, and the course of disorders. Our discussion will be divided into concurrent validity and diagnostic validity.

The factor structure of the DISC, like most comprehensive child interviews, has not been adequately examined, largely due to the exhaustive number of variables. Williams, McGee, Anderson, and Silva (1989) performed a second-order factor analysis on the 13 DISC scales, separately for 391 boys and 360 girls involved in a community study. With a principal factor analysis rotated to an oblique solution, both boys and girls evidenced a similar factor, which suggested an externalizing dimension composed of inattention, impulsivity, hyperactivity, conduct, and oppositional features. Gender differences were found for the rest of the factor structure. Boys appeared to manifest an internalizing dimension composed of the remaining DISC scales with the exception of phobias. In contrast, the factor structure for the girls was divided into an anxiety dimension (separation anxiety, overanxiety, obsessive-compulsive, and phobia) and a depression dimension (affective, suicidal, vegetative, and cognitive). As a second-order factor analysis, the results do not address whether individual symptoms form meaningful dimensions. However, the results provide support for the internalizing/externalizing dimension of child psychopathology and the conceptually logical division of anxiety and depressive scales, at least with girls.

Concurrent Validity. E. J. Costello et al. (1985) performed the original validity study by contrasting differences in DISC scales for 40 psychiatric and 40 nonpsychiatric subjects. Not surprisingly, significant differences were found for almost all the scales. Total symptom scores for the DISC-P were moderately correlated (r = .71) with the CBCL; a similar relationship was not found for the

DISC-C (r = .14 for the psychiatric sample).[6] This study demonstrated that the DISC may be useful in differentiating impaired from nonimpaired samples but did not address its usefulness for specific diagnoses.

Weinstein et al. (1989; also see Aronen, Noam, & Weinstein, 1993) compared admission diagnosis with DISC diagnosis on a consecutive sample of 163 inpatient admissions. Overall, they found that the DISC tended to overdiagnose (M = 3.4) in comparison to clinical diagnosis (M = 1.2),[7] which resulted in a poor concordance between the two methods (κ < .20). The DISC missed few (typically < 20%) of the admission diagnoses, but found many disorders not reported in admitting evaluations. Although the results are dismal, the question remains whether this study is a fair test of concurrent validity. As noted in Chapter 1, mental health professionals tend to stop the diagnostic process after rendering the principal diagnosis.

Piacentini et al. (1993) examined DISC-R diagnosis in comparison to an informant-based clinical diagnosis that utilized the Clinical Assessment Form. Four diagnoses were adequately represented in a sample of 71 children and their parents: oppositional defiant disorder, attention-deficit disorder, conduct disorder, and major depressive episode. Piacentini and his colleagues found moderate convergence across the measures, with a median kappa of .44 (range = .32 – .46). Although the findings are relatively modest in absolute terms, the design is stringent in its assessment across methods (DISC-R and Clinical Assessment Form) and sources of data (child vs. parent informant).

Fisher et al. (1993) tested the clinical usefulness of a very recent DISC version (DISC-2.1) for the identification of rare disorders. Children (ages 11 – 17) were selected from specialized treatment centers which were responsible for establishing clinical diagnosis. Employing a combined DISC-C and DISC-P, Fisher et al. were able to establish high sensitivity rates for the DISC-2.1; these percentages for eight diagnoses ranged from 73% to 100% with a median of 88%. They did not report the corresponding specificity rates, which are likely to be lower. Although not published, Shaffer (1994) reported that promising validity data on the DISC-2.3 are nearing completion.

Haley, Fine, and Marriage (1988) compared DISC symptom scales with clinical diagnoses for 15 adolescents with major depression with psychotic features, 18 depressed without psychotic features, and 21 with other disorders. They found predicted differences on the DISC depression scale and overall severity. Rather unexpectedly, those with psychotic depression were more likely to have hypomanic episodes than were either of the other groups. Although limited in scope, the study provides data supporting the concurrent validity of the DISC with major depressive disorders.

Bird, Gould, and Staghezza (1992) examined the Spanish version of the DISC (see Bird et al., 1987) and clinical diagnoses for a community sample of 386 children. With the use of the DISC-P for five common diagnoses, the kappas

---

[6]The CBCL and the DISC-P constitute a single-source/multiple-method approach. By contrast, the CBCL and DISC-C make up a multiple-source/multiple-method approach. Therefore, the DISC-P should correlate more highly with the CBCL than should the DISC-C.

[7]According to Blashfield (1992), clinicians often stop after making a primary diagnosis. If this is correct for the present study, then admission diagnosis is an improper criterion for judging the validity of the DISC.

were modest, ranging from .24 to .50 (median = .47). Kappa coefficients were very low for the DISC-C, with a range of .04 to .42 and a median of .35. Bearing in mind the Spanish translation, these results by accomplished investigators are still disappointing.

Several studies have addressed the concurrent validity of the DISC in relationship to the CBCL and the teacher's version of the CBCL, namely the TRF. For example, Edelbrock and A. J. Costello (1988, p. 223) found significant biserial correlations between CBCL scales and DISC diagnoses but did not report the magnitude of these correlations. Through an application of multiple regression to dichotomous variables, they reported a linear trend for the diagnoses of attention-deficit disorder, conduct disorder and depression with their respective CBCL scales. In their current form, these data are difficult to evaluate with respect to concurrent validity.

Benjamin, E. J. Costello, and Warren (1990) evaluated 300 children enrolled in a health maintenance organization. They found significant differences in overall ratings (CBCL and TRF) for impaired (i.e., anxiety and behavior disorders) and nonimpaired children. Further evidence was provided regarding the level of social functioning of impaired children. No correlations were presented between diagnosis (presence/absence or number of DISC symptoms) and scale elevations.[8] Weinstein et al. (1989) employed a children's version of the CBCL: Youth Self-Report (YSR; Achenbach & Edelbrock, 1987). They administered the DISC and the YSR to 160 consecutively administered inpatients and compared T scores for subjects with and without specific disorders. Although statistically significant differences were found in the expected direction, their interpretation is tempered by (a) clinically small differences (i.e., < 10 points), and (b) nonselective differences (i.e., significant differences were found for scales not associated with the diagnosis).

In summary, studies of the CBCL and its variations (TRF and YSR) provide, at best, weak evidence of concurrent validity. Several studies report insufficient data to adequately assess validity. The Benjamin et al. study suggested that the DISC and YSR both provide a general index of impairment but did not provide concurrent evidence for specific disorders.

Cohen, O'Conner, Lewis, Veliz, and Malachowski (1987), as described in the validity section of the K-SADS, compared DISC and K-SADS diagnoses administered with a 3- to 4-month interval. As noted, the kappa coefficients were very modest (i.e., all < .40), which may reflect on the low prevalence of several disorders as well as the lengthy interval between administrations.

Diagnostic Validity. An important element of diagnostic validity is the discreteness of diagnoses. In other words, do the inclusion and exclusion criteria identify a relatively distinct constellation of symptoms? This problem is typically addressed within the context of symptom overlap. Anderson et al. (1987) examined diagnostic overlap for a New Zealand sample of 792 community subjects.

---

[8]A related study by McGee, Anderson, Williams, and Silva (1986) found that symptoms of depression and impulsivity on the DISC did not appear to be related to performance on the WISC-R. Symptoms associated with inattention appeared to be slightly correlated ($M r$ = .18) with lower performance. These findings are encouraging, since we would not expect psychopathology, at least in community subjects, to be strongly influencing cognitive abilities.

They found that 55% of the sample qualified for multiple diagnoses. Interestingly, nearly all children with depression/dysthymia also warranted at least two other diagnoses (i.e., most common were anxiety disorders [71.4%] and attention-deficit disorder [57.1%]).[9] Bird et al. (1988) reviewed DISC diagnoses and found that 81.1% of 265 Puerto Rican children qualified for multiple diagnoses. What was particularly troublesome was the degree of overlap across broad diagnostic categories (mood, anxiety, conduct/oppositional, and attention-deficit) with nearly half (46.1%) classified into at least two broad categories.[10] The Bird et al. (1988) study is particularly worrisome, as the DISC diagnoses appeared to be almost a general index of impairment rather than a measure of specific diagnoses.

The longitudinal dimension of diagnostic validity may be conceptualized in terms of (a) risk factors or precursors, and (b) outcome variables, such as the course of the disorder and treatment outcome. A strength of the DISC is its substantial literature on predicting disorders and their outcomes.

Three large community studies have examined risk factors associated with DISC diagnoses. E. J. Costello (1989) assessed risk factors of childhood mental disorders in a sample of 300 children (ages 7 – 11) attending primary care pediatric clinics. With a 12-month follow-up, she found that (a) sociodemographic variables (gender, SES, single parent family) were linked with oppositional and conduct disorders, and (b) children's stress was associated with anxiety disorders.[11]

Velez, Johnson, and Cohen (1989) conducted an elegant study using 776 community children (*M* age = 5.7) of risk factors after 8 and 10 years. Sociodemographic characteristics (particularly low income/parent education) were predictive of externalizing disorders (oppositional, conduct, and attention deficit) and one internalizing disorder (separation anxiety). Parental characteristics were logically related to risk factors (i.e., sociopathy with externalizing disorders, emotional problems with internalizing problems). Childhood problems (academic failure, mental health intervention, and stressful life events) formed a general risk factor at the 10-year follow-up.[12]

Bird, Gould, Yager, Staghezza, and Canino (1989) examined risk factors linked to 386 Puerto Rican children with DISC diagnoses. Unlike the other two studies, Bird et al. used a cross-sectional design, relying on retrospective reporting of family history variables. Socio-economic status appeared to be a general factor associated with mental disorders. In general, family dysfunction, stressful events, and parents' psychiatric history tended not to increase the likelihood of childhood diagnoses; the notable exception was depression.

The three general studies of risk factors, when taken together, offer limited support for the diagnostic validity of the DISC. Most encouraging are the

---

[9]Diagnostic overlap between closely related disorders (e.g., dysthymia and depression) is often expected and suggests a constellation of disorders. In contrast, this study found overlap across diverse diagnostic categories.

[10]Inclusion criteria for nine separate disorders were summed individually and compared; these ratings are not, of course, independent, since they include two subtypes of both conduct disorder and attention deficit disorder.

[11]Benjamin, E. J. Costello, & Warren (1990) performed a further analysis that addressed specifically the risk factors for anxiety and behavioral disorders but added little to the previous findings.

[12]The only exception was separation anxiety disorder, which typically has a relatively early onset (i.e., mid-childhood).

differences between (a) externalizing disorders, which are associated with disadvantaged and disrupted families, and (b) internalizing disorders, which are linked to stress and familial histories of mental illness. Because of the nonspecific nature of these risk factors, we cannot expect to identify precise precursors to particular mental disorders.

Borst, Noam, and Bartok (1991) examined risk factors for suicide attempts for 219 adolescent inpatients. They found DISC diagnosis (especially a combined mood and conduct disorder), gender (female), and a measure of ego development (social conformity) predicted suicidal attempts. Use of inpatients limits generalizability of these results to adolescent psychiatric groups.

Diagnostic validity has also been evaluated by studying the course of the disorder and its differential response to treatment. For example, McGee and Stanton (1990) utilized DISC diagnoses on 733 13-year-old adolescents. They selected five diagnostic groups ($n = 82$; attention deficit, conduct, anxiety, depression, and mixed) and compared them to those without a disorder ($n = 651$). In a 2-year follow-up, they found distinct patterns of disability associated with attention-deficit disorder (multiple deficits including communication and disruptive behavior), but not with other disorders. Depression was more likely than other disorders to result in psychiatric hospitalization.

Greenbaum, Prange, Friedman, and Silver (1991) conducted a 7-year study of 547 emotionally disturbed adolescents. They reported that substance abuse disorder with either alcohol or marijuana (regardless of its severity) dramatically increased the likelihood of DISC mental disorders (conduct, depression, attention deficit, and anxiety). Similarly, Rubio-Stipec, Bird, Canino, Bravo, and Alegria (1991) combined epidemiological data on the DISC (Bird et al., 1988) with the DIS (Canino, Bird, Shrout, Rubio-Stipec, Bravo, Martinez, Sesman, Guzman, & Guevara, 1987) to study the effects of parental alcoholism on childhood adjustment. They found that children of alcoholics evidenced overall impairment which was on par with children of mentally ill parents. While interesting in their own right, these studies offer only indirect evidence of diagnostic validity due to the nonspecificity of their results.

The remaining facet of diagnostic validity is the review of familial patterns for corroborative evidence of specific disorders. Studies have addressed either patterns of family functioning or the presence of mental disorders, particularly in parents. Prange et al. (1992) examined patterns of family functioning and DISC diagnoses for 353 emotionally disturbed adolescents and their parents. They probed parents' cohesiveness and adaptability (Family Adaptability and Cohesion Evaluation Scale or FACES; Olson, Portner, & Lavee, 1985) in relationship to three common DISC diagnoses (conduct, alcohol/marijuana, and depression). In a hierarchical regression, they found that conduct disorder was related to parent's substance abuse and lack of family cohesiveness. Both substance abuse and depression were predicted by the lack of family cohesiveness. Interestingly, the family's adaptability was unrelated to DISC disorders.

Two studies have explored the parallels between specific parent and child disorders. Breslau, Davis, and Prabucki (1987) examined 331 mothers with the DIS and one child per family with the DISC. They found 101 mothers who qualified for generalized anxiety disorder (GAD) and 52 who qualified for major depression. They evaluated patterns of disorders in younger (ages 8 – 17) and older (18 – 23) offspring and found that mother's GAD did not increase the risk of anxiety or mood disorders in offspring. In contrast, depressed mothers were more likely to have overanxious disorder in younger and major depression in older offspring. Review of anxiety and mood symptoms from the DISC indicated no differences for younger offspring. However, the older offspring of depressed mothers evidenced more depressive symptomatology, including vegetative and suicidal symptoms. This study does not establish familial patterns for GAD, but provides some evidence, at least in older offspring, for major depression. Lahey et al. (1990) conducted DISC interviews on 177 boys (ages 7 – 12) who were involved in outpatient treatment. They found that APD in biological fathers increased the probability of *DSM-III-R* conduct disorders by three-fold (i.e., 35.5% vs. 11.1%). Moreover, a jail sentence by any first or second degree biological relative doubled the likelihood (i.e., 43.3% vs. 20.0%) of conduct disorders. The Lahey et al. study provides evidence of a specific diagnosis (conduct) being linked to a father's disorder (APD).

In summary, studies of diagnostic validity have addressed the overlap of DISC disorders, risk factors, course of particular disorders, and familial patterns. For the most part, studies offer general evidence of the DISC's assessment of psychopathology but lack specific data on particular disorders. This limitation is typically methodological. If only global precursors of DISC disorders are studied, then it is unrealistic to expect that unique or distinctive patterns can emerge.

Overlap of child disorders affects the clarity of inclusion/exclusion criteria, especially when the overlap exceeds 50% (e.g., depression and anxiety disorders; Anderson et al., 1987). Moreover, Bird et al. (1988) found overlap between broad diagnostic groups, which militates against the ability to establish distinct and recognizable outcome criteria. Studies of outcome criteria (E. J. Costello, 1989; Velez et al., 1989) have provided useful data that differentiate externalizing (disadvantaged and conflictual homes) and internalizing (parents' mental illness and childhood stress) disorders. DISC diagnoses can be linked to specific outcomes (suicide attempts, hospitalization, and the emergence of other disorders), although these links are typically only low to moderate in magnitude. Finally, familial patterns suggest a nonspecific dimension (i.e., noncohesiveness) that may contribute to child psychopathology as well as a familial connection for major depression in mothers and APD in fathers. As this review suggests, much more research is needed on each facet of diagnostic validity. Still, the current studies offer general support of the DISC-derived diagnoses, plus specific evidence with several disorders.

Spanish Version

A Spanish version of the DISC is available through the University of Puerto Rico School of Medicine (see Bird et al., 1988). Unlike the DIS, the DISC offers no published studies on either the reliability of its Spanish version or its comparability to the English version. Without reliability studies, the reproducibility of results is called into question. Without research on comparability, the generalizability of the DISC to Spanish populations remains unknown.

Available DISC research has established risk factors (Bird et al., 1989; Rubio-Stipec et al., 1991) and prevalence rates (Bird et al., 1988) for Puerto Rican children. Bird et al. (1992) addressed parent-child agreement with 222 children selected from a community sample because of suspected psychiatric problems. Unfortunately, the concordance between the two groups was very modest, with a median kappa coefficient of .18 (range = −.05 – .47).[13] Although cross-informant measures of consistency are typically modest, these estimates are substantially lower than comparable studies with the K-SADS (Apter et al., 1989; Chambers et al., 1985) and the CAS (Hodges, Gordon, & Lennon, 1990). Bird et al. (1992) found low to moderate agreement (DISC-P κ = .24 – .50; DISC-C κ = .04 – .37) between DISC diagnoses and a comprehensive diagnosis.

The usefulness of the Spanish version is constrained by the lack of reliability and comparability data and the limited research on its validity. As discussed below, psychologists with Spanish-speaking children have few viable alternatives and may consider the possible use of the Hispanic DISC, despite its manifold limitations.

Response Styles

Zahner (1991) conducted an important study using 138 preadolescents, 95 of whom were identified on the CBCL with elevated scores. She examined the quality of responses to the DISC-R based on interviewer ratings. She found that 8.3% of children engaged in "yea-saying," while 10.1% responded with "nay-saying." In addition, 12.0% of the younger children (ages 6 – 8) tended to present themselves in an ideal light. Other response problems included attempts to please the interviewer (8.0%) and guarded responses (14.0%). She also pilot-tested a 10-item social desirability scale which appears to have promise with defensiveness and other response sets.

Clinical Applications

The DISC is a reliable diagnostic interview for children, with extensive validity data drawn primarily from outpatient and community settings. The DISC is certainly useful clinically in assessing risk factors, patterns of psychopathology, and overall impairment. In the following paragraphs, I will expand on its applications and limitations.

A strength of the DISC is its interrater reliability, which has been well established on large outpatient samples. The work of Edelbrock et al. (1985) is particularly notable, since it allows clinicians to estimate reliability of DISC scales on the basis of the source (DISC-C or DISC-P) and the age of the child. They found, for example, that younger children (< 10 years) were generally unreliable in reporting many symptoms, but that older children and parents of all children had satisfactory reliability. Even data on individual symptoms (see Anderson et al., 1987) appear to be satisfactory. Psychologists should therefore feel comfortable in describing scales and overall impairment on the DISC. Substantially less research is available on diagnostic reliability, but its results appear promising (Anderson et al., 1987; Lahey et al., 1990).

---

[13]Data are reported only on the four most common disorders; reliability estimates are likely to be even smaller if less frequent symptoms were included.

Validity studies clearly demonstrate the usefulness of the DISC as a measure of impairment and offer substantial findings on internalizing and externalizing disorders. This conceptualization of internalizing and externalizing disorders, which incorporates the more common childhood disorders, appears to have a well-defined factor structure (Williams et al., 1989) and be significantly related to the emergence of mental disorders (see discussion of risk factors in Costello, 1989, and Velez et al., 1989).

Surprisingly little research has examined the usefulness of the DISC in establishing specific *DSM-III-R* diagnoses. Available studies (Bird et al., 1992; Cohen et al., 1987; Piacentini et al., 1993) addressing the DISC in relationship to clinical and SADS-based diagnoses offer only modest evidence of discriminant validity. Therefore, in cases in which specific diagnoses are essential, psychologists may wish to consider other structured interviews.

An important facet of the DISC is its utility in making clinical predictions. Available data suggest that diagnosis and DISC scores may assist in predicting suicide attempts (Borst et al., 1991), overall disability and need for hospitalization (McGee & Stanton, 1990), and future arrests (Lahey et al., 1990). Clinical cases which involve these important treatment/management considerations would benefit from the use of the DISC.

The Hispanic version has limited clinical applicability. This version has not been tested in the United States and does not have established reliability. Moreover, no evidence was found concerning its comparability with the English DIS, and only meager confirmation of its diagnostic validity exists. However, the Hispanic DISC is the only available Spanish-structured interview for Axis I disorders in children. Psychologists with monolingual Hispanic children are placed in the untenable situation of using the DISC or no standardized interview at all. One less-than-ideal alternative is to employ the DISC as a structure for diagnostic interviewing and to place explicit caveats in clinical reports.

Response styles are often overlooked in general structured interviews, either for children or adults. Two findings are particularly relevant from the Zahner (1991) study: (a) substantial numbers of children distort their answers by adopting a response set (yea- and nay-saying) or exhibit defensiveness, and (b) a 10-item social desirability scale has promise in identifying these children. Since this scale had not been cross-validated, psychologists may wish to include a social desirability scale (e.g., the Crown-Marlowe) in the DISC assessments.

In summary, the DISC is clinically useful for the reliable assessment of psychopathology and impairment. Its effectiveness in inpatient settings and with *DSM-III-R* diagnoses is not well established and, thus, should be deemphasized. The DISC may be especially useful in addressing highly problematic questions regarding the course of a disorder and suicidal/antisocial behaviors.

Children's Assessment Schedule (CAS)

Description

Hodges, Kline, et al. (1982), in a collaborative arrangement between the University of Missouri and NIMH, developed the CAS as a semistructured diagnostic interview intended for clinical use with children and adolescents (age range = 7 – 16 years). Its authors attempted to address what was considered a substantial problem with earlier measures, namely lengthy formats that are organized by symptom constellations which form a barrier to rapport-building. In addition, Hodges, Kline, et al. sought to remedy what they considered were unrealistically fine distinctions regarding symptom characteristics.

The CAS was first developed in 1978 and became available in 1981 (Hodges, Kline, Fitch, McKnew, & Cytryn, 1981). Little information is available on its actual development. Hodges, Kline, et al. (1982) reported that they modeled the organization of the CAS after the PSS. The structure of the clinical inquiries apparently corresponds to questions customarily employed by the investigators in their interviewing of children. In addition, Hodges, Kline, et al. constructed the clinical inquiries and ratings in order to match the *DSM-III* and subsequent *DSM-III-R* diagnostic criteria. Apparently, because of its rational construction and reliance on the *DSM-III* and *DSM-III-R*, the authors relied primarily on informal (nonstatistical) means of item selection and refinement.

The CAS, like most structured interviews for children, is composed of two parallel forms, one for children and one for a parent serving as an informant. To improve user friendliness, the CAS is organized around 11 topic areas, beginning with general topics (i.e., school, friends, activities, and family) and proceeding to more personal matters (i.e., fears, worries/anxieties, self-image, mood/behavior, physical complaints, acting out, and reality testing). Each form has slightly more than 250 clinical ratings which differ only slightly in structure (e.g., the child form often begins with the stem "Do you...," which is altered in the parent form to "Does your child..."). An important feature of the CAS is that diagnostic criteria are embedded in topical questions, so as to improve the flow of the interview.

The great majority of clinical inquiries are standard questions which are asked of each respondent. In addition, the CAS utilizes optional probes under two conditions, either an affirmative response that requires an additional follow-up or elective questions that gather ancillary information. In the latter case, interviewers may choose to probe further with elective questions designated by *"If desired:"*.

Responses to individual items are organized on a 3-point rating: 0 for "false or no," 1 for "an ambiguous response," and 2 for "true or yes." In addition, 9 is reserved for not-scored items. The CAS differs from other structured interviews in its use of the intermediate score (1) for responses which are not clearly present or absent. In contrast, most other structured interviews use the intermediate score as a positive endorsement, either at a subclinical or clinical level. Given its explicitly equivocal nature, the 1 rating on the CAS appears less interpretable than on other more common alternatives.

CAS items are organized into content scales, symptom scales, and total symptom scores. As described above, the 11 content scales address overall functioning and psychopathology. These scales (see Hodges & Saunders, 1989) appear to have a moderate level of internal consistency (median α = .68) when administered to 116 inpatient and outpatient children. However, two scales evidenced low levels of internal consistency (Activities = .09 and Reality-testing = .58). The parent version appeared to fare slightly less well (median α = .64) with three scales at low levels (Activities = .27, Reality-testing = .47, and Fears = .57). Attempts to reduce the number of variables to those that are diagnostically significant appeared to have a negligible effect on alpha coefficients.

Reliability

Hodges and her colleagues conducted four studies (Hodges, Cools, & McKnew, 1989; Hodges, Gordon, & Lennon, 1990; Hodges, Kline, et al., 1982; Hodges, McKnew, Cytryn, Stern, & Kline, 1982) of the CAS's interrater and test-retest reliability (see Table 6.3). The original study (Hodges, Kline, et al., 1982) examined interrater reliability of the CAS on 53 children, utilizing videotaped

Table 6.3
Reliability Studies of the Child Assessment Interview (CAS)

Study	Agreement
Hodges, Kline, Stern, Cytryn, & McKnew (1982) Interrater reliability was investigated with interviewing by four psychology staff using a mixed (clinical and normal) sample of 53 children (7 – 14 years old).	Dimensional ratings, r = .72. Symptom agreement, κ = .60
Hodges, McKnew, Cytryn, Stern, & Klein (1982) Interrater reliability was examined with 10 children interviewed by two raters.	Interrater, total symptom score, r = .91[a]. Interrater, content scores, r = .94[a]. symptom scale scores, r = .94[a]
Verhulst, Berden, & Sanders-Woudstra (1985) Videotaped interrater reliability study used 20 children with psychological problems.	Interrater, total symptom score, ICC = .94. Interrater, content scores, ICC = .85
Hodges, Cools, & McKnew (1989) Test-retest reliability was assessed on 32 psychiatric inpatients (ages 6 – 12); *M* interval was 9 days.	Diagnostic categories, κ = .72. Symptom scale scores, r = .80
Hodges, Gordon, & Lennon (1990) Parent-child concordance study by three mental health professionals used 48 psychiatric inpatients; the sample excluded psychotic and mentally retarded children.	Total symptom score, r = .41[b]. Diagnostic scores, r = .45[b]. Content scores, r = .35[b]

Note. κ = unweighted kappas; r = product-moment correlations. Except where otherwise noted, median statistics are reported.
[a]Although it was not specifically stated, I assumed these were correlations based on a parallel study (Hodges, Kline, et al., 1982). [b]Cross-informant correlations (see Achenbach et al., 1987) extend beyond reliability to measure consistency across different sources of data.

interviews. Product-moment correlations were computed for the total CAS score (r = .90), content scales (median r = .75) and dimensional ratings of diagnostic groupings (median r = .68). Levels of diagnostic agreement were not reported. Overall, the Hodges, Kline, et al. study suggests acceptable, although not exceptional, estimates of interrater reliability.

Hodges, McKnew, et al. (1982) reported reliability estimates on the basis of 10 psychiatric patients. They found high interrater reliabilities (rs > .90) for scale scores and total symptom scores. Hodges et al. (1989) conducted a test-retest reliability study on the CAS, employing 32 inpatient children (ages 6 – 12) with an interval averaging 9 days. They found good correlations for the CAS scales (median r = .80) and satisfactory reliability for common diagnoses (median κ = .72).

In their fourth and final study, Hodges et al. (1990) examined the concordance between child and parent versions of the CAS. Although not strictly a measure of reliability, this study provides evidence of reproducibility of symptomatology across parallel forms.[14] They used a sample of 48 nonpsychotic and non-retarded inpatient children assessed independently by a team of three experienced clinicians. For content scales, the correlations were very modest, with a range from .08 to .58 and a median of .35. These correlations improved marginally for diagnostic groupings (.12 – .63, median = .45) but remained low across the entire CAS (r = .41). As found with other child diagnostic interviews, the association between child and parent parallel forms appears to be a very stringent and difficult-to-achieve standard for the reproducibility of clinical data.

Investigation of the CAS's reliability has been limited almost exclusively to its originators. One exception is a study by Verhulst, Althaus, and Berden (1987), which examined interrater reliability on 20 videotaped interviews and found good reliability for 10 content scales (Reality-testing was not reported; median r = .85) and excellent agreement on total scores (r = .94). For diagnoses, the kappa was described as exceeding .70 for five of the six disorders, the sole exception being conduct disorder at .50.

The emphasis of CAS reliability research has been on dimensional ratings of content areas and diagnostic groupings. In contrast, relatively little attention has been paid to diagnostic agreement, both in terms of number of studies and range of disorders. Therefore, psychologists may feel more comfortable in utilizing the CAS for the assessment of severity of psychopathology rather than diagnosis per se.

Validity

Hodges, Kline, et al. (1982) conducted the original validity study of the CAS, which combined known-groups design (i.e., comparisons of 18 inpatients, 32 outpatients, and 37 controls) with convergent measures. Of nine symptom scales, six met the predicted severity (inpatient > outpatient > controls). For the content scales, more variability was observed; however, the clinical groups had

---

[14]In adults, similar studies would likely be categorized as convergent validity. In the case of children, however, these virtually identical versions are intended to be integrated into a single assessment of the child. From this perspective, I might argue that comparison of the two parallel versions is roughly analogous to split-half reliability.

greater impairment than controls on all but two scales (i.e., Fears and Worries). Use of the CAS total score in a discriminant model predicted clinical status in 65.5% of the subjects which was comparable to the CBCL. The CAS evidenced moderate correlations with convergent measures: .53 for the total CAS and the CBCL, .53 for CAS depression scale and the Children's Depression Inventory (CDI; Kovacs, 1978), and .54 for the CAS overanxious scale and the State-Trait Anxiety Inventory for Children (STAIC; Spielberger, 1973).

Verhulst et al. (1987) examined CAS scores for 371 8- and 11-year-old Dutch children with a parent interview (Isle of Wight Inventory), the CBCL, and the Teacher Report Form (TRF; Achenbach & Edelbrock, 1986). They found a moderate correlation on total score (r = .58) between the Isle of Wight Inventory and the CAS, but low agreement on individual scales (median r = .30). For a subsample of 116 children, the CBCL/TPF showed a modest correlation for those with significant symptoms ("high" scorers; r = .36), which was substantially lower for those with few symptoms ("low" scorers; r = .26). Taken together, the Verhulst et al. study underscores the difficulty in obtaining high agreement rates among convergent measures of child psychopathology.

Verhulst, Bieman, Ende, Berden, and Sanders-Woudstra (1990) conducted a further study of 65 impaired and 67 well-adjusted 14-year-old children with the CAS. They employed the CBCL and TRF, and compared these results with summary diagnoses and severity of impairment that relied heavily on the CAS. They found a moderate correlation among sources of clinical data of .63. Moreover, the number of problems reported on the CBCL was negatively related to the severity of impairment (r = –.45).

Hodges et al. (1987) carried out an important study that compared the CAS with the K-SADS. On a sample of 29 children referred for outpatient services and their mothers, both measures were administered in a counterbalanced order. Diagnoses were examined for four common diagnoses: attention deficit, conduct, anxiety, and affective. Interestingly, when diagnosis was based on the child interview alone, nearly half the disorders were missed by both the CAS (48.8%) and the K-SADS (42.3%). When based on the parent interview alone or a consensus between the parent and child interviews the kappas were moderate (range = .51 – .75, median = .60). One caveat that must be borne in mind, however, is that these reliability estimates are for only four general diagnostic categories, and that these categories subsume multiple disorders.

Several studies are limited in their relevance to CAS validity. For example, Hodges and Craighead (1990) found that CAS-diagnosed depressed children had significantly higher scores than nondepressed children on the CDI for three factors: dysphoric mood, loss of interest, and self-deprecation. Hodges and Plow (1990) found that CAS-based disorders were not generally associated with tested intelligence on a sample of 76 inpatient children. The sole exception appeared to be anxiety disordered children, who scored lower; whether this difference reflects test anxiety/impairment or underlying cognitive deficits remains to be investigated.

In summary, the CAS validity studies have focused primarily on patient status (inpatient, outpatient, or control) or select diagnostic categories. Substantially less information is available on specific disorders and convergence between diagnostic measures. Instead, attention has been paid to the CAS and its relationship to self-report measures, such as the CBCL, TRF, and CDI. In this regard, the CAS evidences a moderate level of convergence.

Clinical Applications

The CAS was specifically designed to assess nonpsychotic *DSM-III-R* disorders in intellectually normal children. It, therefore, has not been validated with psychotic or mentally retarded samples. This limitation imposes two important restrictions on the use of the CAS in clinical settings: (a) psychotic disorders cannot be diagnosed, and (b) other mental disorders cannot be diagnosed in psychotic or retarded individuals. In the latter case, validity data are not available on how the presence of these disorders would affect self-reporting in the CAS interviews.

The CAS may lend itself to outpatient evaluations, particularly in clinics where common childhood disorders (conduct, attention-deficit, anxiety) are prevalent. The CAS may be used in conjunction with standardized self-report measures for parents (CBCL) and teacher (TRF). The CAS, like other child-interview measures, should not be administered to the child alone. Research findings strongly suggest that child-only interviews substantially underdiagnose mental disorders. When combined with the parent interview (see Hodges et al., 1987), the CAS may offer diagnostically useful information.

An important feature of the CAS is its problem-oriented approach. Through its 11 content scales, clinicians can easily identify (a) troublesome problems, and (b) discrepancies in child and parent perspectives. Within a treatment framework, both problems and discrepancies are important dimensions for clarification of treatment goals and improved communication. The CAS offers a systematic approach to common child and family problems that may assist in the treatment process.

For differential diagnosis, the CAS is circumscribed in its clinical usefulness. In addition to the above noted restriction with psychotic disorders, the reliability and concurrent validity of specific disorders has received only limited attention. In cases where diagnosis is paramount, clinicians may wish to consider other interview-based measures. The CAS is better utilized in clinical settings where the focus is on dimensions of psychopathology rather than diagnosis and where assessment becomes a problem-oriented basis for intervention.

Diagnostic Interview for Children and Adolescents (DICA)

Description

Herjanic et al. (1975; also see Herjanic & Campbell, 1977), as described in the introduction to this chapter, were responsible for developing one of the very first structured interviews for children[15] that was subsequently refined and

---

[15]According to Welner, Reich, Herjanic, Jung, and Amado (1987, p. 649), the very first version of the DICA appeared in 1969 and was patterned after the Renard Diagnostic Interview (RDI). This statement is puzzling, as the RDI was apparently developed in 1977 (see Robins & Helzer, 1991).

named the Diagnostic Interview for Children and Adolescents (DICA). What modifications were made from the 1975 version were unclear. Initial studies of the DICA appeared in 1982 (Herjanic & Reich, 1982; Reich, Herjanic, Welner, & Gandby, 1982) with the first referenced version in the following year (Herjanic & Reich, 1983a, 1983b).

The DICA was developed in line with the RDI and the DIS (Reich, 1992b) and was intended for use by lay interviewers with modest levels of training. According to Hodges (1993), the DICA was first designed to assess childhood diagnoses in pediatric and psychiatric samples for children from 6 to 17 years old. The DICA has subsequently been employed in epidemiological as well as clinical studies. Despite the intent that the DICA be administered by lay interviewers, the majority of the investigations have utilized mental health professionals (Hodges, 1993).

The DICA was modified in accordance with *DSM-III-R* criteria, which resulted in the DICA–Revised or DICA-R. As described by Kaplan and Reich (1991), the DICA-R differs from its predecessor in rewording of questions and addition of further inquiries. DICA-R questions were rephrased to achieve a much more conversational style and were pretested for comprehension on children, adolescents, and their parents. In addition, questions were added for more comprehensive coverage of *DSM-III-R* criteria. Subsequent descriptions will be limited to the most recent version of the DICA-R, namely draft 7.3, which is available for children, adolescents, and parents (Reich, Shayka, & Taibleson, 1991a, 1991b, 1991c).

The DICA-R is typically described as a structured interview, since the questions and sequence of probing are clearly specified. However, this description is not entirely accurate, since clinicians are allowed "on rare occasions" to supplement the interview with their own unstructured questions (see Kaplan & Reich, 1991, p. 8).

The basic structure of the DICA-R is standard questions followed by optional probes. Standard questions are presented in bold print and should be asked verbatim. In cases where the answer is "yes" or even a tentative "no," the interviewer follows up with one or more probes. Probes are organized into three types: (a) question-specific probes, (b) standard probes, and (c) open-ended probes. Question-specific probes (presented in upper-case type immediately following most standard questions) allow the interviewer to clarify or verify whether a particular diagnostic criterion is met. In contrast, standard probes (presented in lower-case type at the beginning of some sections) assist primarily in establishing the magnitude of the problem. Examples of standard probes include: "Does this happen a lot?" "Was this a big problem for you?" Open-ended probes are described in the test manual and are intended to elicit an example of the diagnostic criterion (e.g., "Can you give me an example of that?"). Generally, standard and open-ended probes are used only when the interviewer remains unclear about the diagnostic criterion.

The DICA is comprehensive in its coverage through standard questions and probes. Approximately 900 items are presented in branching format, with screening questions for many sections (Sylvester, Hyde, & Reichler, 1987). As a result of this screening, the DICA-R-C is administered in approximately 40 minutes and the DICA-R-P in 45 minutes.

The DICA-R is scored on a 4-point scale that is organized primarily by the frequency of symptoms. The basic scoring is 1 for "no," 2 for "rarely," 3 for "sometimes or somewhat," and 5 for "yes." Additional scores included RF for refusing to answer a question and 9 for "don't know." Unless otherwise specified, symptoms are scored for lifetime occurrence.

The DICA-R is organized into 15 major sections. The first two sections cover general and sociodemographic information. A total of 11 sections address mental disorders and symptomatology: behavior disorders (e.g., ADHD, conduct disorders, and substance abuse), mood disorders (e.g., symptoms of major depression and mania), dysthymic disorder, anxiety disorders, obsessive-compulsive disorder, post-traumatic stress disorder, eating disorders, elimination disorders, gender identity, somatization, and psychotic symptoms. Other sections focus on menstruation, psychosocial stressors, and clinical observations. Parallel formats are found for the child, adolescent, and parent versions. The parent version, DICA-R-P, allows the interviewer to evaluate up to three children during the same assessment. The DICA-R-P also includes the DICA-R Pregnancy, Birth and Preschool Questionnaire (Reich, 1992a) that surveys problems with pregnancy, birth, and early development. In addition, the questionnaire includes a brief medical history not only for the child being evaluated but also for other siblings in the family.

Care has been taken to make the DICA understandable and a positive experience for children and parents. Reich and Kaplan (in press) surveyed 50 parents and their children (n = 72). Nearly all the subjects ($\geq$ 90%) reported the interviewing as a positive experience from which they learned more about themselves. When children were asked about specific topics (e.g., school and family life), the majority were more neutral, reporting that they "didn't mind."

Reich and Earls (1990) tested the efficacy of telephone interviews in eliciting information on the DICA. Using matched samples (age, sex, alcohol status of parents), they compared elicited information on the DICA for 25 in-person and 25 telephone interviews. They found that in-person interviews resulted in slightly more symptoms being reported, although comparable numbers were found for "sensitive" questions (e.g., those related to drug use and sexual relations).

The basic procedure is to administer the DICA-R-C and DICA-R-P separately. As with all childhood interviews, the natural question is, How should interviewers integrate the sometimes discrepant findings in achieving a diagnosis? Reich and Earls (1987), following a severe flood in rural Missouri, administered the DICA to 32 mother-child pairs and combined these data with teachers' ratings (TRF) and a second set of interviews, which included Home Environment Interview for Children (HEIC; Reich & Earls, 1984). In developing a composite diagnosis, Reich and Earls (1987) concluded that the children's reports often had fewer symptoms reported, but in sufficient numbers to make most diagnoses. Interestingly, the children appeared much more accurate than parents and teachers in identifying symptoms associated with separation anxiety and over-anxious disorders. Reich and Earls provide guidelines for how to integrate discrepant data (child, parent, and teacher) for specific disorders.

A self-administered computerized version of the DICA was developed and pilot-tested for adolescents and parents (Stein, 1987). Preliminary data on 23 adolescents suggested that this format may have potential usefulness as an ancillary data source. However, supplementary findings of Stavrakaki, Williams, Walker, Rogers, and Kotsopoulos (1991) suggested that a computerized and self-administered DICA may be less effective than other self-report measures. Without any formal validation (comparability with in-person evaluations; reliability and validity studies), the computerized version should be used only for research purposes.

Reliability

The original study of the DICA, unlike studies for most structured interviews, did not address reliability specifically but focused on cross-informant consistency. As has been documented with other child interviews, agreement across parents and children is a stringent test of consistency that often yields disappointing results. The original research on the DICA (Herjanic & Reich, 1982; Reich, Herjanic, Welner, & Gandhy, 1982) is no exception. These investigators examined 307 children, most of whom were psychiatric referrals from low-SES families. Agreement was assessed for 168 individual symptoms that were reported on at least 10 occasions. The resulting kappas were very low, with a range from .00 to .75 and a median of .19. Good agreement was found on important external events (e.g., hospitalization and suspension from school). For diagnosis, the kappas remained low, with a range from .15 to .58 and a median of .37 (see Table 6.4).

Sylvester et al. (1987) examined two aspects of cross-informant consistency: parent-child and parent-parent agreement. She and her colleagues compared the DICA with the DICA-P for 91 children who participated in an ongoing proband study for anxiety and depression. They found consistently low kappas that ranged from .11 to .42 (median = .24). In addition, they compared DICA-Ps completed separately with each parent for 74 children. The overall concordance rate was substantially higher, with a median kappa of .54 (range = .33 – .61).

Welner, Reich, Herjanic, Jung, and Amado (1987) conducted a test-retest reliability study using 27 consecutive inpatients and established a high level of agreement (κ = .76 – 1.00, median = .86). In a separate study of 84 outpatients, they achieved a good level of cross-informant consistency (κ = .49 – .80, median = .63). This latter finding is exceptionally high, both for the DICA and for other child interviews.

Earls, Reich, Jung, and Cloninger (1988) examined cross-informant agreement in a study of parents with alcoholic, antisocial, or medical histories. In 93 comparisons of DICA and DICA-P, the kappas were generally modest (range = .11 – .50, median = .28). Unlike several earlier studies, in this investigation children appeared to report almost as many disorders as did their parents. This finding raises the tantalizing notion that disordered parents may be "blind" to their own problems when manifested in their children.[16]

---

[16]For example, the parents, which included a substantial minority with APD, reported 14.3% fewer oppositional disorders and 140.0% fewer conduct disorders. Since only aggregate data were presented, we cannot explore whether APD parents tended to underreport symptoms associated with oppositional and conduct disorders.

Table 6.4
Reliability Studies of the Diagnostic Interview for Children and Adolescents (DICA)

Study	Agreement
Herjanic & Reich (1982) Cross-informant study used 307 children (ages 6 – 16), of whom 222 were referrals for psychiatric services; 15 interviewers conducted independent interviews.	Individual symptoms, κ = .19
Reich, Herjanic, Welner, & Gandby (1982) Further analysis of Herjanic & Reich (1982) study was performed.	Diagnoses, κ = .37
Sylvester, Hyde, & Reichler (1987) Cross-informant study was conducted as part of a proband study on parents' anxiety and depression; independent DICA interviews yielded comparisons for both mother-father reports on the same child (*n* = 74) and parent-child agreement (*n* = 91).	Mother-father agreement, diagnosis, κ = .54; parent-child agreement, diagnosis, κ = .24
Welner, Reich, Herjanic, Jung, & Amado (1987) Test-retest reliability study assessed 27 psychiatric inpatients (ages 7 – 17) with four lay interviewers at an interval of 1 to 7 days; mother-child concordance study was conducted on 84 outpatients with nine professional and lay interviewers.	Test-retest, diagnosis, κ = .86. Child-parent agreement, diagnosis, κ = .63
Earls, Reich, Jung, & Cloninger (1988) Children (*n* = 91) of parents involved in a long-term family/genetics study of alcoholism were interviewed; parent-child agreement on five common disorders was investigated.	Child-parent agreement, diagnosis, κ = .28

Note. κ = unweighted kappas; *r* = product-moment correlations. Except where otherwise noted, median statistics are reported.

Several studies have reported high interrater reliabilities but provide insufficient information to evaluate the quality of the data. For example, Bartlett, Schleifer, Johnson, and Keller (1991, p. 317) reported a kappa above .90 for DICA interviews with community adolescents, although the size of the sample and range of diagnoses (probably only depression) were not described. Similarly, Biederman et al. (1990) reported an overall kappa of .88, but failed to specify sample size or diagnostic range.

In summary, available research would suggest that the DICA is likely to have acceptable interrater reliability for diagnosis, although current data are presented in insufficient detail. An apparent oversight is the lack of test-retest reliability. The only exception is Welner et al. (1987), who found good reliability estimates based on a rather small sample. Without cross-validation, the stability of child diagnoses based on the DICA remains in question. Finally, studies of cross-informant agreement (except for Welner et al.) yielded poor levels of agreement between parents and children. However, Sylvester et al. (1987) were able to establish a moderate level of parent-parent agreement. Two important cautions must temper the interpretation of these findings. First, we have no data on the reliability of individual symptoms. Second, the majority of studies cluster diagnoses (e.g., subsuming specific anxiety disorders under one category).

Validity

Validation research with the DICA has focused primarily on concurrent and diagnostic validity. Studies of concurrent validity have compared DICA diagnosis with clinical diagnosis and self-report measures. Studies of diagnostic validity have emphasized risk and familial factors for mental disorders, particularly alcohol abuse/dependence, and laboratory correlates.

Concurrent Validity. Welner et al. (1987) compared DICA diagnoses with chart diagnoses for 27 inpatients. Although the level of agreement was highly variable ($\kappa = -.18 - .52$, median = .43), one reason for disagreement was that treating psychiatrists often reported fewer disorders ($M = 1.4$) than the DICA-based assessments ($M = 3.6$). The greatest number of disagreements were found with anxiety and adjustment disorders.

Several studies have examined DICA diagnosis in relationship to other psychometric measures. For example, Brunshaw and Szatmari (1988) compared DICA diagnosis to results on the Survey Diagnostic Instrument (SDI; Boyle, Byles, Offord et al., 1987), which was derived from the CBCL. When parent SDI was correlated with DICA and DICA–P, moderate kappas (.41 – .50) were generated for five common disorders in a sample of 100 children referred for outpatient treatment. In contrast, teacher SDIs evidenced little correspondence (.08 – .27) to diagnoses. As a further example, Sylvester et al. (1987) examined the DICA in relationship to diagnostic patterns on the Personality Inventory for Children (PIC; Lachar & Gdowski, 1979) for 74 children. Kappa coefficients, as commonly found between multiscale inventories and diagnosis, were very modest and ranged from .11 to .30 for four common disorders.

Two additional studies (Kashini, Strober, Rosenberg, & Reid, 1988; Marton, Churchard, Kutcher, & Korenblum, 1991) explored the relationship of the DICA to other measures of psychopathology and overall functioning. Kashini et al. compared the DICA to the Millon Adolescent Personality Inventory (Millon, Green, & Meagher, 1972). In a study of 150 community adolescents, they found that adolescents with disorders had higher elevations on four Millon scales (Sensitive, Self-Concept, Personal Esteem, and Family Rapport) than those who were well-adjusted. Marton et al. (1991) found predicted differences between DICA depressed ($n = 60$) and nondepressed ($n = 59$) adolescents on the Beck Depression Inventory.

Research on the DICA has also examined its concurrent and convergent validity with specific disorders. Several studies have addressed attention-deficit disorders (ADD). For example, Shapiro and Garfinkel (1986) compared 27 ADD with 276 non-ADD children, as identified by the Conners' Teacher Rating Scale (CTRS; Conners, 1969). They found highly significant differences for the majority of individual ADD symptoms on the DICA. Moreover, these differences appeared to be associated with measures of attentional deficits (e.g., continuous performance task). Livingston, Dykman, and Ackerman (1990) attempted to differentiate subtypes of ADD based on hyperactivity and aggression. They found notable differences for 115 White ADD boys on the CBCL and teacher ratings. Finally, Biederman, Keenan, and Farone (1990) compared DICA-P diagnoses of ADD with teacher checklists and found very modest agreement on individual symptoms ($M \phi$ coefficient = .21). However, the concordance rate on the diagnosis itself was quite high (90.2%).[17]

Allen-Meares (1991) investigated the concurrent validity of DICA-diagnosed depression in a sample of 41 behaviorally disordered children. Interestingly, the DICA correlated with the CDI (r = .49), but not with other measures of depression. Given the fact that the study used a very early (1975) version of the DICA, its findings have little relevance to the current measure.

Diagnostic Validity. DICA studies have focused on the onset (particularly risk factors), course of the disorder, and familial/laboratory correlates. Of these studies, the majority have addressed risk factors, especially those associated with alcoholic parents.

Reich, Earls, and Powell (1988) conducted the first study of risk factors associated with alcoholic parents and DICA diagnoses in their children. In a 5-year follow-up study of 22 children without and 32 with alcoholic parents, they found a pronounced risk for disorders in children of alcoholic parents. This risk increased dramatically for behavior disorders (65.6% vs. 0.0%). In a more recent study, Reich, Earls, Frankel, and Shayka (1993) contrasted childhood diagnoses across three groups: (a) neither parent alcoholic; n = 51, (b) one parent alcoholic; n = 82, and (c) both parents alcoholic; n = 22. They found highly significant differences in the predicted direction for oppositional and conduct disorders. In addition, children of alcoholic parents were at greater risk of warranting substance abuse diagnoses. This finding that children of alcoholics are at greater risk for behavior disorders appears to be very robust (see also Earls, Smith, Reich, & Jung, 1988).

Researchers have also investigated the relationship of parental mood and anxiety disorders to childhood diagnoses. In a study of 53 families, Sylvester et al. (1987) found that panic-disordered and depressed parents had increased likelihood of similar disorders in their children, although the data do not suggest any specific risk (e.g., parent to childhood depression).[18] Kashini, Beck, & Burk (1987) reported that factors increasing the risk of childhood disorders in depressed parents included (a) documented child abuse, (b) fear of future abuse, and (c) learning disorders.

---

[17]Since the study was limited to ADD children, this high level of agreement is not surprising.

[18]Based on the DICA, children appear to be at greater overall risk of mental disorders if their parents have panic disorders. In contrast, results of the DICA-P suggest that children of depressed parents are at greater risk for mental illness than those of panic-disordered parents.

Earls et al. (1988) investigated risk factors associated with a natural disaster, namely a devastating flood in rural Missouri. Of interest, they found that 1 year later children's symptoms did not appear to be associated with the intensity of their flood experiences. Instead, presence of preexisting disorders appeared to significantly increase the likelihood of flood-related symptoms (i.e., prior diagnosis, 47.4% flood symptoms; no prior diagnosis, 0.0% flood symptoms).

Livingston and Bracha (1992) examined the risk factors for suicide in 62 inpatient children who were diagnosed with the DICA. Predictably, they found that children with the diagnosis of major depression were more likely than others to have suicidal ideation. Surprisingly, certain psychotic symptoms, particularly visual hallucinations, appeared to increase the likelihood of suicidal ideation.

The relationship of medical diseases to increased prevalence of mental disorders has received relatively little attention, at least with respect to diagnostic interviews. One exception is a study by Kashini, Konig, Shepperd, Wilfley, and Morris (1988) that examined DICA diagnoses for 56 asthmatic and 56 control children. Although few differences were observed, asthmatic children appeared to have more anxiety symptoms on the DICA-P than did their healthy counterparts.

Beyond risk factors, studies have examined biological correlates and treatment response of specific disorders. Gillis, Gilger, Pennington, and DeFries (1992) evaluated the genetic etiology for the DICA diagnosis of ADHD with 37 identical and 37 fraternal twin pairs. Concordance rates were significantly higher for identical (79%) than for fraternal (32%) twins. These results are sustained when adjusted for age, intelligence, and reading level. Biederman et al. (1993) examined behavioral inhibition (highly constricted behavior that is assumed to be the result of low thresholds of limbic arousal) across young children with mentally disordered parents. They found much greater risks of DICA diagnosis (particularly anxiety disorders) for inhibited children than for either uninhibited children or controls with healthy parents. Livingston, Dykman, and Ackerman (1992) found a differential treatment response, dependent on dosage, for ADHD children with concomitant disorders. ADHD children with both mood and oppositional/conduct disorders responded more effectively to higher dosages of psychostimulants.

In summary, relatively few studies have examined the concurrent validity of the DICA, and these have yielded mixed results. Perhaps the most promising results were reported by Brunshaw and Szatmari (1988), who reported moderate kappa coefficients. Other studies have described modest correlations with external measures (i.e., < .40). From the perspective of diagnostic validity, a substantial body of literature has examined risk factors associated with mental disorders in parents and other variables (e.g., child abuse and natural disasters). In light of other diagnostic interviews, more research is needed on concurrent validity with structured interviews and well-established parent and teacher ratings (i.e., CBCL and TRF).

Clinical Applications

The relatively few DICA studies of interrater reliability and less-than-optimal findings with respect to concurrent validity are both likely to lead psychologists to actively consider alternative interviews. Clearly, additional research is needed to address these important facets of the DICA-R. The development of the DICA-R suggests careful crafting of questions and sequencing of sections to facilitate the interviewing of youth. In clinical cases where the identification of particular diagnosis is not the paramount issue, the DICA-R should be seriously considered as a comprehensive measure that is user-friendly.

One advantage of the DICA-R over other structured interviews is the availability of an adolescent version, with a slight rewording of some questions to make them more appropriate to this population. As yet, no validational studies have been published on this version, apparently based on the assumption that the changes were not so substantial as to require separate evidence of reliability and validity. Still, psychologists may find merit in using the adolescent version, because of its tighter focus.

A distinguishing characteristic of the DICA-R is its emphasis on the child's or adolescent's confidentiality. In the introduction to the interview (Reich et al., 1991a, p. 2), the child is assured, "I won't tell anyone what you tell me—not even your parent(s), unless we find out that somebody might be getting hurt in some way." The likely trade-off is that (a) children and especially adolescents will be more likely to divulge personal problems and problematic behaviors, but (b) psychologists, particularly those employing family interventions, may be hampered in their treatment by an inability to address openly any problems raised by the child or adolescent. In contrast, the K-SADS encourages an open discussion of disparities between parent and child versions. In choosing the DICA-R, psychologists should be aware of both the positive and negative implications of confidentiality. For example, Famularo, Kinscherff, and Fenton (1992) employed the DICA-R in the evaluation of maltreated children. They found that the children reported nearly twice as many cases of PTSD as their abusive parents. We might safely assume that the assurance of confidentiality facilitated the children's self-disclosure.

The DICA, perhaps more than other measures, has been used in studies of children with alcoholic parents. Although these studies provide only a general understanding of risk factors associated with alcoholism and antisocial behavior, clinicians may feel comfortable in using the DICA-R in the assessment of these populations because of the available comparative data.

Myers and his colleagues (Myers & Kemph, 1990; Myers, Burket, Lyles, Stone, & Kemph, 1990) have found the DICA-R useful in the assessment of juvenile delinquents. As expected, these samples revealed a predominance of conduct and substance abuse disorders.[19] The authors concluded that the DICA-R was helpful in eliciting clinical data from delinquents, even when parent interviews were not possible.

---

[19]An unexpected finding across these two small samples (combined $n = 29$) was the proportion of delinquents (34.5%) with prior histories of separation anxiety.

Research reports have suggested the feasibility of employing the DICA-R with a range of clinical populations. Investigators have advocated its use with common disorders: adolescent depression (Kashini, Sherman, Parker, & Reid, 1990), borderline personality disorder (Famularo, Kinscherff, & Fenton, 1992) and obsessive-compulsive disorders (Grad, Pelcovitz, Olson, Matthews, & Grad, 1987).

Other Diagnostic Interviews

Interview Schedule for Children (ISC)

Kovacs (1983) developed the Interview Schedule for Children (ISC) as a semistructured interview on which symptoms are rated on a 9-point scale. The ISC is designed to be used in conjunction with the *DSM-III* and consists of parallel interviews, the first with a parent and the second with the child. When discrepancies occur, the parents' data are given greater weight than children's. Reliability data reported by Last, Strauss, and Francis (1987) suggest good to excellent diagnostic agreement (median $\kappa = .81$, range $= .64 - 1.00$) on 11 disorders.

Kovacs and her colleagues (Kovacs, Feinberg, Crouse-Novak, Paulauskas, & Finkelstein, 1984; Kovacs, Feinberg, Crouse-Novak, Paulauskas, Pollock, & Finkelstein, 1984) conducted several longitudinal studies on childhood depression employing the ISC. Kovacs, Feinberg, Crouse-Novak, Paulauskas, and Finkelstein (1984) examined 65 outpatient children diagnosed with the ISC as depressed. In subsequent follow-up, major depression and adjustment disorder with depressed mood evidenced greater recovery than "double depression" (i.e., major depression superimposed on dysthymia). Kovacs, Feinberg, Crouse-Novak, Paulauskas, Pollock, and Finkelstein (1984), using the same sample, attempted to predict further episodes of depression. Subsequent follow-up, spanning upwards to 12 years, has demonstrated the outcome criteria for depression and dysthymia (Kovacs, Akiskal, Gatsonis, & Parrone, 1994).

Autism Diagnostic Interview (ADI)

Le Couteur et al.(1989) constructed the Autism Diagnostic Interview (ADI) to accurately classify autism by ICD-10 standards. The interview is intended for patients, ages 5 to early adulthood, in which a pervasive developmental disorder is suspected. The diagnostic questioning focuses principally on parent's or caretaker's observations of the patient, with a concentration on three related areas: (a) reciprocal social interaction, (b) use of language, and (c) repetitive or stereotyped behaviors. Interrater reliability on the basis of four experienced raters was evaluated with most weighted kappas for individual items exceeding .70. In addition, the intraclass coefficients for the three areas described previously were excellent, ranging from .94 to .97. Comparisons of 16 autistic and 16 mentally retarded patients indicated highly significant differences on symptomatic basis, leading to a perfect discrimination between the two groups. While in need of cross-validation, the results of this initial study appear highly promising. With the publication of *DSM-IV*, further refinements will be needed to differentiate autistic disorder from Rett's, Asperger's, and childhood disintegrative disorders.

Home Environment Interview for Children (HEIC)

A structured interview was designed to complement the DICA in assessing family/home conflicts and stresses. This interview was named the Home Environment Interview for Children (HEIC; Reich & Earls, 1984) and is available in parallel forms for parents and children. Unpublished data (cited in Reich, Earls, and Powell, 1988) suggest good mother-child agreement and test-retest reliability. Content areas addressed by the HEIC include family and peer relationships as well as school adjustment. The HEIC may be particularly useful in assessing dysfunctional behaviors at home and school, and may serve as a useful adjunct to diagnostic interviews (Reich & Earls, 1987).

Child and Adolescent Psychiatric Assessment Scale (CAPA)

The Child and Adolescent Psychiatric Assessment Scale (CAPA; Angold, Cox, Prendergast, Rutter, & Simonoff, 1987) was recently developed for use in the clinical assessment of children's disorders and level of impairment. The CAPA interviews are administered by lay interviewers. Psychometric data are not yet available on the reliability and validity of this measure (see Hodges, 1993). Pending further validation, the CAPA is not recommended for clinical use.

Part II

Differential Diagnosis for Axis II Disorders

7

Structured Interview for *DSM-III* Personality Disorders (SIDP)

Description, Rationale, and Development

The Structured Interview for *DSM-III* Personality Disorders (SIDP; Pfohl, Stangl, & Zimmerman, 1982) and the revised version (SIDP-R; Pfohl, Blum, Zimmerman, & Stangl, 1989) were constructed to assess Axis II disorders. A new SIDP-IV version will be available in late 1994; this version was not reviewed since final modifications were being carried out and validity studies had yet to be conducted as this book was written.

The SIDP is composed of 160 clinical inquiries/ratings that entail the inclusion criteria for personality disorders. The items are organized into 17 topical sections which progress from relatively nonthreatening components, such as general interests and activities, to more potentially intrusive components that address disordered perceptions and thinking. The design of the SIDP is intended to parallel a psychiatric interview in its progression through topical sections. The advantages of this organization are that (a) questions have a natural flow, and (b) patients may have greater difficulty in modifying their response styles, since diagnostic criteria are not necessarily clustered together. The chief disadvantage of this approach is that rescoring patient responses on the basis of *DSM-III-R* criteria is a convoluted process.

Consistent with the *DSM* model of personality disorders, the format of the SIDP is designed to emphasize patients' characteristic functioning. Instructions ask patients to respond to questions "according to the way you are when you are your usual self" (Pfohl, Blum, et al., 1989, p. 4). With these directions, the authors hope to minimize any undue influence because of situational (e.g., marital crisis) or psychopathological (e.g., major depressive episode) factors. In cases where the patient reports significant personality changes, the patient is instructed to respond in the manner which has been typical for the greatest amount of time in the last 5 years.

Pfohl and his colleagues also recognized that Axis II patients are sometimes inaccurate in their self-appraisals as well as their self-reporting. To this end, mental health professionals attempt to secure permission from each patient for an "informant" interview with a family member or close friend. A subset of clinical inquiries (approximately one-half) form the basis for the informant interview; these questions are marked with asterisks. Additional inquiries are employed to clarify informants' responses. Pfohl, Blum, et al. (1989) reported that the use of informant interviews tends to reveal personality disorders that might otherwise be missed. Moreover, clinicians should integrate clinical records into their rendering of Axis II diagnoses.

The SIDP, like many structured interviews, employs a 3-point rating scale: 0 for "not present," 1 for "moderately present," and 2 for "severely present." Psychologists should note that a rating of 1 is deemed sufficient to meet *DSM-III-R* criteria. In this respect, the SIDP is substantially different from other diagnostic interviews, such as the SADS and the SCID, for which the intermediate rating is considered "subthreshold." For diagnostic purposes, a rating of 1 on the SIDP is the functional equivalent of a rating of 2 on the SCID. In this regard, the SIDP forces clinicians to choose between "not present" and "moderately present" and avoids subthreshold ratings altogether. Whether this polarization of ratings improves diagnostic reliability remains to be investigated.[1]

The scoring of individual items also includes descriptive statements to assist in specific ratings. For ratings of 2, descriptions of symptoms are stated in terms of frequency (e.g., "constantly," "almost never") or severity (e.g., "preoccupied," "desperate"). Scored items are then transposed to a two-page SIDP-R Rating Sheet. Clinicians are asked to use the most valid information from patient's answers, informant's responses, and other clinical data. No guidelines are offered on how to reconcile disparities among clinical sources. The Rating Sheet provides *DSM-III-R* criteria for the diagnosis of personality disorders.

Interviewers record the patient's and informant's responses to the SIDP. Since many questions are open-ended, clinicians may find it necessary to follow the standard questions with optional probes that are provided for clarification. These probes are highlighted by conditional clauses presented in capital letters (e.g., "IF YES,..." and "IF HAS NOT HAPPENED..."). The clinician is also asked periodically to make clinical observations regarding verbal and nonverbal behaviors. Responses to specific questions may inform more than one item rating. Finally, clinicians are asked to make judgments, often complex, on whether symptoms for certain personality disorders occurred exclusively during the course of specified Axis I disorders.

Pfohl and his colleagues reported that a typical SIDP interview requires 60 to 90 minutes to complete, with an additional 30 minutes for an informant interview. Green (1987, 1989) considered these time estimates to be optimistic, since the clinician is obliged to take detailed notes during both interviews. To facilitate the selective use of the SIDP, Pfohl (1993) has developed a 6-item screen (the Iowa Personality Disorder Screen) that may identify as many as 80% of psychiatric patients who have Axis II disorders.

One valuable and possibly overlooked feature of the SIDP-R is its clarity in the diagnosis of mixed personality disorder. As noted in Chapter 1, psychologists and other mental health professionals may apply mixed personality disorder to cover characterological features of varying dysfunction and distress. In this regard, the SIDP-R imposes a stringent standard. The mixed personality diagnosis

---

[1]On the other hand, the presence of subthreshold ratings creates a quandary for clinicians who may find such clinical data difficult to ignore.

is invoked only when the patient (a) does not meet any specific personality disorder, and (b) has one less than the necessary inclusion criteria for two or more personality disorders. I would argue for the adoption of this standard to reduce the diagnostic slippage common in current practice.

The rationale and development of the SIDP is not described in detail. In the original study of the SIDP, Stangl, Pfohl, Zimmerman, Bowers, and Corenthal (1985) offer only a passing comment on the rationale for its development by stating that perennial problems in the assessment of personality disorders had been observed: (a) marked variations in traditional interviewing, (b) lack of differentiation between time-limited crises and stable personality characteristics, and (c) variable thresholds for meeting inclusion criteria. Presumably, the SIDP was developed to reduce substantially the considerable Axis II problems with information and criterion variances.

Stangl et al. (1985) reported that the development of the SIDP involved three major revisions over an 18-month period. Although early versions of the SIDP were "field tested," no details are provided for how this process was carried out. Apparently, "confusing" and "ineffective" questions were modified or replaced. The lack of any formal description of this refinement would suggest an intuitive, nonempirical approach. Similarly, no description is offered on the changes between SIDP and SIDP-R, except to note that the revision is keyed to the *DSM-III-R*.

Validation of the SIDP

The SIDP and subsequent Axis II interviews capitalized on the emergence of *DSM-III* to provide the criteria and conceptual underpinnings for the systematic assessment of personality disorders. In this sense, the SIDP, at least in its early development, relied solely on the *DSM-III* inclusion criteria as its gold standard. Pfohl and his colleagues saw their primary task as the standardization of clinical inquiries and the establishment of reliability. More recent studies have investigated more fully the SIDP's diagnostic validity.

Diagnostic Reliability

Pfohl and his colleagues conducted the first reliability study of the SIDP (Stangl et al., 1985; Pfohl, Coryell, Zimmerman, & Stangl, 1986) and participated in three further studies (Zimmerman & Coryell, 1989; Zimmerman, Coryell, Pfohl, Corenthal, & Stangl, 1986; Zimmerman, Pfohl, Coryell, Stangl, & Corenthal, 1986). In addition, the reliability of the SIDP has been investigated by a handful of other researchers who were not associated with its development (see Table 7.1).

In the original reliability study, Stangl et al. (1985) employed an adult psychiatric sample ($N = 63$) that consisted primarily of inpatients (90%) and females (76%), and excluded patients with diagnosis of schizophrenia, mental retardation, or organic brain syndrome. For the five personality disorders that were adequately represented (> 10 subjects), the kappa coefficients ranged from .45 to .90, with a median of .75. Pfohl et al. (1986) performed a further analysis of these data and computed kappas for each diagnostic criterion. They found an extraordinary range (–.04 – .90), with most items evidencing modest to moderate agreement (> .40). Several items related to interpersonal feelings (e.g., absence of tender feelings, emotional coldness, and lack of empathy) were completely unreliable. On the other hand, several personality disorders (dependent, avoidant, and borderline) evidenced high levels of agreement, with reliabilities for individual criteria at a uniformly satisfactory level ($\geq$ .50).

Table 7.1

Reliability Studies of the Structured Interview for DSM-III Personality Disorders (SIDP)

Study	Agreement
Stangl, Pfohl, Zimmerman, Bowers, & Corenthal (1985) Combined study of interrater (*n* = 43) and test-retest (*n* = 20; interval < 1 week) reliability used a primarily inpatient sample (90%) that excluded schizophrenic and organic brain syndrome; five interviewers from varied backgrounds were employed.	Diagnosis, κ = .75
Pfohl, Coryell, Zimmerman, & Stangl (1986) Further analysis of Stangl et al. (1985) on individual symptoms was performed.	Symptoms, κ = .55
Zimmerman, Coryell, Pfohl, Corenthal, & Stangl (1986) Combined sample of interrater and test-retest reliability (total *N* = 25; details not provided) used 25 inpatients with major depression; the authors tested only for the presence or absence of *any* personality disorder.	Interrater, κ = .71. Test-retest, κ = .66
Zimmerman, Pfohl, Coryell, Stangl, & Corenthal (1986) Combined sample of interrater (*n* = 27) and test-retest (*n* = 19) reliability used depressed and other psychiatric patients; diagnoses were rendered by the same clinicians on (a) the patient interview alone, and subsequently (b) the patient plus an informant interview.	Patient-only, diagnosis, κ = .68. Patient + informant, diagnosis, κ = .71
Zimmerman & Coryell (1988) Interrater reliability study used 104 first-degree relatives of patient and normal controls. Most evaluations were accomplished by telephone interview (86.5%) with audiotapes rated by a second interviewer.	Dimensional scores, *M* ICC = .91. Any personality disorder, κ = .93[a]

Table 7.1   (continued)
Reliability Studies of the Structured Interview for DSM-III Personality Disorders (SIDP)

Study	Agreement
Baer et al. (1990) Interrater reliability was studied with 16 patients referred to clinic for obsessive-compulsive disorders; two research assistants conducted interviews.	Any personality disorder, κ = .88
Brent, Zelenak, Busstein, & Brown (1990) Videotaped interrater reliability study used 17 mood-disordered adolescent patients.	Presence/absence of personality traits, κ = .58[b]
Hogg, Jackson, Rudd, & Edwards (1990) Interrater reliability study compared results for 21 recent-onset schizophrenic inpatients by two raters.	Any personality disorder, κ = .59. Dimensional scores, r = .54
Jackson et al. (1991) Interrater reliability study of 39 inpatients (schizophrenic or mood-disordered) had two independent raters.	Diagnosis, κ = .72
Trull (1992) Interrater reliability study of 18 psychiatric outpatients utilized five raters.	Dimensional scores, ICC = .86
Serper et al. (1993) Interrater reliability study of 45 VA inpatients with borderline, schizotypal, and combined disorders compared results for two raters.	Diagnosis, κ = .81

Note. κ = unweighted kappas; ICC = intraclass coefficients. Except where otherwise noted, median statistics are reported.
[a]The kappas for individual personality disorders were also high (median = .90) despite very low frequencies (i.e., ≤ 6). [b]Instead of using dimensional ratings, the investigators simply dichotomized each personality disorder into "no traits" and "one or more traits."

Zimmerman and his colleagues (Zimmerman & Coryell, 1989; Zimmerman, Coryell, et al., 1986; Zimmerman, Pfohl, et al., 1986) conducted three additional studies of the SIDP's reliability. In the first of these studies, Zimmerman, Pfohl, et al. (1986) recruited subjects with major depression and a smaller number with other mental disorders (excluding schizophrenia, mental retardation, and organic brain syndrome) in a reliability study of the SIDP. Reliability estimates were made by the same clinicians in two stages: (a) after a SIDP interview with the patient alone, and (b) after separate SIDP interviews with the patient and his/her informant. The SIDP maintained approximately the same reliability across the two conditions (median κs = .68 and .71). However, Zimmerman, Pfohl, Coryell, Stangl, and Corenthal (1988), in a study of 66 nonpsychotic depressed patients, found virtually no convergence between totally independent patient and informant interviews for dimensional scores (rs = .15 – .61; median = .29) and categorical diagnosis ($κs$ = –.06 – .32; median = .00). Use of consensus ratings suggested that patients were either unaware of or chose not to report many symptoms associated with personality disorders. When symptoms were reported by the patient but not the informant, consensus ratings tended to support the accuracy of the patient.[2] A similar study by Pica, Edwards, Jackson, Bell, Bates, and Rudd (1990) also found an increase in reported symptoms when informant and patient interviews were integrated. Together, these studies would suggest that informant interviews are vital in confirming unreported personality disorders but less necessary in confirming patient-reported personality disorders.

Zimmerman and Coryell (1989) investigated the interrater reliability of audiotaped telephone interviews of a nonclinical sample. They computed dimensional scores for each of the personality disorders and found a very high level of agreement (M ICC = .91 with all but one ICC > .85). Moreover, the kappas were moderately high despite the low frequency ($≤$ 6 subjects per category) of specific personality disorders. Finally, Zimmerman, Coryell, et al. (1986) conducted a small study of 25 depressed patients and found moderate agreement on the presence or absence of any personality disorder.

Studies by other investigators have largely been limited in their scope. For example, research by Baer et al. (1990); Brent, Zelenak, Busstein, and Brown (1990); and Hogg, Jackson, Rudd, and Edwards (1990) were restricted both in terms of sample size and Axis I diagnosis. Because of these limitations, the studies were unable to report reliabilities for specific personality disorders. Of the two, Hogg et al. (1990) reported modest results for both diagnosis ($κ$ = .59)[3] and dimensional scores (r = .54). Colleagues of Hogg et al. conducted a further study at the same British hospital (Jackson et al., 1991; also see Bell & Jackson, 1992). Interestingly, they reported substantially higher kappas than Hogg et al. while employing a more stringent standard (specific personality disorders vs. any personality disorder). Jackson, Whiteside, et al. (1991) found for seven personality disorders ($≥$ 5 subjects) a median kappa of .72 (range = .48 – 1.00).

Trull (1992) examined SIDP dimensional scores on a modest sample of 16 outpatients. He found good to excellent agreement on dimensional scores that ranged from ICCs of .61 to .91 (median = .86). Given the circumscribed sample, the numbers were insufficient to compute reliability coefficients for specific disorders. With a diagnostically restricted sample (borderline, schizotypal, borderline/schizotypal patients), Serper et al. (1993) established good agreement ($κs$ = .73 – .82).

In summary, the reliability estimates of the SIDP are generally comparable to those of other Axis II measures (see Chapter 9), although the Personality Disorder Examination (PDE) has superior reliability (see Chapter 8). One major limitation of the SIDP is the general absence of test-retest reliability studies. The

---

[2]Of course, the researchers could have had the bias (implicit or explicit) that reported psychopathology, regardless of the source, was likely to be true.

[3]I describe this kappa as modest not only because of its absolute value, but because the level of discrimination (presence or absence of any personality disorder) is so basic that we would expect a higher value.

sole exception[4] is the study by Zimmerman, Coryell, et al. (1986), who established a moderate reliability of .66 on 25 depressed patients. Certainly, further research on the stability of the SIDP vis-a-vis a test-retest design would be very helpful. The second limitation of the SIDP is that the reliabilities of categorical diagnoses have not been established for schizoid and narcissistic personality disorders. With both disorders, however, dimensional ratings offer at least indirect evidence of diagnostic reliability. A third limitation of the SIDP is that the available research addresses the SIDP and not the recently revised SIDP-R.[5]

An advantage of the SIDP is the detailed examination by Pfohl et al. (1986) of individual diagnostic criteria. Psychologists and other mental health professionals can review the reported symptomatology and concomitant observations for particular patients. By examining item reliabilities, a psychologist can establish his/her own level of certainty for a specific diagnosis, based on a unique array of symptoms. In addition, these item reliabilities are invaluable for applied research which often involves specific psychopathology in addition to psychiatric diagnoses.

Validity

Validational studies of the SIDP have approached this onerous task from several perspectives. As evidence of construct validity, studies have explored the discreteness of SIDP-diagnosed personality disorders (i.e., Do inclusion/exclusion criteria distinguish specific disorders?) and their general relationship to personality. Moreover, a substantial body of research has examined SIDP convergent validity with comparisons to self-report measures of personality disorders. From a very different avenue of research, investigations of SIDP personality disorders have addressed their effects on treatment outcome in selected groups of Axis I patients.

Zimmerman and Coryell (1989) conducted an important investigation regarding the boundaries and diagnostic overlap of personality disorders, as measured by the SIDP. In a nonreferred sample[6] of 797 community-based adults, they examined the comorbidity of Axis II disorders. They found that "pure" SIDP personality disorders ranged from 14.3% for paranoid to 71.4% for dependent and schizoid personality disorders (median = 47.9%).[7] With reference to dimensional scores, two scales (schizoid and dependent) appeared largely uncorrelated ($rs <$ .40) with other scales. Conversely, two pairs of scales (i.e., paranoid and schizotypal; histrionic and borderline) appear highly correlated ($\geq$ .60) and may lack sufficient discriminability. As might be expected, borderline personality disorder appeared to be moderately correlated ($rs \geq$ .50 with four other scales).

---

[4]Several studies have combined an interrater design with small numbers of test-retest subjects. For example, Stangl et al. (1985) reported that they administered the SIDP to 20 patients in a test-retest design; however, they did not report any specific reliability coefficients, although the concordance rate appeared to be modest (i.e., 19 of 33 diagnoses or 57.8%).

[5]Preliminary data on concordance rates appear promising (Syrakic, Whitehead, Przybeck, & Cloninger, 1993).

[6]Most subjects were recruited as first-degree relatives in a family proband study of psychiatric disorders. When administered the DIS as part of this study, substantial numbers evidenced a lifetime prevalence for mood, anxiety, and substance abuse disorders.

[7]An unexpected finding was that none of the 797 subjects warranted the diagnosis of narcissistic personality disorder.

Perhaps the best way to understand Zimmerman and Coryell (1989) results is to compare these SIDP findings to other research. As noted in Chapter 1, research on Axis II disorders has yielded pure personality disorders in as few as 1% of clinical cases (Blashfield, 1992). In contrast, the SIDP yielded pure diagnoses in roughly one-half of the cases. Likewise, when the SIDP data are compared to the Personality Diagnostic Questionnaire–Revised (PDQ-R) on the same community sample (see Zimmerman & Coryell, 1990), the SIDP continues to have substantially less overlap. Moreover, research by Reich and Noyes (1987) suggested that SIDP-based personality disorders have less comorbidity with panic and depressed disorders than is found with the PDQ and the MCMI (i.e., 24% less overlap). With the exception of the specific overlaps noted above, the SIDP scales appear to be relatively discrete.

The SIDP has also been employed to test the diagnostic overlap of newly proposed personality disorders with established disorders. Spitzer, Feister, Gay, and Pfohl (1991) examined whether the proposed criteria for sadistic personality disorder would discriminate patients exhibiting these features from other SIDP personality disordered patients. According to Spitzer et al. (1991), the inclusion criteria would form a constellation of symptoms that are not shared by other Axis II patients.

Trull (1992) approached the construct validity of the SIDP by examining its relationship to the five-factor model of personality (i.e., neuroticism, extraversion, openness to experience, agreeableness, and conscientiousness). He compared SIDP dimensional scores for 54 psychiatric outpatients with these five factors as measured by NEO Personality Inventory (NEO-PI; Costa & McCrae, 1985). He found relationships which made conceptual sense and were consistent with other measures of personality disorders, namely, the MMPI personality disorder scales (Morey, Waugh, & Blashfield, 1985) and the PDQ-R (Hyler & Rieder, 1987). From a psychoanalytic perspective, Torgersen and Alnaes (1989) attempted to relate, with modest success, SIDP diagnoses to characterological dimensions, as measured by Basic Character Inventory (Torgersen, 1980).

Bell and Jackson (1992) explored the structure of SIDP-derived diagnoses and their relationship to three clusters proposed by *DSM-III-R*. Using data described previously (Hogg et al., 1990), these investigators established only moderate correspondence with *DSM-III-R*, partly due to the overlap of five specific personality disorders with two clusters. These findings are encouraging, since most patients also had Axis I disorders which were likely to obscure the observed structure of Axis II disorders.

Gasperini et al. (1989) attempted to explore cognitive differences for personality-disordered affective patients. Regrettably, the factor analysis was based on an insufficient number of subjects (i.e., 40 variables and 52 subjects). Possible differences in cognitive style among clusters A, B, and C personality disorders, as measured by the SIDP, deserve further investigation.

Little research has attempted to establish biological markers or familial patterns that would be associated with specific SIDP personality disorders. One exception is a study by Siever and his associates (Siever et al., 1990). They examined eye-tracking ability in 26 schizotypal patients who were compared to controls with other personality disorders, normal controls, and schizophrenic patients. The researchers found that schizotypal patients were less impaired than schizophrenic patients and more impaired than controls, including those with personality disorders. In a proband study, Coryell and Zimmerman (1989) did not find predicted results. For example, schizophrenic patients did not have an increased prevalence of schizotypal disorders in their family members.

Reich (1986) studied early childhood events in 82 outpatients who had personality disorders in addition to an Axis I diagnosis (typically depression or anxiety). He found that Cluster B patients had a higher frequency than Clusters A or C of parent's death or parent's absence. The etiological significance of this finding is not understood, although understandably APD patients frequently had an absent parent. Obviously, much more research is needed on the antecedent events for specific personality disorders.

Convergent Validity with Other Psychological Measures. Stangl et al. (1985) performed the first convergent validity study by comparing SIDP personality disorder clusters to MMPI elevations. While significant differences were found, interpretation of the results is hampered by small group sizes and by the fact that most differences were nonspecific (i.e., between nonpersonality-disordered and personality-disordered subjects).

The majority of convergent validity studies have compared diagnosis with the SIDP to the PDQ, a self-administered questionnaire, and/or the Millon Clinical Multiaxial Inventory-II (MCMI-II; Millon, 1982), a multiscale inventory. Comparisons are most often made simply on the concordance of diagnoses across measures. Less frequently, investigators have examined dimensional scores across measures (see Table 7.2). I have described the validity of these studies as "convergent" rather than "criterion-related" since self-report scales for personality disorders often evidence only a modest relationship with clinical diagnosis (e.g., Widiger & Sanderson, 1987) or other structured interviews, such as the Personality Disorder Examination (PDE; see Chapter 8).

Riech and his colleagues have carried out a program of research on the SIDP and its relationship to the PDQ and MCMI-II (Reich, 1987a, 1987b, 1988a, 1988b, 1990; Reich & Noyes, 1987; Rcich, Noyes, & Troughton, 1987). Riech examined concordance of personality disorders on 170 psychiatric outpatients (approximately one-half with panic disorders). In a subsample of 108 females, he found only a modest consensus among the three measures, with the SIDP tending to be the most conservative at diagnosing disorders. Despite the multiple studies, Reich and his colleagues report little data on the specific relationships among the three measures.

Zimmerman and Coryell (1990) conducted an interesting study of the SIDP and its concordance with the PDQ. On a large sample of 697 community subjects, they found virtually no agreement on categorical diagnoses (κs = .00 – .38; median = .13), which is due in part to the low prevalence (13.5% for any personality) in this community sample. Even so, dimensional ratings yielded relatively modest results (see Table 7.2), with a median r of .37.

Three studies have directly compared dimensional scores on the SIDP with elevations on the MCMI-II, all with disappointing results. Samples included 40 schizophrenic inpatients (Hogg et al., 1990), 272 psychiatric outpatients (Torgersen & Alnaes, 1990), and 82 inpatients (Jackson, Grazis, Rudd, &

Edwards, 1991). Modest but consistent correlations (≥ .30) were found for schizoid, avoidant, and borderline. In contrast, slight negative correlations were found for compulsive personality disorder. As previously noted, the relationship of MCMI-II to personality disorders is not well established. Therefore, these negative results should not be alarming.

Dubro, Wetzler, and Kahn (1988) compared SIDP diagnoses to the MCMI-II, the PDQ, and the Personality Disorder Scales of the MMPI (PDS; Morey, Waugh, & Blashfield, 1985) in a sample of 20 medical and 36 psychiatric inpatients. For the four personality disorders that were adequately represented (histrionic, borderline, avoidant, and dependent), the MCMI-II and the PDQ evidenced moderate sensitivity (.70 and .71, respectively), with excellent specificity (.87 and .91, respectively). In contrast, the MMPI PDS scales yielded poor sensitivity (.33) for the four personality disorders. These results provide moderate support for the convergent validity of SIDP diagnoses.

Serper et al. (1993) compared SIDP-diagnosed borderline, schizotypal, and borderline/schizotypal patients on the MMPI. Interestingly, patients with combined diagnoses had higher elevations on scales 1, 7, and 8. As might be expected, borderline patients scored higher than schizotypal patients on scale 4. While informative, these findings provide only circumscribed evidence of convergent validity.

Table 7.2

Convergent Validity Studies between the Structured Interview for DSM-III Personality Disorders (SIDP), the MCMI, and the PDQ

SIDP personality disorder	Hogg (MCMI)	Torg (MCMI)	Jack (MCMI)	Zimm (PDQ)
Paranoid	.03	.22	.20	.43
Schizoid	.47	.39	.31	.24
Schizotypal	.39	.37	.23	.34
Compulsive	.04	.18	.00	.47
Histrionic	.26	.20	.07	.42
Dependent	.21	.38	.31	.35
Antisocial	.23	—[a]	.14	.55
Narcissistic	.34	.18	.26	.26
Avoidant	.60	.42	.56	.30
Borderline	.33	.32	.63	.39
Passive-aggressive	.17	.14	.41	.37

Note. Hogg = Hogg, Jackson, Rudd, & Edwards (1990; N = 37); Torg = Torgersen & Alnaes (1990; N = 272); Jack = Jackson, Grazis, Rudd, & Edwards (1991); Zimm = Zimmerman & Coryell (1990; N = 697).
[a]Not reported in Table 3 of Torgersen & Alnaes (1990).

Treatment Outcome Studies With Axis I Patients. An important dimension of diagnostic validity is the longitudinal perspective, which is typically assessed in terms of either the course of the disorder or its response to treatment. More than other Axis II measures, the SIDP has paid close attention to treatment outcome. However, the studies have addressed the issue only indirectly by examining the effects of comorbidity (Axis I and II interactions) on the treatment of Axis I disorders. Ideally, studies of specific personality disorders and tailored treatment programs would allow the investigation of theory-driven treatment outcome. For example, we might speculate that persons with avoidant personality disorders might benefit more than other personality-disordered individuals from social skills training focused on their general deficits. In contrast, the existing studies, summarized below, simply evaluate their nonspecific effects on treatment.

The effects of SIDP-diagnosed personality disorders on the treatment of mood- and panic-disordered patients are summarized in Table 7.3. In general, the presence of personality disorders tends to complicate treatment and reduce its effectiveness. Studies of depressed patients (Mellman et al., 1992; Pfohl, Stangl, & Zimmerman, 1984, 1987; Reich & Troughton, 1988a; Zimmerman, Coryell, et al., 1986; Barrash, Pfohl, & Blum, 1993) have yielded mixed results. On a short-term basis, Pfohl et al. (1984) found that depressed patients with personality disorders were less likely to improve than their counterparts. Most studies have found that the mere presence of an Axis II disorder does not reduce the effectiveness of treatment for depression, although dimensional scores reflecting the total character pathology may reflect on poor treatment outcome (Pfohl, Coryell, Zimmerman, & Stangl, 1987). Results also suggest (a) that depressed patients with certain personality disorders (i.e., "anxious" cluster) may respond better to treatment (Reich & Troughton, 1988a), (b) that older Cluster B (primarily borderline) patients may have more episodes of depression and suicide attempts (both serious and manipulative), and (c) that ECT may be more effective than antidepressant medication for those with personality disorders (Pfohl et al., 1987).

Four studies with panic-disordered patients have established few differences between those with and without personality disorders. Although personality-disordered panic patients are more likely to drop out of placebo treatment (Reich, 1990), these results are difficult to interpret.[8] Interestingly, Reich (1988a) found that patients with personality disorders from the "dramatic" cluster tended to have more situational panic attacks than others. Mellman et al. (1992) found essentially no differences between panic patients with and without personality disorders.

---

[8]This finding should not be taken as evidence that personality-disordered patients are less treatment-compliant than others for at least two reasons: (a) the samples are very small (i.e., only seven drop-outs across both groups), and (b) panic patients in the placebo condition were not likely to be blind to condition (i. e., in the absence of medication effects, they were likely to be aware that they were in a control or "non-treatment" group).

Table 7.3
Treatment Outcome Studies with the Structured Interview for DSM-III Personality Disorders (SIDP)

Pfohl, Stangl, & Zimmerman (1984)

Design. Follow-up of 78 inpatients with major depression was conducted at time of discharge (approximately 4 weeks). Outcome measures included the HDRS and the GAS.

Results. Although hospital stay was nearly identical, depressed patients with personality disorders evidenced less improvement on the Hamilton and the GAS than those without. Interestingly, the personality-disordered patients were more depressed prior to the beginning of the study and were more likely to be suppressors on the dexamethasone suppression test (DST).

Zimmerman, Coryell, Pfohl, Corenthal, & Stangl (1986)

Design. Six-month follow-up was conducted on 25 inpatients treated for major depression with ECT. Outcome measures included the HDRS and the GAS.

Results. Nonsignificant trend toward a poorer outcome was determined for personality-disordered subjects.

Pfohl, Coryell, Zimmerman, & Stangl (1987)

Design. Six-month follow-up was conducted on 65 inpatients with major depression with outcome measured on multiple indices, including the HDRS and absence of symptoms.

Results. The presence of a personality disorder by itself did not appear to affect outcome. However, either the diagnosis of mixed personality disorder or the total number on personality disorder criteria (> 19) decreased the likelihood of a positive outcome. In general, patients with personality disorders evidenced poorer response to antidepressant medication (16% vs. 50%) but similar response to ECT (see Pfohl et al., 1984).

Reich (1988a)

Design. Eight-week follow-up was conducted on 52 panic patients receiving anxiolytic treatment. Outcome measures included number of panic attacks and Hamilton ratings on depression and anxiety.

Results. Relatively few differences were found for SIDP personality disorder, except that Cluster B patients had more situational panic attacks than others.

Reich & Troughton (1988a)

Design. Recovered panic-disordered (*n* = 57) and depressed (*n* = 19) patients were compared to controls without Axis I disorders (*n* = 40).

Results. Recovered patients evidenced more personality disorders (particularly in Cluster C) than did controls.

Table 7.3   (continued)
Treatment Outcome Studies with the Structured Interview for DSM-III Personality Disorders (SIDP)

Pfohl, Barrash, True, & Alexander (1989)
Design. One-year follow-up was conducted on 42 hypertensive patients' compliance with medication.
Results. No significant differences on the basis of personality disorders.

Reich (1990)
Design. Panic patients (N = 28) in a placebo condition who dropped out of "treatment" were compared to those who completed at least 3 weeks.
Results. A greater proportion of patients with personality disorders dropped out as compared to those without (41.7% vs. 12.5%).

Baer et al. (1992)
Design. A sample of 55 patients with obsessive-compulsive disorder were followed in a 10-week double-blind, placebo-controlled study of clomipramine, with comparisons of treatment outcome for 33 subjects with and 22 subjects without personality disorders. The primary baseline and outcome measure was the Yale-Brown Obsessive-Compulsive Scale (YBOC; Goodman et al., 1989).
Results. No differences were found between the presence of a single personality disorder and no personality disorder. However, the presence of multiple Axis II disorders was related to more impairment on baseline and less improvement on follow-up.

Mellman et al. (1992)
Design. Variable follow-up period (9 – 101 weeks) was based on duration of hospitalization of 46 patients (panic- and mood-disordered).
Results. No differences in outcome as measured by episodes or duration. Mood-disordered patients with personality disorders had a significantly earlier onset that those without (M ages = 15.8 vs. 28.3 years).

Barrash, Pfohl, & Blum (1993)
Design. A sample of 69 depressed inpatients from the Zimmerman, Coryell, et al. (1986) were reassessed at a 4-year follow-up interval.
Results. Eighteen patients with Cluster B personality disorders (mostly borderline combined with other disorders) were compared to 16 patients without Cluster B personality disorders. Only for older patients did the unstable features of Cluster B appear to affect depressive episodes and suicidal behavior.

Baer et al. (1992) examined the differences in treatment outcome for 55 obsessive-compulsive (OCD) patients. They found that while a single personality disorder did not appear to affect treatment outcome, the presence of more than one personality disorder affected both baseline measure (i.e., more impairment) and treatment outcome (i.e., less improvement). Baer et al. speculated that severe OCD may be expressed as Axis II symptomatology. If this were true for other Axis I disorders, then the comorbidity of Axis I and multiple Axis II disorders might reflect generalized distress rather than multiaxial diagnoses. This perspective would run contrary to the more popular view that personality disorders are an independent and possibly negative factor in treatment studies.

Pfohl, Barrash, True, and Alexander (1989) examined whether personality disorders would affect treatment compliance in a group of 173 hypertensive patients. They found no differences on the basis of personality disorders regarding which patients followed the treatment regimen. No other studies have addressed SIDP diagnoses in relationship to treatment compliance and/or outcome for Axis III disorders (i.e., medical conditions).

An important oversight of these treatment outcome studies is their lack of SIDP follow-up. Given the complex interactions of Axis I and II disorders, treatment intended to address mood and panic disorders may have a positive effect on personality disorders. Although investigators have typically assumed the stability of "traits," studies have not necessarily supported this assertion (e.g., even APD has proven relatively unstable; see Rogers, Duncan, Lynett, & Sewell, in press). Furthermore, there is evidence that current Axis I episodes may result in an over-endorsement of personality traits/symptoms (e.g., see Hirschfeld et al., 1988). If treatment of Axis I disorders has a beneficial effect of Axis II symptomatology, then clinicians may need to reevaluate their generally negative attitudes towards personality-disordered Axis I patients.

A reanalysis of previously reported data by Reich and Troughton (1988b) further illustrates the interactions between Axis I and II disorders. Dysphoric mood, not depression, was the strongest predictor of all three personality disorder clusters. Diagnosis of alcohol abuse and panic disorder were slight predictors of Clusters B and C, respectively. These findings raise interesting possibilities. For instance, does subclinical depression form a substrate of personality disorders, or is this dysphoria simply an effect of long-standing personality disorders? Irrespective of etiology, would treatment of the subclinical depression improve patients' Axis II disorders?

In summary, these studies suggest personality disorders may affect the onset of Axis I disorders (see Mellman et al., 1992) and have important implications for medication and other forms of treatment. In addition, certain clusters appear to be related to treatment outcome, although the relatively small numbers argue against any firm conclusions. Of particular interest are biological differences (e.g., responses to DST; see Pfhol et al., 1984) in personality-disordered depressed patients. Although not well defined, studies offer preliminary evidence that personality disorders, as measured by SIDP, may have a differential course and treatment response.

Clinical Applications

The emergence of *DSM-IV* has relatively little impact on the clinical usefulness of the SIDP and the SIDP-R. Of the three major changes for *DSM-IV* personality disorders, two involve the simplification of criteria (i.e., APD) and elimination of the disorder (i.e., passive-aggressive). The only addition is a single inclusion criterion to borderline personality disorder. Psychologists will need to assess transient paranoid and dissociative symptoms in marginal cases for borderlines.

The SIDP is clearly a worthy measure for the assessment of personality disorders. It is organized topically to address important facets of patients' day-to-day functioning as it relates to Axis II disorders. I would recommend its use in clinical settings, particularly with patients with concomitant Axis I disorders. In subsequent paragraphs, I will outline response-style issues with the SIDP and its major advantages and disadvantages for clinical use (see Table 7.4).

Table 7.4
Advantages and Disadvantages of the Structured Interview for DSM-III Personality Disorders (SIDP)

Advantages

1. Good interrater reliability

   Particularly for dimensional scores, the SIDP has demonstrated excellent agreement. For diagnosis, the coefficients of agreement tend to be in the moderate range, although these estimates are negatively affected by small sample sizes and poor representation of specific personality disorders.

2. Clear boundaries for personality disorders

   The SIDP distinguishes itself from other Axis II measures in the discreteness of specific personality disorders, with as many as 50% of subjects qualifying for a single or "pure" Axis II disorder.

3. Relationship to treatment

   The SIDP has investigated the role of Axis II disorders in the treatment of Axis I patients. Studies offer preliminary data on how treatment might be tailored to interventions for comorbidity.

Disadvantages

1. Little evidence of test-retest reliability

   Although small samples of patients were evaluated in a test-retest design (see Table 7.1), their amalgamation with interrater-reliability subjects prevents any accurate estimates.

2. Modest evidence of convergent validity

   In general, studies of the SIDP in relationship to the PDQ and MCMI-II have yielded disappointing results. As described in the accompanying text, paper-and-pencil measures are often limited in accurately portraying diagnosis. What is needed, however, is a comparison of the SIDP to other Axis II diagnostic interviews, including the PDE and SCID-II.

3. Lack of cultural and cross-cultural studies

   Research on the SIDP, unlike the PDE, has not focused on minority and cultural issues.

Zimmerman and Coryell (1990), in an attempt to explain the disparities between the SIDP and the PDQ, examined the relationship of these discrepancies to the Lie and Social Desirability subscales of the PDQ. Despite the limitations of these indices,[9] discrepancies appear to be slightly correlated ($r \geq$ .20) with deviant response style for 4 of the 11 scales. Although not clinically useful by themselves, the results suggest that clinicians must attempt to assess response styles and their effect on reported personality symptoms.

Three options for addressing response style on the SIDP include: (a) requiring examples before rating symptoms, (b) using informant interviews, and (c) administering a self-report measure with validity indices. Psychologists should be aware that there are limitations to each option. The primary limitation of the first option is that patients denying or minimizing symptoms will not be detected by this approach. Limitations of the second option are that the patient selects the informant, and that the informant often does not have any independent source of information. The limitation of the third option is that patients' response styles often change, depending on whether the measure is paper-and-pencil or interview-based. Despite these limitations, the use of examples and collateral interviews is likely to improve the quality of clinical data. For example, patients who realize that an informant will also be utilized may be more careful and accurate in their responses. Since the PDQ-R tends to yield a substantially higher endorsement of symptomatology, it may serve as a useful screen to ensure that all potential personality disorders are fully investigated.

The major advantages of the SIDP are summarized in Table 7.4. The real hallmark of the SIDP is its clear diagnostic boundaries that allow both clinicians and researchers to investigate single ("pure"), multiple, and mixed personality disorders in a systematic and reliable manner. Whether SIDP diagnoses represent "true" disorders is an entirely different matter. With the absence of a gold standard, however, the SIDP provides an unparalleled opportunity to evaluate pure Axis II diagnoses.

A second major advantage of the SIDP is the concerted efforts to understand the role of personality disorders in the treatment of Axis I disorders. While research is needed on Axis II disorders alone, the comorbidity of Axis I and II disorders deserves our serious attention. The SIDP, more than any other Axis II measure, offers us this opportunity.

The SIDP also has several notable limitations in clinical practice (see Table 7.4). As noted previously, little work has been accomplished on test-retest reliability. This oversight, easily remedied, curtails the current usefulness of the SIDP for treatment outcome on Axis II disorder.

A second and serious limitation is the dearth of research addressing minority and cultural issues. One exception is research by Borgherini, Bernasconi, and Magni (1992) on an Italian version of the SIDP. At present, the SIDP is not recommended with minority patients.

---

[9]Neither the original or more recent research (e.g. Hyler, Skodol, Kellman, Oldham, & Rosnick, 1990; Hyler, Skodol, Oldham, Kellman, & Doidge, 1992) offers any description of the development and validation of these indices.

The SIDP lacks convergent validity data with other diagnostic measures. As noted in Chapter 1, diagnostic validation is typically a bootstrapping operation, with small but incremental improvements in validation. Whether comforting or not, it must also be noted that the PDE (see Chapter 8) faces similar problems in the absence of a gold standard.

In summary, I see the SIDP as a top contender with the PDE for the complicated task of assessing personality disorders. In this regard, the SIDP offers a reliable diagnosis with clear diagnostic boundaries and preliminary evidence to treatment efficacy in Axis I patients.

8

Personality Disorder Examination (PDE)

Overview

Description

The Personality Disorder Examination (PDE; Loranger, Susman, Oldham, & Russakoff, 1987; Loranger, 1988) is an extensive semistructured interview for the assessment of personality disorders. The PDE is composed of 126 criteria that are organized into six major categories to facilitate the interview flow: work, self, interpersonal relations, affects, reality testing, and impulse control. Because of the overlapping nature of this categorization, the organizing principle for ordering individual symptoms was the promotion of "user friendliness" through the logical sequencing of clinical inquiries.

Each of the six major categories begins with open-ended inquiries for eliciting a general discussion of potential problems and issues. For example, the work category commences with such inquiries as, "How well do you function?" and "What annoyances or problems keep occurring?" Responses to these introductory questions provide points of comparison for the structured questions that follow.

Structured questions are organized by *DSM-III* criteria. Typically, several clinical inquiries form the basis for making a decision regarding each criterion. The clinical inquiries themselves are occasionally composed of multiple questions, with an additional probe presented for an affirmative response. The responses to the clinical inquiries are rated on a 3-point scale: 0 when the behavior is absent or not clinically significant, 1 when the behavior is present but of uncertain clinical significance, and 2 when the behavior is present and clinically significant. For purposes of clarity, clinicians must distinguish whether the onset was in early adulthood (< 25 years of age). Loranger (1988) provided detailed scoring instructions for specific questions. Responses to these clinical inquiries are then integrated into a single rating of the *DSM-III* criterion by one of two methods: (a) numerical (i.e., the individual clinical inquiries are summed and compared to a predetermined cutting score) and (b) clinical judgment (i.e., the mental health professional provides his/her own weighting of the responses subsumed under each criterion).

Loranger et al. (1987) operationalized *DSM-III* requirements that personality disorder features represent "current" and "long-term" functioning. After considerable experimentation, Loranger et al. determined that defining "current" as a brief period of time (e.g., 3 months) yielded unstable results. Instead, they opted to define "current" as the last 12 months. In addition, they designated "long-term" as characteristic behavior during the last 5 years.

The PDE is designed for both categorical and dimensional scoring. The categorical scoring corresponds to the *DSM-III* inclusion criteria. When sufficient inclusion criteria are met in the absence of exclusion criteria, then the specific disorder is diagnosed. Dimensional scoring is composed of two elements: (a) the summing of clinical inquiries for each the 11 personality disorders, and (b) the transformation of these raw scores into standard scores ($M = 50$, $SD = 10$). Standard scores allow direct comparisons of personality dimensions across both scales and samples.

Rationale and Development

The introduction of the *DSM-III* had a profound effect on psychiatric diagnosis in general and personality disorders in particular. Due to the multiaxial structure of the *DSM-III* and greater specification of Axis II disorders, more attention is now paid to personality disorders. For example, Loranger (1990), in a study of 10,914 psychiatric inpatients, found a remarkable increase with the advent of *DSM-III* in the diagnosis of personality disorders, from 19.1% (*DSM-II*) to 49.2% (*DSM-III*). With this increased attention came growing concerns regarding the diagnostic reliability and validity of Axis II disorders. These validational concerns have spawned more rigorous diagnostic measures, including structured interviews (Skodol, Rosnick, Kellman, Oldman, & Hyler, 1991).

Loranger et al. (1987) developed the PDE to address several methodological problems with Axis II diagnoses. First and foremost, Loranger and his colleagues recognized the limitations in diagnostic reliability for personality disorders, with most kappa coefficients not meeting the .70 benchmark of good agreement. Second, they believed that personality disorders represented a continuum of maladaptive traits that would be best measured by a dimensional system. Third, they expressed concern over information variance and the lack of assessment techniques for standardizing the assessment process.

Loranger and his colleagues first attempted to modify existing measures in order to address these methodological issues (Loranger, Oldham, Russakoff, & Susman, 1984). Not satisfied with the results, this research team created the PDE to "systematically survey the phenomenology and life experiences relevant to the diagnosis of the personality disorders in *DSM-III*" (Loranger et al., 1989, p. 3). As observed by Green (1989), the actual development and refinement of the PDE is not adequately described. According to Loranger et al. (1987), they wrote for the PDE as many items as "deemed necessary" to establish reliability and validity. Again, test materials do not comment on what criteria were imposed and which procedures were followed for test item creation and revision.

The original form of the PDE was pilot-tested by pairs of clinicians on 25 psychiatric patients. Although specific data are not reported, the primary goal of pilot testing was to improve the content, phrasing, and sequencing of clinical inquiries. Over a 5-year period from 1983 to 1988, two preliminary drafts and a final version were created (Loranger, Hirschfeld, Sartorius, & Regier, 1991). The second draft of the PDE, which was completed and made available in May 1985, consisted of 249 questions and 79 clinician ratings of verbal and nonverbal behavior (Loranger, Susman, Oldham, & Russakoff, 1985). The bulk of the published research employs the 1985 version. Modifications since the 1985 version are essentially minor in nature and incorporate changes found in *DSM-III-R*.

A new revision of the PDE is currently underway that should incorporate changes found in *DSM-IV* (A. W. Loranger, personal communication, March 22, 1994). As with other *DSM-IV* revisions, this version of the PDE will require substantial time for rigorous testing of its validation. However, only a few diagnoses are substantially affected by *DSM-IV*.

Validation of the PDE

Diagnostic Reliability

Reliability estimates with the PDE must take into account its dual scoring system with intraclass coefficients (ICC) for dimensional scores and kappa coefficients for categorical diagnoses. Table 8.1 provides a distillation of the major reliability studies.

Loranger and his colleagues have conducted three substantial reliability studies of the PDE; a fourth study was underway at the time this book was being written. Loranger et al. (1987) conducted the first interrater reliability study with 60 nonpsychotic inpatients who suffered primarily from mood disorders (53.3%), substance abuse (38.3%), eating disorders (16.7%), and anxiety disorders (13.3%).[1] The ICCs for the dimensional scales were uniformly high, with a median of .97 and a range of .84 to .99. Diagnostic agreement was computed for five personality disorders that had sufficient representation (≥ 5 cases) with a median kappa of .80. As noted in Chapter 1, kappas take into account low base rates; the actual percentage of diagnostic agreement across 11 personality disorders was very high, ranging from 92% to 100%.

Loranger (1988) expanded this sample to include outpatients for a total sample of 129. He found correlations that ranged from .77 to .97 for dimensional scores (median r = .96). Moreover, the agreement of *DSM-III* personality disorders was generally satisfactory (median κ = .78, range = .54 – .93). Test-retest reliabilities were apparently poor, but were unreported in the test manual.

Loranger et al. (1991) tested 84 patients at intake and discharge to assess the reliability and stability of Axis II diagnoses. Patients were excluded from the study if they had a history of psychotic, bipolar, or organic disorders. At both time periods, the PDE evidenced very high reliability for dimensional scores (median ICCs = .93 and .94) and excellent agreement on diagnosis (median κs = .87 and .88). Test-retest reliability was estimated through comparisons of intake to discharge. Kappas for five diagnoses, which were adequately represented,

---

[1]Inexplicably, this "nonpsychotic" sample included one patient with schizophrenia and two with schizoaffective disorders.

were moderate (median = .57, range = .26 – .57). With the exception of schizoid and antisocial personality disorders, patients experienced a significant reduction in Axis II symptoms by the time of discharge. Obviously, the intervening treatment complicates the interpretation of this finding.[2]

Table 8.1
Reliability Studies of the Personality Disorder Examination (PDE)

Study	Agreement
Loranger, Susman, Oldham, & Russakoff (1987) Interrater reliability study with 60 nonpsychotic inpatients used four clinicians combined in different pairs.	Dimensional scores, ICC = .97. Diagnosis, κ = .80
Loranger (1988) Interrater reliability study was conducted on 129 nonpsychotic inpatients and outpatients; test-retest reliability estimates were not reported.	Interrater dimensional scores, ICC = .96. Interrater diagnosis, κ = .78. Test-retest diagnosis, κ = .49
Standhage & Ladha (1988) Interrater reliability study used 20 inpatients (most with concurrent substance abuse disorders) who were jointly evaluated by two psychiatrists.	Dimensional scores, ICC = .92. Diagnosis, κ = .63
Edell, Joy, & Yehuda (1990) Interrater reliability study used 21 inpatients with psychotic and neurological patients excluded. Evaluation was by two raters.	Interrater on dimensional scores, κ > .89[a]
Schmidt & Telch (1990) Interrater reliability study was performed on 15 bulimic women.	Interrater on individual symptoms, κ = .93
Pilkonis, Heape, Ruddy, & Serrao (1991) Interrater reliability study was carried out on 40 depressed patients; three estimates of interrater reliability were calculated: intake evaluations (n = 29), 6-month follow-up evaluation (n = 30), and intake evaluations with the same patients using an informant (n = 28). Test-retest reliability (n = 31) is reported only for the presence/absence of any personality disorder and not for specific disorders.	Interrater intake diagnosis, κ = .79. Interrater follow up diagnosis, κ = .84. Interrater informant diagnosis, κ = .76. Test-retest diagnosis, κ = .52

---

[2]The notable exception was passive-aggressive personality disorder, which was deleted as a diagnosis in *DSM-IV*. Without passive-aggressive personality disorder, patients reported twice as many disorders as did informants.

Table 8.1   (continued)
Reliability Studies of the Personality Disorder Examination (PDE)

Study	Agreement
Loranger, Lenzenweger, et al. (1991) This reliability study was carried out on 84 patients without histories of psychotic, bipolar, or organic disorders. Various pairs of seven clinicians were employed for interrater reliability at intake and follow-up. Test-retest reliability varied in intervals from 1 week to 6 months.	Interrater dimensional scores at intake, ICC = .93; interrater dimensional scores at follow up, ICC = .94. Interrater diagnosis at intake, κ = .87; interrater diagnosis at follow up, κ = .88. Test-retest, diagnosis, κ = .57
Loranger (1992) This is the preliminary report on the IPDE administered to 243 patients using different translations of the PDE in 11 countries. The study reevaluated patients at a 6-month interval with the use of the same interviewer.	Temporal stability of diagnosis, κ = .56
Loranger et al. (in press) Combined interrater (*n* = 141) and temporal stability (i.e., same interviewer on both occasions; *n* = 243) design was based on 12 international research sites and 58 clinicians; retest occurred at a 6-month interval.	Individual symptoms, interrater, ICC > .80[b]; individual symptoms, temporal stability, ICC = .59[c]. Dimensional scores, interrater, ICC = .89; dimensional scores, temporal stability, ICC = .77. Diagnosis, interrater, κ = .73; diagnosis, temporal stability, κ = .62

Note. κ = unweighted kappas; ICC = intraclass coefficients. Except where otherwise noted, median statistics are reported.
[a]Not all reliabilities are presented; however, 10 of the 12 kappas are greater than .89. [b]Data are reported for 157 IPDE items. [c]Data on temporal stability include probable and definite diagnoses.

Several investigators beyond Loranger's team have examined PDE reliability. Standage and Ladha (1988) reported excellent ICCs (median = .92) for PDE dimensional scores on 20 inpatients, 17 of whom also carried substance abuse diagnosis. The only exception was schizoid personality disorder (ICC = .52), which may have been constrained by the limited range of scores. Five personality disorders had sufficient representation ($\geq$ 5); the median kappa coefficient of .63 suggested a moderate level of agreement. Similarly, Edell, Joy, and Yehuda (1990) conducted an interrater reliability study of the PDE with 21 psychiatric inpatients. Although complete data are not available, their results mirrored those of Standage and Ladha, with very high reliabilities ($\geq$ .89) for all personality disorders except schizoid (κ = .60).

Pilkonis, Heape, Ruddy, and Serrao (1991) administered the PDE to 40 patients with major depression in an interrater reliability design. Like Loranger,

Lenzenweger, et al., they administered the PDE on two occasions: intake and follow-up at a 6-month interval. Pilkonis et al. found good reliability estimates on both occasions (κs = .79 and .84). Moreover, they were able to establish the PDE's reliability on this same sample with the use of significant others as informants. Even with the use of informants, the reliability remained good (κ = .76). Test-retest reliability was generally unimpressive; the kappa for the presence of any personality disorder was only .52. Pilkonis et al. did not report the kappas for individual disorders.

Several additional studies have addressed the PDE's reliability with relatively small samples. Schmidt and Telch (1990) examined the interrater reliability of the PDE with 15 bulimic women. They calculated reliability coefficients for individual item responses, which yielded a kappa of .93. Angus and Marziali (1988) examined the diagnostic agreement of the PDE on six borderline patients and found a perfect concordance on borderline personality disorder and an overall kappa for personality disorders of .78. O'Boyle and Self (1990) reported a moderate level of agreement for the PDE's interrater reliability but had too few cases to draw a meaningful conclusion.

Mauri et al. (1992) cited earlier research on an Italian version of the PDE. They report achieving a reliability estimate of .80 for the presence/absence of any personality disorder, but do not furnish any further details. Research on the reliability of the international version, IPDE, is summarized in the section on generalizability below.

Riso, Klein, Anderson, Ouimette, and Lizardi (1994) examined patient-informant consistency and found virtually no agreement for diagnosis[3] (median κ = –.01) and modest correlations for dimensional scores (median ICC = .36). While this was not a formal test of reliability, the results caution against overreliance on either source without corroboration. In particular, the results suggest that informants may underreport symptoms of personality disorder.

Criterion–Related Validity

Criterion-related validity studies have compared the PDE to Axis II diagnoses generated either by clinicians or by other structured interviews, such as the Structured Clinical Interview for *DSM-III-R* Personality Disorders (SCID-II; Spitzer, Williams, & Gibbon, 1987b) and the Personality Assessment Form (PAF; Pilkonis & Frank, 1988; Shea, Glass, Pilkonis, Watkins, & Docherty, 1987). Other studies have examined the relationship of the PDE to self-report measures (e.g., the Personality Disorder Questionnaire–Revised [PDQ-R; Hyler & Rieder, 1987]) and other indices of psychopathology.

Pilkonis et al. (1991) conducted the most comprehensive validity study of the PDE. As previously described, 40 depressed patients were evaluated at intake and follow-up. In addition to the standard administration of the PDE, the investigators used informants' PDE data, the PAF, the SCL-90 (Derogatis, 1977), the Beck Depression Scale (Beck et al., 1961), and the Hamilton Depression Rating

---

[3]Research on cross-informant consistency has generally been disappointing in both children and adults.

Scale (Hamilton, 1960). They followed Spitzer's LEAD model (Longitudinal Expert Evaluation using All Data; Spitzer, 1983) for establishing personality disorders with the readministration of most measures at a 6-month interval.

Pilkonis et al. (1991) found complete correspondence between the clinical diagnosis, PDE, and PAF in 50.0% of the cases. The PDE appeared slightly more conservative than either of the other two measures in rendering diagnoses. Using the clinical diagnosis as the gold standard, the PDE had a sensitivity of 71% and a specificity of 58%. Interestingly, PDE diagnoses at intake appeared to predict treatment outcome as measured by the Global Assessment Scale of the SADS; patients with PDE personality disorders and depression evidenced less recovery than those with depression alone.

Hyler, Skodol, Kellman, Oldham, and Rosnick (1990) administered the SCID-II, PDQ-R, and PDE to 87 psychiatric inpatients, many of whom warranted Axis I diagnoses of mood, anxiety, substance abuse, and eating disorders. A low to moderate level of agreement was found between the SCID-II and the PDE (median κ = .46). Interestingly, Cluster A (paranoid, schizoid, and schizotypal disorders; median κ = .27) performed more poorly than Clusters B and C (median κs = .54 and .52, respectively). Moreover, the PDE evidenced only a modest level of agreement with the self-administered PDQ-R (median κ = .38). In a replication study, Hyler, Skodol, Oldham, Kellman, and Doidge (1992) administered the same three measures to 59 applicants for psychoanalysis and found only modest agreement between the PDE and the SCID (median κ = .36), which is likely an artifact of the low prevalence of Axis II disorders in this sample.

Hunt and Andrews (1992) administered the PDE and the PDQ-R to 40 outpatients with anxiety disorders. As expected of a screening measure, the PDQ-R elicited a much higher level of symptom endorsement than the PDE. Overall, correlations between the measures for the 40 anxiety patients were very modest (median ICC = .25, range = .05 – .61).

Soldz, Budman, Demby, and Merry (1993) examined 97 outpatients referred for the treatment of personality disorders. They compared the results of the PDE with the MCMI-II (Millon, 1987) with disappointing results. For the six diagnoses with adequate representation ($\geq$ 5 cases), the kappas ranged from –.06 to .41, with a median of .24. Of interest, the MCMI-II tended to overdiagnose personality disorders (total of 191 Axis II disorders) compared to the PDE (total of 67 Axis II disorders). To put these findings in perspective, however, I should point out that both the SIDP and clinical interviews have also shown a relatively poor correspondence with the MCMI-II.

Studies by Angus and Marziali (1988) and O'Boyle and Self (1990), while addressing the convergent validity of the PDE, are severely limited by their sample sizes. Angus and Marziali (1988) compared the scores on the PDE, the PDQ, and the Diagnostic Interview for Borderlines (DIB; Gunderson, 1982; Gunderson, Kolb, & Austin, 1981) for 22 patients including 20 borderlines. The level of diagnostic agreement was generally poor on borderline personality disorder (PDE and DIB, κ = .08; PDE and PDQ, κ = .25). O'Boyle and Self (1990) compared the PDE and the SCID on 20 depressed inpatients. Although a high concordance rate (90.0%) was found, the degree of association for the presence/absence of any personality disorder was modest (κ = .38). The study was constrained by the limited sample and range of disorders (i.e., 36 diagnoses across 11 disorders).

Korenblum, Marton, Golombek, and Stein (1990) employed teacher and parent behavior rating scales (Arnold & Smeltzer, 1974; Conners, 1969) to 36 highly disturbed and 36 well-adjusted youth. Korenblum et al. followed these samples for an 8-year period and found that disturbed adolescents had much higher scores on most PDE scales. They did not provide data, however, on specific disturbances in childhood and their relationship to particular Axis II disorders.

Studies have examined the differences in PDE dimensional scores and diagnoses for clinical samples. Schmidt and Telch (1990) found, consistent with the literature, that bulimic patients exhibited more impairment and greater frequency of personality disorders on the PDE than did binge eaters or controls. Similar results were found by McCann, Rossiter, King, and Agras (1991) on subtypes of bulimia. Squires-Wheeler, Skodol, Bassett, and Erlenmeyer-Kimling (1990) reported that the offspring of schizophrenic parent(s) had substantially more schizotypal features on the PDE than did the children of parents with affective disorders or no mental disorders, although none of the individual symptoms differed between the schizophrenic and affective disorder probands. Hayward and King (1990) found a striking relationship between somatization and PDE personality disorders. More specifically, high scores on somatization for males were highly correlated with Cluster B disorders (median $r = .72$) but not with other clusters (median $r = .18$) or females with any cluster (median $r = .17$).

Research (e.g., Pfohl et al., 1984) has suggested that the presence of personality disorders may decrease treatment effectiveness. As evidence of construct validity, several studies have found that the presence and severity of PDE criteria were related to treatment outcome. For example, Gartner, Marcus, Halmi, and Loranger (1989), in a study of 35 patients with eating disorders, found that the presence of Axis II disorders was related to greater depression and anxiety at initial and repeat examinations. Similarly, Turner (1989) found that the PDE effectively measured treatment change in borderline patients.

Abrams, Alexopoulos, and Young (1987) examined PDE scores for 36 elderly persons, of whom 21 had recovered from depression and 16 were normal controls. In an ANCOVA, they controlled for any residual depression, as measured by the HDRS, and still found that recovered depressives had much higher PDE dimensional scores on 9 of 11 scales. They suggested that the existence of personality dysfunction may increase the vulnerability for late-onset depression. Of course, an alternate explanation is that personality disorders, as they were recently defined by *DSM-III-R* and assessed by the PDE, do not constitute discrete entities, but represent correlates or sequelae to major mental illness (also see Marin, Kocsis, Frances, & Klerman, 1993).

Loranger, Lenzenweger, et al. (1991) expressed concern that reported personality traits might reflect distorted perceptions resulting from an Axis I disorder such as anxiety and depression. To address this issue, they administered the PDE to 71 inpatients and 13 outpatients, the majority of whom had depressive, anxiety, or eating disorders. Following treatment, they found that most PDE dimensional scores had decreased. Because the reduction of personality-disorder symptoms did not differ significantly on several clinical measures, including the HDRS, the BDI, and the GAS, the investigators concluded that personality traits were independent of these disorders.[4]

I do not finding the reasoning of Loranger, Lenzenweger, et al. (1991) to be compelling. First and foremost, we cannot prove the null hypothesis; the fact that no significant differences were found on three of the four measures does not demonstrate that these differences did not occur. Second, if we hypothesize that most hospital admissions were for the treatment of pressing Axis I conditions, how do we explain the large main effect of treatment on personality disorder features with an average of 4.7 fewer Axis II symptoms? The concerns raised by the Loranger, Lenzenweger, et al. (1991) study extend beyond the PDE. They suggest, consistent with the generally poor test-retest reliability (see Pilkonis et al., 1991), that "stable" personality traits may fluctuate substantially. Indeed, the existing data might serve as an impetus for a radical rethinking of many personality disorders, since they do not appear to reflect deeply ingrained and inflexible characteristics.

Antecedent conditions that may be associated with PDE personality disorders have rarely been investigated. One exception is a small study by Raczek (1992) of adult survivors of child abuse (n = 16) compared to nonabused adults (n = 34), all 50 of whom were referred to a military mental health clinic. They found that members of the abused group qualified for more Cluster B disorders, particularly borderline and antisocial. This line of research is promising in the advancement of our understanding of precursors to specific personality disorders.

In summary, the PDE validity literature leaves many questions unanswered. As noted in Chapter 1, the use of Syndeham's model is complicated by Axis II disorders, since the outcome is generally predicted to be nonspecific and static. In general, studies suggest that a subsample of personality-disordered patients can be identified who appear to have prototypical characteristics. For example, Pilkonis et al. (1991) was able to identify 50% of their sample as clearly meeting personality disorder diagnoses, irrespective of the method. Perhaps the next step is to reexamine the cardinal features of these patients towards the refinement of our inclusion criteria. Hyler et al. (1990) offer the best data on the PDE's convergent validity. Even employing a liberal standard ($\kappa \geq .50$), Cluster A disorders lack convergent validation, while Clusters B and C are only marginal. Other small convergent validity studies (Angus & Marziali, 1988; O'Boyle & Self, 1990) provide only modest support. While other research documents the potentially negative effects of PDE dimensional scores on overall functioning and treatment outcome, these findings are nonspecific and cannot be related to specific personality disorders.

The validation of Axis II disorders is a bootstrapping operation in the absence of any gold standard. One heartening result of the Pilkonis et al. (1991) study was that the PDE appeared more conservative than either the PAF or clinical diagnosis in evaluating personality disorders. Given the diagnostic slippage apparent in Axis II disorders, this conservatism is welcomed.

---

[4]Differences were found, however, on the Clinical Anxiety Scale (CAS; Snaith, Baugh, Clayden, Husain, & Sipple, 1982) with treatment apparently reducing the number of avoidant symptoms.

Generalizability and International Version of the PDE

Under the aegis of the World Health Organization, an International Personality Disorder Examination (IPDE; Loranger, Hirschfeld, Sartorius, & Regier, 1991) was developed. The format was modified to include both *DSM-III-R* and ICD-10 criteria for personality disorders. Some questions were reformulated to address ICD-10 disorders; the scoring manual also incorporated ICD-10 inclusion criteria so that both diagnostic systems could be implemented. The expanded IPDE requires 3 to 4 hours to administer.

The English version of the IPDE has been translated into 10 languages: Dutch, French, German, Hindi, Italian, Japanese, Kannada, Norwegian, Swahili, and Tamil. In each case, the IPDE translation was followed by a back-translation by a psychiatrist or psychologist who was blind to the English version of the IPDE. Discrepancies in translations were reviewed by additional translators. The authors recognized that cultural issues may contaminate certain personality-disorder characteristics. However, standardized administrations are now suggested so that these cultural differences may be systematically assessed.

Loranger, Hirschfeld, et al. in 1991 reported that an international field trial was underway in 11 countries. In each country, samples of 50 were being compiled (i.e., 30 with personality disorders and 20 with other common mental disorders). Reliability was being assessed in several forms: interrater reliability (10 per site), intercenter reliability through the use of videotapes, and test-retest reliability at 6-month intervals. As summarized in Table 8.1, preliminary data from the IPDE study (Loranger, 1992) suggested moderate stability of diagnosis (median $\kappa = .56$).

Loranger et al. (in press) have conducted an impressive study of the IPDE's reliability. They compiled data from 14 participating centers with 38 clinicians and a total of 714 patients. Of these, 141 patients were involved in an interrater reliability study.[5] The interrater reliability was generally satisfactory for *DSM-III-R* diagnosis (κs = .51 – .87, median = .73), but were superior for dimensional scores (.79 – .94, median =.89) and individual symptoms (median > .80).

These investigators also examined the consistency of personality disorders over time on 242 patients. The use of 6-month interval (actual range was 2 – 12 months) makes this actually a test of temporal stability, not test-retest reliability.[6] Personality disorders (minimum of 5 years duration) should evidence only modest changes in symptoms across time. Loranger et al. (in press) found a marked range of kappas for the stability of *DSM-III-R* diagnoses (.28 – .72, median = .62). Several personality disorders evidenced only modest (< .50) stability: paranoid, histrionic, dependent, and passive-aggressive. As a measure of individual symptoms, the IPDE yielded a superior level of consistency, with a

---

[5]Videotapes were made to monitor scoring practices during the course of the study were conducted in English. The methodology does not make it clear how many of the reliability interviews were conducted in English and how many in other languages.

[6]When the statistics are corrected for attenuation, the ICCs increase slightly (.74 – .95, median = .83).

median ICC of approximately .59. Moreover, dimensional scores were generally excellent, with a range from .68 to .92 and a median of .77.[7]

Clinicians from the research sites, located in 11 different countries, were surveyed regarding the cultural acceptability of the IPDE. Surprisingly, only two items (monogamous relationships and harsh treatment of spouse/children) were viewed as culturally bound. Therefore, the preliminary evidence suggest that the IPDE may be applicable to diverse cultures.

The Loranger et al. (in press) study is important both to the IPDE and as a standard for personality disorders. The authors were able to establish cross-culturally excellent reliability estimates for symptoms and dimensions. Temporal stability was sustained over a 6-month period. The interrater reliabilities are based on a large clinically diverse sample of inpatients and outpatients. The results compare favorably to many Axis I studies. More variability was found in temporal stability after a 6-month interval.[8]

Clinical Applications

The emergence of *DSM-IV* has relatively little impact on the clinical usefulness of the PDE and the IPDE. Of the three major changes for *DSM-IV* personality disorders, two involve the simplification of criteria (i.e., APD) and elimination of one disorder (i.e., passive-aggressive). The only addition is a single inclusion criterion to borderline personality disorder. Psychologists will need to assess transient paranoid and dissociative symptoms in marginal cases for borderlines.

The PDE and its international version, IPDE, offer significant advantages to psychologists in the systematic assessment of personality disorders. The interview format is "user friendly," with clinical inquiries organized into six major categories. In addition, psychologists are permitted a range of clinical inquiries that begin with open-ended questions and proceed with structured questions and optional probes. Unlike other Axis II interviews such as the SCID-II, most of the *DSM-III-R* are evaluated through the use of multiple questions, which should facilitate data gathering and clinical judgment. From this perspective alone, mental health professionals may consider the PDE a valuable asset to their clinical assessment.

One hallmark of the PDE is its interrater reliability. Studies as reported in Table 8.1 suggest good to superb coefficients of agreement. One likely contribution to its excellent reliability is its detailed scoring manual, which provides specific criteria for each clinical rating. Moreover, studies of test-retest reliability suggest a moderate level of consistency over time. The most recent study of the IPDE indicated, however, excellent diagnostic stability for both symptoms and dimensions.

Predictions of treatment outcome in personality-disordered patients must be tempered by the fact that these patients frequently evidence fewer characterological symptoms when offered treatment of an even more general nature.

---

[7]Most of the interviewers reinterviewed the same patients on both occasions, which confounds the use of this study for test-retest reliability.

[8]Data are also available for ICD-10 diagnoses; they appear roughly comparable to *DSM-III-R*. For interrater reliability, the κs range from .43 to 1.00 (median = .71); for temporal stability, the κs range from .30 to .65 (median = .60).

Encouragingly, studies have generally found a gradual decrease in symptoms over time. Whether this decrease is the direct result of treatment is, of course, a matter deserving investigation. Alternative explanations would include (a) an habituation to the symptoms, (b) an overall decrease in general distress making marginal symptoms less important, and (c) natural changes in the course of the disorder. Irrespective of the explanation, the data would seem to question conventional wisdom that characterological symptoms gradually become more deeply ingrained with more pervasive impairment. Longitudinal studies of specific personality disorders with the PDE and similar measures are clearly needed.

The PDE and IPDE offer several advantages from a diagnostic perspective. The PDE provides for both dimensional scores and categorical diagnoses. Depending on the clinical question, dimensions of personality disorders may be more germane to selection of treatment methods and measuring treatment outcome than the relatively crude distinction between the presence and absence of an Axis II disorder. However, the option of producing a *DSM-IV* diagnosis is important for epidemiological research and administrative purposes. As noted by Loranger (1991), the provision of both forms of classification is an important feature. In addition, the IPDE provides a singular opportunity to directly compare the two major diagnostic systems: the *DSM-III-R* and the ICD-10.

The final advantage of the IPDE is its international focus. With translated versions, the possibility exists that personality disorders may be understood from both intracultural and transcultural perspectives. One unfortunate oversight, at least from an American viewpoint, is the lack of a Spanish version to the IPDE. The Loranger et al. (in press) study is likely to be followed by additional reports which will specify its effectiveness by countries/languages. For the reader's convenience, Table 8.2 summarizes the major advantages of the PDE and IPDE.

Most studies of the PDE have employed mostly inpatients, the bulk of whom have concomitant Axis I disorders. Clinically, of course, the complicated interactions between Axis I and Axis II disorders are a matter of considerable importance for treatment choice and subsequent outcome (Widiger & Hyler, 1987). Studies are also needed, beyond borderline and antisocial personality disorders, of specific Axis II disorders and well-articulated treatment methods (e.g., see Kocsis & Mann, 1985). Additionally, the employment of either target symptoms or dimensional scores may serve as useful outcome measures.

I would recommend use of the PDE in following inpatients and outpatients, given its excellent interrater reliability and satisfactory diagnostic stability. The most thorough approach would be the employment of a multimethod assessment, perhaps incorporating a self-report measure. Judging from research by Hyler et al. (1990, 1992), the PDQ-R might be a useful adjunct measure, since this questionnaire might help to identify missed diagnoses. Hyler and his colleagues found that the PDQ had a much broader scope than the PDE, generally identifying two to three times more patients with specific personality disorders. In cases where the PDQ suggests a possible personality disorder, a thorough follow-up PDE evaluation that included significant others would be warranted.

Table 8.2
*Advantages of the Personality Disorder Examination (PDE)
in the Assessment of Axis II Disorders*

1. Ease of use

   Clinical inquiries are conveniently organized into six major categories. A range of clinical inquiries is used, including open-ended questions, standard questions, and optional probes.

2. High interrater reliability

   Studies have consistently shown good to superb interrater reliability for both dimensional scores and categorical diagnoses (see Table 7.1).

3. Dimensional and categorical scores

   The PDE distinguishes itself by making available both dimensional scales and DSM-III-R diagnoses.

4. International version with translations

   The IPDE offers a direct opportunity for assessment and research to assess patients from different nationalities. In the future, international emphasis is likely to provide crucial data on cultural influences on personality disorders.

5. Direct comparisons of DSM-III-R and ICD-10 personality disorders

   The IPDE offers an unparalleled opportunity to compare the two major diagnostic systems.

9

Other Structured Interviews for Axis II Disorders

This composite chapter provides a detailed description of three promising Axis II interviews: the Structured Clinical Interview for *DSM-III-R* Personality Disorders (SCID-II), the Personality Disorder Interview–IV (PDI-IV), and the Standardized Assessment of Personality (SAP). Despite a substantial body of often-encouraging research, all three measures have important limitations that circumscribe their clinical usefulness. In addition, two other less-researched structured interviews are briefly summarized: the Diagnostic Interview of Personality Disorders (DIPD) and the Personality Assessment Schedule (PAS).

The advent of *DSM-IV* does not really affect the clinical usefulness of these Axis II measures for two distinct reasons. First, the SCID-II, PDI-IV, and SAP require more complete validation, whether the standard be *DSM-III-R* or *DSM-IV*. Second, as noted in previous chapters on the SIDP and the PDE, *DSM-IV* changes add only one additional Axis II inclusion criterion (borderline personality disorder); thus, nearly all personality disorders can continue to be diagnosed.

Structured Clinical Interview for *DSM-III-R* Personality Disorders (SCID-II)

Description and Rationale

Spitzer, Williams, and Gibbon (1987c) constructed, as a complementary measure to the SCID, an Axis II interview named the SCID-II. The combined use of the SCID and SCID-II was designed to provide a comprehensive assessment of both Axis I and II disorders. A slightly revised version of the SCID is now commercially available (Spitzer, Williams, Gibbon, & First, 1990c).

Like the SCID, the SCID-II is organized by diagnosis and has an identical 3-point rating system: 1 for "absent or false," 2 for "subthreshold," and 3 for "threshold or true." For each of the diagnostic criteria, the patient is typically asked one or two standard questions. If an affirmative response is given, the patient is then asked to provide examples. As is the case with many structured interviews, all items are unidirectional, so that all endorsements are indicative of psychological impairment. The advantage of this approach is the ease of evaluating criteria which are grouped by diagnosis and scored in the same direction. The inherent limitation is the transparency of the interview format, making it vulnerable to manipulation and distortion.

Spitzer, Williams, and Gibbon (1987a) also developed a self-report screen. Originally named the SCID Personality Questionnaire, it was later revised and renamed the SCID-II Questionnaire (SCID-II-Q; Spitzer, Williams, Gibbon, & First, 1990a). The SCID-II-Q is composed of one item per diagnostic criterion and parallels the SCID-II in its sequencing of criteria. The sole exception is the diagnosis of APD; in this case, the SCID-II-Q provides questions only with respect to conduct symptoms, based on the apparent assumption that patients are more likely to acknowledge childhood than adult antisocial behavior.[1] The answers for the SCID-II-Q are dichotomous ("no" or "yes") and are completed by the patient as he or she has "usually felt or behaved over the past several years."

Reliability and Validity Studies

Few studies have systematically investigated SCID-II reliability. Renneberg, Chambless, Dowdall, Fauerbach, and Gracely (1992) cited unpublished Dutch data on the SCID-II for 32 patients diagnosed with anxiety disorders that reported highly variable estimates of interrater reliability (κs = .52 – 1.00). Brooks, Baltazar, McDowell, Munjack, and Bruns (1991) conducted an interrater reliability study with three clinicians, utilizing videotaped interviews and a 3-month pilot/training program. They evaluated 30 patients referred for a panic disorder study and found three disorders (paranoid, avoidant, and obsessive-compulsive) which had sufficient representation (> 5). These disorders evidenced only a moderate level of agreement with a generalized kappa with coefficients of .77 for paranoid, .56 for avoidant, and .66 for obsessive-compulsive disorder.[2] Renneberg et al. (1992) examined the interrater reliability for 32 patients with panic disorders who were referred for outpatient treatment. For the four personality disorders with even minimal representation (≥ 3), the kappa coefficients ranged from .61 to .83, with a median of .67. Most recently, Vaglum, Friis, Karterud, Mehlum, and Vaglum (1993) employed the SCID-II in an interrater reliability study of 29 audiotaped interviews, yielding a moderate kappa of .63; however, this reliability estimate was simply for the presence or absence of any severe personality disorder.

Reliability studies have tended to emphasize only diagnostic agreement. As an exception, O'Boyle and Self (1990), in a pilot study of eight depressed patients, suggested high agreement on dimensional scores. Likewise, Clarkin, Hull, and Hurt (1993) found good agreement in a very circumscribed study of borderline symptoms. A fruitful avenue for research would be large-scale studies of dimensional scores.

The reliability of the SCID has not yet been sufficiently established for the majority of diagnoses. In the cases where interrater reliability estimates are available, the coefficients are often lower than what has been established for the SIDP and the PDE. Moreover, test-retest reliability and the temporal stability of its personality disorders have yet to be investigated for the SCID-II.

---

[1]However, the *DSM-III-R* child conduct symptoms are much more violent than their adult counterparts.

[2]The generalized kappa is a very stringent estimate of reliability based on polychotomous data and differentiating among absent, subthreshold, and threshold ratings. When ICCs were computed on the presence or absence of personality disorders, the coefficients were substantially higher (i.e., > .75).

Torgersen, Skre, Onstad, Edvardsen, and Kringlen (1993) conducted an elaborate first-order factor analysis with an early draft of the SCID-II on 445 subjects from an ongoing twin-family study of psychiatric patients. They factor-analyzed on SCID-II items, with the exception of APD conduct symptoms, and established 12 factors. Items on factors were summed to yield factor scores, which were examined for each personality disorder. The results were strongly supportive of the current SCID-II typology, with fully two-thirds of the symptoms loading on the predicted personality disorder. Moreover, the majority of the remaining symptoms loaded on factor scores which were conceptually meaningful. The Torgersen et al. study offers strong evidence for the construct validity of the SCID-II.

Three studies have directly examined the concurrent validity of SCID-II diagnoses with the PDE. As reported in Chapter 8, Hyler et al. (1990, 1992) found only moderate levels of agreement between the SCID-II and the PDE, with median kappas of .46 and .36. These findings are consistent with those of O'Boyle and Self (1990), who found low agreement (κs = .18, .23, and .63) on three personality disorders with adequate representation.

Rennenberg et al. (1992) examined the convergent validity of the SCID-II with the MCMI-II. On a sample of 52 agoraphobic outpatients, they found relatively low correspondence between SCID-II diagnoses and MCMI-II elevations (i.e., > 74). For nine diagnosis, the range of kappas was from .14 to .51, with a median of .25. Unfortunately, the authors did not report dimensional scores, which may have been more useful in comparing the two measures.

Studies have also employed the SCID-II to establish normative data on personality disorders. For example, Maier, Lichertermann, Klingler, Heun, and Hallmayer (1992) combined a sample of normal controls with psychiatric inpatients and their first-degree relatives (N = 452). They found relatively consistent prevalence rates for personality disorders across gender and age. One exception was older ($\geq$ 40 years old) males who appeared to have a lower overall prevalence (6.7%) than their younger counterparts (13.5%). In contrast, females remained relatively stable for both older (9.2%) and younger (11.5%) groups. Finally, W. H. Berman, E. R. Berman, Heymsfield, Fauci, and Ackerman (1992) explored the incidence of personality disorders in a small sample of 56 obese outpatients. They found a high prevalence of both Axis I and Axis II disorders.

Clinical Applications

The SCID-II is a user-friendly structured interview for the assessment of personality disorders. Because of its parallel format with the SCID, the SCID-II can be employed selectively to examine specific personality disorders. Its organization and scoring facilitate its application to personality-disordered individuals. Indeed, psychologists need relatively little training to apply the SCID-II to clinical populations.

A major advantage of the SCID-II is the availability of the SCID-II-Q, which provides an item-by-item screening of Axis II criteria. Preliminary research by Nussbaum and Rogers (1992) has indicated that employing lower cutting scores for personality disorders (i.e., one less than criterion) enables psychologists to effectively screen for personality disorders while maintaining high sensitivity and moderate specificity rates.

A major disadvantage of the SCID-II is the lack of large-scale reliability studies. Available data do not adequately address reliability for the majority of personality disorders. Even those disorders which are addressed have only moderate reliability estimates. A very serious omission is the lack of test-retest reliability. We simply do not know whether SCID-II results will remain consistent from one day to another.

Other limitations of the SCID-II are related to the quality of information obtained. The SCID-II relies solely on the patient; in contrast, the SIDP requires and the PDE recommends collateral interviews. This limitation can, of course, be easily resolved by the use of informant interviews. In addition, the face validity of the items makes the SCID-II vulnerable to response styles. Again, the use of informant interviews would largely address this concern.

Psychologists must also consider the lack of validity data in deciding whether to use the SCID-II in clinical settings. Other measures, such as the SIDP and PDE, have demonstrated substantially more concurrent and convergent validity. Most encouraging, however, is the construct validity research by Torgersen et al. (1993) on the underlying dimensions of SCID-II personality disorders.

The question remains on whether the SCID-II has sufficient validity for clinical practice. In my opinion, the chief stumbling block is the lack of demonstrated reliability. When examined the two major reliability studies are examined (Brooks et al., 1991; Renneberg et al., 1992), obsessive-compulsive disorders appear to be the most reliable, although even this finding may be inflated since both samples were composed of anxiety-disordered patients. Recognizing this fundamental limitation, I believe that psychologists would be on safer ground employing the PDQ-R/SIDP or PDQ-R/PDE assessments of personality disorders. At present, the SCID-II may be effectively employed in clinical research for studying elements of a specific personality disorder (e.g., Gallager, Flye, Hurt, Stone, & Hull, 1992), particularly when SCID-II reliability is established by the investigators themselves.

In summary, the SCID-II, in conjunction with the SCID-II-Q, offers considerable promise as an effective structured interview of personality disorders. However, until further reliability and validity research is conducted, I would not recommend the SCID-II for clinical practice.

Personality Disorder Interview-IV (PDI-IV)

Description and Rationale

Widiger (1985) began the initial development of an Axis II interview which eventually evolved into the PDI-IV (Widiger, Mangine, Corbitt, Ellis, & Thomas, in press). In the original version, Widiger called the measure the Personality Interview Questions (PIQ). One feature of the PIQ, unique among Axis II measures, was its use of nonprofessional interviewers. Curiously, the author (see Widiger & Frances, 1987, p. 53) made the assumption that "the use of lay interviewers minimizes the effect of clinical biases and expectations." This assumption does not appear to be tenable, since the lay interviewers were trained by mental health professionals and, therefore, were likely to have been inculcated with these same biases.

The PIQ was distinguished from other Axis II interviews in that symptoms and traits were rated on a 10-point scale of increasing severity. As reported by Trull, Widiger, and Frances (1987), the degree of severity was organized according to the following format: 1 for "absent," 2–4 for "symptom is present but to a subclinical level," 5–9 for "increasing severity in the clinical range." Initial data on 67 audiotaped interviews of nonpsychotic inpatients suggested that the PIQ was reliable, with median kappa for diagnosis of .71 (Widiger, Frances, Warner, & Bluhm, 1986) and a median r for the number of symptoms per disorder of .80 (Widiger, Trull, Hurt, Clarkin, & Frances, 1987).

The PIQ-II (Widiger, 1987) was developed to incorporate changes made in *DSM-III-R*. These modifications did not significantly affect its interrater reliability. For example, Widiger, Freiman, and Bailey (1990) assessed the reliability of the PIQ-II using two highly trained interviewers[3] and a sample of 47 inpatients which excluded mental retardation and schizophrenic and organic disorders. Kappa coefficients for PIQ-II personality disorders ranged from .45 (schizotypal) to .92 (passive-aggressive), with a median of .73. In addition, the number of reported symptoms for each disorder was highly correlated across the two interviewers (rs = .75 – .96, median r = .88).

The final revision consisted of two closely related stages. In anticipation of *DSM-IV*, the PIQ-III (Widiger, Corbitt, Ellis, & Thomas, 1992) was refined to address changes in diagnostic criteria. Then the structure of the PIQ-III was further modified, resulting in the current measure, which has been renamed the Personality Disorder Interview–IV (PDI-IV; Widiger et al., 1995).

The PDI-IV, similar to other Axis II interviews, is scored on a 3-point scale, with 0 for "not present," 1 for "meets *DSM-IV* criteria," and 2 for "severe, exceeds *DSM-IV* criteria." The PDI-IV assesses each of the 94 diagnostic criteria for 10 established and 2 proposed personality disorders. The PDI-IV is organized into two formats: by theme and by disorder. For the thematic format, the 94 diagnostic criteria address nine themes: attitudes towards self, attitudes towards others, security or comfort with others, friendships and relationships, conflicts and disagreements, work and leisure, social norms, mood, and appearance and perception. For the disorder format, the criteria are organized by specific personality disorders. Validational studies appear to be based on the thematic format.

DSM-IV criteria are evaluated with 317 standard questions which are utilized to assess particular diagnostic criteria. With the exception of observational items, each criterion is assessed by at least two and generally three or four standard questions. In addition, a small number of branching questions are presented. The PDI-IV is a semistructured interview; the interviewer is encouraged to ask unstructured questions to clarify responses. Scoring issues and conventions are presented in separate chapters devoted to each disorder.

The PDI-IV emphasizes extensive questioning of the patient; as a result, administration time is approximately 2 hours. Unlike the SIDP and the PDE, the PDI-IV places little emphasis on collateral data and offers no instruction on integrating informant data.

---

[3]Interviewers completed a 3-month training program with Widiger, and continued discussions of problematic items that occurred throughout data collection.

Reliability and Validity Studies

Widiger, as a chief architect of the *DSM-IV* personality disorders, devoted a sustained attention to congruence between *DSM-IV* diagnostic criteria and the development of PDI-IV questions that closely reflected their meaning and intent. To a large extent, the validation of the PDI-IV has been a matter of face validity. Important issues remain with respect to validity:

1. *Concurrent validity.* The results of PDI-IV should substantially agree with clinical diagnosis and other Axis II structured interviews (especially the SIDP and PDE).

2. *Convergent validity.* The PDI-IV should evidence predicted associations, in a theoretically coherent manner with measures of personality and psychopathology.

3. *Concordance between professional and lay interviewers.* Despite assumptions regarding possible clinical bias, psychologists and other mental health professionals are the mainstay of psychiatric diagnosis. If highly divergent findings occur between psychologists and college student interviewers, then the validity of the PDI-IV is brought into question.

4. *Generalizability across settings/training.* The PDI-IV should be tested across a variety of settings (inpatient, outpatient, and nonclinical). In addition, testing the usefulness of the PDI-IV with interviewers not extensively trained and supervised by its developer would be most helpful.

Important first steps have already occurred in the validation of the PDI-IV. I will discuss this research with respect to PDI-IV reliability and validity. I will then summarize additional studies that are needed to address these four points.

The reliability of the PIQ-II was summarized in the earlier section on the development of the PDI-IV. With respect to interrater reliability, research by Widiger, Frieman, and Bailey (1990) indicated that the PIQ-II had satisfactory diagnostic reliability when employed by two highly trained doctoral students. Moreover, the use of dimensional scores appeared to yield very promising results.

Widiger et al. (1994) presented relatively little information on PDI-IV reliability. They report finding (on an unspecified sample) excellent interrater reliability for personality disorders, with kappas ranging from .72 to .93, with a median of .87. As of yet, the test-retest reliability of the PDI-IV has not been investigated. Given the chronic nature of personality disorders, the test-retest reliability and temporal stability of PDI-IV personality disorders would appear to be critical components of its validity.

Several validity studies have been reported on the PIQ and the PIQ-II. For example, Trull, Widiger, and Frances (1987) examined intercorrelation of symptoms for three PIQ disorders (avoidant, schizoid, and dependent) on 84 inpatients. They found moderate correlations between avoidant and dependent symptoms, which raises questions regarding diagnostic boundaries and comorbidity. They also mentioned a moderate correlation ($r = .53$) between the MCMI avoidant scale and the number of PIQ avoidant symptoms.

Widiger et al. (1986) evaluated the PIQ-II criteria for borderline and schizotypal disorders in a sample of 84 inpatients (diagnoses of schizophrenia, major mood disorders, and organic mental disorders had been excluded). They found that borderline symptoms had moderate item-scale correlations (.15 – .46, median = .32) but that schizotypal symptoms did not appear to be correlated (-.21 – .35, median = .07). One concern expressed in the study was the substantial diagnostic overlap, with an average of 3.75 personality disorders per patient.

Widiger, Freiman, et al. (1990) compared PIQ-II disorders to prototypical behaviors for schizoid, histrionic, and compulsive personality disorders for 50 psychiatric inpatients. They found that (a) three histrionic prototypic acts were significantly correlated with histrionic personality disorder, (b) none of the schizoid prototypic acts were significantly correlated with schizoid personality disorder, and (c) several other personality disorders were significantly correlated with these prototypic acts. Finally, PIQ-II schizoid criteria were significantly correlated with the Interpersonal Sensitivity scale of the SCL-90-R (median r = .46) and the Aloof-Introverted scale of the Interpersonal Adjective Scales or IAS (Wiggins & Broughton, 1985; median r = .40). Unfortunately, the authors do not present convergent and discriminant validity data for other personality disorders based on the SCL-90-R and the IAS.

Bailey, West, Widiger, and Freiman (1993) addressed the convergent and discriminant validity of five Schizotypia scales (Chapman & Chapman, 1987) with PIQ-II ratings. They found that these scales were moderately correlated (rs = .49 – .68, median = .56) with schizotypal criteria. In contrast, only a few of the other disorders (e.g., schizoid and avoidant) were correlated at all, although these correlations were conceptually meaningful. In sum, the study provides useful convergent and discriminant validity for schizotypal personality disorder.

Kruedelbach, McCormick, Schulz, and Grueneich (1993) employed the PIQ-II in a study of borderline and nonborderline substance abusers seeking treatment from the VA. They established significant differences between the two groups on the NEO Personality Inventory (Costa & McCrae, 1985) on anxiety, impulsivity, depression, and hostility. These data, as well as findings on research scales, provided convergent validity of the PIQ-II differentiation between borderlines and nonborderlines.

No validity studies have yet been reported on the PDI-IV. The critical issue is whether the PIQ-II studies can be employed in the validation of the PDI-IV. According to Widiger et al. (1994), *DSM-IV* criteria differ substantially from *DSM-III-R* criteria, with only 17% remaining virtually unchanged. Of those modified, significant modifications were made in 50 criteria (52%), and an additional 9 criteria (9%) were added. Since the PIQ-II is based on the *DSM-III-R* and the PDI-IV on the *DSM-IV*, the generalizability across measures in seriously questioned. Although Widiger et al. (1994) report a good correspondence (median κ = .77) between PIQ-III and PDI-IV, they do not report any research between the PIQ-II and the PDI-IV.

In summary, validity information on the PDI-IV and its predecessors is sparse. The best available research is devoted to the PIQ-II, on which a handful of studies have found convergent validity for borderline, schizotypal, schizoid, and histrionic personality disorders. Regrettably, other Axis II disorders have been only peripherally addressed. As previously noted, the comparability of the PIQ-II to the PDI-IV has yet to be established.

In reviewing the major facets of PDI-IV validity, it is clear that considerable work remains to be completed. Although the interrater reliability appears to be satisfactory, only a very small number of interviewers were employed, and these were extensively trained and personally supervised by the test's developer. Critical evidence of test-retest reliability has yet to be provided. Moreover, the temporal stability of diagnoses has not been investigated.

A major shortcoming of the PDI-IV is that no studies have been reported on its concurrent validity with other established measures, such as the SIDP and the PDE. Additionally, matters of generalizability require careful attention. For example, does the PDI-IV yield comparable results when employed by psychologists and nonprofessionals? Furthermore, can the PDI-IV be used effectively in outpatient psychiatric settings, other health care facilities, and community agencies? What happens when the PDI-IV is used with patients with schizophrenic and other psychotic disorders?

Clinical Applications

A primary use of the PDI-IV at the present time is as a valuable source book on *DSM-IV* disorders. The PDI-IV manual provides extensive and authoritative reviews of each of the personality disorders, with a thorough discussion of every Axis II diagnostic criterion. In addition, the PDI-IV provides a valuable template for evaluation of personality disorders and the provision of standard questions which closely reflect the diagnostic criteria.

The PDI-IV is not sufficiently validated for clinical practice. As noted in the previous sections, crucial questions remain with respect to its reliability and validity. Although it was intended for use with nonprofessionals, reliability studies on the PIQ-II (and presumably on the PDI-IV) were conducted exclusively with highly trained psychology staff. Therefore, the PDI-IV remains virtually untested with respect to its stated use with lay interviewers.

One practical concern with the PDI-IV is the complexity of some of its inquiries, especially for APD, and the sophistication of its language. Its demands for concentration and complex understanding may undermine its usefulness among the chronically mentally ill and intellectually limited. These matters are likely to be addressed in further refinements of the PDI-IV. A second practical concern is the sheer number of clinical inquiries. Given the competing demands on clinicians, a distillation of key questions, followed by a greater number of optional probes, may be an efficient alternative.

In conclusion, the PDI-IV has considerable promise, both as a diagnostic resource and as a future structured interview. Widiger and his colleagues are actively working on its validation and are likely to address many of its limitations in the coming years.

Standardized Assessment of Personality (SAP)

Description and Rationale

The SAP was originally developed by Mann, Jenkins, Cutting, and Cowen (1981) as a brief measure of personality disorders that could easily be applied to large-scale studies. The three goals of the SAP were composed of (a) evaluation of premorbid personality and its effects on the course and treatment of Axis I disorders, (b) standardization of personality assessment, and (c) development of a user-friendly measure that could be applied to clinical and nonclinical populations.

The SAP is distinguished from other Axis II interviews on several grounds. First and foremost, the SAP does not rely on the accuracy of self-reports by personality-disordered individuals. Instead, the SAP is based entirely on informant interview. In contradistinction to the SIDP and PDE, which require (SIDP) or recommend (PDE) a combination of patient and informant interviews, the SAP forgoes the patient interview altogether in favor of an informant's observations. Second, the SAP was developed in Great Britain and is based on the ICD-9 and ICD-10 diagnostic standards. Compatible with ICD-10 criteria, the SAP covers eight diagnoses: paranoid, schizoid, dyssocial, impulsive, histrionic, anankastic (i.e., similar to obsessive-compulsive), anxious, and dependent. In addition, Mann and Pilgrim (1992) report that a *DSM-III-R* version has been prepared.[4]

A newly modified version of the SAP (SAD-ICD-10 Version or SAP/10; Mann & Pilgrim, 1992) is now available. The SAP/10 is utilized with an informant who has known the patient for at least 5 years. First, questions are asked of the informant concerning periods of time when the patient was "illness-free." The unstructured portion of the interview requires the informant to provide a free-flowing description of the patient. Any relevant Axis II descriptors from a list of 72 are recorded. Following the unstructured portion, 10 general probes are asked verbatim. Again, any relevant descriptors are recorded.

The next step in the SAP/10 interview is a systematic review, in a run-on sentence format, of all the criteria for any personality disorder for which any descriptors were endorsed. The number of criteria vary with the disorder, ranging from six to nine. For any personality disorder with three or more criteria endorsed, the clinician completes the final step, namely, the assessment of impairment. Impairment is evaluated on three separate indices: personal distress for the patient, occupational problems, and social problems.

The final classification for each disorder is a trichotomy. Patients with fewer than three criteria are classified as not having that trait accentuation or personality disorder. Patients with three or more criteria but no impairment are classified as having that trait accentuation. Patients with three or more criteria *and* significant impairment are classified as having that personality disorder.

The administration of the SAP can be completed in 10 to 15 minutes (Pilgrim, Mellers, Boothby, & Mann, 1993). Because of its simplicity, the training required for reliable use of the SAP/10 is relatively brief. According to Pilgrim and Mann (1990), sufficient training typically requires a single 2-hour session.

The rationale for the SAP/10 was the need for a brief but standardized structured interview that would circumvent problems of self-report by personality-disordered individuals. Moreover, the SAP was intended for use with inpatients as well as outpatients. Pilgrim and Mann (1990) expressed a concern that

---

[4]I have described only the ICD-10 version, because no validity data are reported on the *DSM-III-R* version.

customary evaluations of hospitalized patients (i.e., self-report and observation) may result in an overestimation of personality disorders among chronic populations, since their clinical presentation may cloud the true diagnostic picture. Finally, the SAP/10 was developed to address the obvious need for a structured interview that was consistent with ICD-10 standards.

Reliability and Validity Studies

Mann, Jenkins, et al. (1981) examined the interrater reliability of the original SAP on a small sample (N = 24) of psychiatric inpatients. Employing pairs of psychiatrists, they established satisfactory reliability estimates with weighted kappas for four personality disorders ranging from .60 to .85 (median = .64). Test-retest reliabilities after a 1-year interval were relatively modest, with reliability coefficients ranging from .13 to .74, with a median of .42. McKeon, Roa, and Mann (1984) assessed the interrater reliability and test-retest reliability (12-month interval) for 25 obsessive-compulsive patients. Utilizing close relatives, clinicians found a high level of agreement on three personality disorders, both on estimates of interrater (.88 – .93) and test-retest (.76 – .88) reliabilities.

Pilgrim et al. (1993) investigated the reliability of the SAP/10. For interrater reliability, they studied 16 elderly subjects suspected of dementia and 36 psychiatric patients. For the six disorders with sufficient representation (≥ 5 cases), the kappa coefficients ranged from .60 to .82, with a median of .80. For test-retest reliability, they examined a consecutive sample of 77 inpatients. For the seven disorders with adequate representation, the range of kappas was .54 to .79, with a median of .69. In addition, they found that females and family members tended to be the most accurate in reporting personality disorders. In contrast, males and friends tended to be much more variable in their accounts of the same patient.

The diagnostic validity of the SAP/10, like that of many diagnostic interviews, is largely assumed, based on the face validity of its items and their correspondence to ICD-10. Towards this end, Pilgrim and Mann (1990) assessed the prevalence rates of SAP personality disorders for 120 inpatients. Among personality disordered individuals (n = 43), the SAP/10 produced relatively little diagnostic overlap, with subjects qualifying for an average of 1.74 personality disorders. This number appears quite low for an Axis II structured interview, although direct comparisons cannot be made with measures based on *DSM-III-R* and *DSM-IV*. Interestingly, significant gender differences were observed, with 50.0% of women and only 25.8% of men warranting a single personality disorder.

Initial validation of the SAP has focused on its relationship to overall functioning. For example, Mann, Jenkins, and Belsey (1981) followed 100 nonpsychotic outpatients for a 1-year period. Interestingly, they found that psychiatric morbidity was determined chiefly by estimates of psychological and social functioning. SAP personality dimensions appeared to play a peripheral role in predicting future mental disorders, although they proved significant in establishing future needs for psychotropic medication.[5]

---

[5]Interpretation of these data is constrained in two ways: (a) the authors used abnormal traits rather than personality disorders, and (b) discriminant analysis allowed for only the entry of presence or absence of any personality trait. A fairer test would be to assess separately dimensional scores for each personality disorder.

McKeon et al. (1984) examined 25 obsessive-compulsive patients involved in a behavior treatment program. Surprisingly, those patients with premorbid personality disorders, as measured by the SAP, had fewer significant life events than their counterparts without personality disorders. This finding defies simple explanation. One possible reason is that personality-disordered patients require fewer traumatic events before the onset of an additional disorder, in this case obsessive-compulsive neurosis. A second possibility is that obsessive-compulsive neurosis and the reported constellation of personality traits (obsessional, anxious, and self-conscious) are etiologically linked and unrelated to stressful events. A third explanation might be that the presence of these personality disorders insulated patients from substantial involvement in social and work spheres, thereby decreasing the likelihood of stressful events.

Validation of the SAP, as noted in the above distillation of research findings, has focused largely on its reliability, with relatively little attention given to establishing validity. Available studies have addressed matters of diagnostic validity only indirectly and have yielded equivocal results. Certainly, concurrent and convergent validity studies of the SAP are strongly recommended.

Clinical Applications

The SAP/10 clearly merits further attention, because of its distinctive attributes. By focusing on critical descriptors that are followed by standardized criteria and impairment probes, the SAP/10 provides a rapid and efficient method of assessing personality traits. For American psychologists, however, the SAP/10 cannot be employed for diagnostic purposes, given its lack of diagnostic validity and the lack of demonstrated convergence between ICD-10 and *DSM-IV* for personality disorders. Moreover, further attention is needed to the comprehensiveness of the descriptor list as an effective screen for personality disorders (Widiger & Frances, 1987).

Mental health professionals who work with personality-disordered patients may choose to use the SAP/DSM version as a secondary screen. In other words, a self-report screen, such as the PDQ-R, could easily be supplemented by the SAP/DSM version. In such cases the SAP would provide valuable information about personality dimensions observed by others. In addition, the SAP may provide information regarding treatment issues. For example, if the patient's spouse perceives overall problems in interpersonal functioning, these issues could become a focus of individual and/or marital therapy.

The choice of informant appears to be critical to the reliable use of the SAP/10. The ideal choice would be a close family member, preferably female. Use of nonfamily informants may lead to unacceptably inconsistent data. Of course, the use of multiple informants would appreciably improve the value of convergent data.

Other Axis II Interviews

Personality Assessment Schedule (PAS)

Tyrer and Alexander (1979) developed one of the earliest semistructured interviews for the assessment of personality disorder, the PAS. As noted by

Widiger and Frances (1987), the PAS is composed of personality traits rated on a 9-point scale. Based on ICD classification, the PAS employs standard questions to assess, from the patient and an informant, the following personality disorders: explosive, asthenic, paranoid-aggressive, histrionic, anankastic, and schizoid. Available studies suggest that the PAS may have adequate interrater reliability but only modest test-retest reliability (see Tyrer, Alexander, Cicchetti, Cohen, & Remington, 1979; Tyrer, Strauss, & Cicchetti, 1983). Although it has been used occasionally in British research (e.g., Casey, Tyrer, & Platt, 1985), extensive validation studies have not been forthcoming. The PAS is not recommended for clinical practice.

Diagnostic Interview of Personality Disorders (DIPD)

Zanarini, Frankenburg, Chauncey, and Gunderson (1987) constructed the DIPD to systematically assess *DSM-III* personality disorders. The DIPD comprises 252 standard questions organized by disorder and scored on a 3-point scale: 0 for "absent or clinically insignificant," 1 for "present and probably clinically significant," and 2 for "present and definitely clinically significant." In addition, optional probes are provided for many questions, and unstructured questions are encouraged in cases of ambiguity. Although the DIPD was developed in 1982, Zanarini et al. (1987) provided the first study of its validity.[6]

Reliability was assessed in a study of nonpsychotic inpatients that employed three raters for both interrater (n = 43) and test-retest (n = 54) reliability. The resulting kappa coefficients were excellent for interrater reliability (> .85, median = .92) with the exception of paranoid personality disorder (κ = .52). Moreover, the test-retest reliabilities tended to be relatively robust, with a range from .46 to .84 and a median of .68.

Comparatively little research has been conducted on the DIPD since its development. For example, Zanarini, Gunderson, Frankenburg, and Chauncey (1989) employed a revised version of the DIPD in research on borderlines (see Chapter 10) but offered little evidence of validity. Regrettably, the DIPD appears to be a reliable Axis II interview that has faltered not because of its psychometrics, which appear to be very encouraging, but because of lack of sustained research effort. Alternative Axis II interviews offer much more substantial validation to justify their use in clinical practice.

---

[6]Despite repeated attempts, I have been unable to secure a copy of the DIPD from Zanarini or her colleagues.

Part III

Focused
Structured Interviews

10

Diagnostic Interview for Borderlines (DIB)

The connotations and denotations of "borderline" vary widely by clinical setting, diagnostic standard, and theoretical formulation. As observed by Stone (1985), six distinct usages can be found for the term borderline in current clinical practice: (a) psychic organization, (b) syndrome, (c) personality disorder, (d) dynamic constellation, (e) prognostic statement, and (f) descriptor for interjacent states of spectrum psychoses. From these multiple sources, two perspectives have emerged as the most influential, namely those of Kernberg and Gunderson.[1]

Kernberg (1967) postulated that borderline organizations represent severe impairment of ego-integration and disturbed interpersonal relationships. He delineated the relatively primitive use of defense mechanisms (e.g., denial, splitting, projective identification), impulsivity, and instability of identity. In contrast, Gunderson and Singer (1975) offered a syndromal approach that was characterized by lowered achievement, impulsivity, manipulative suicidal threats, mild or brief psychotic episodes, good socialization, and disturbed relationships. Perry and Klerman (1978) provided a penetrating analysis of the two systems. They concluded that the two systems were highly divergent with respect to affect and cognitive processes, although they found some similarities in interview behavior (e.g., angry, manipulative, and devaluative) and thought content (e.g., depersonalization, derealization, and intolerance of anxiety). In addition, both systems described (a) personal histories marked by unpredictable behavior, self-mutilation, and substance abuse, and (b) profound problems in establishing interpersonal relationships.

Spitzer, Endicott, and Gibbon (1979) attempted to amalgamate the Kernberg and Gunderson systems by the identification of schizotypal and unstable criteria with 808 borderline and 808 control patients. Of these, the eight unstable criteria became the basis for *DSM-III* borderline personality disorder (BPD; see Stone, 1985), with two criteria specifically from Kernberg (identity disturbance and chronic feelings of emptiness and boredom), five from Gunderson (unstable and intense relationships, inappropriate and intense anger, physically damaging acts, affective instability, and intolerance of being alone),

---

[1]Other influential models are those offered by Knight (1953) and Grinker, Werble, and Drye (1968).

and one criterion shared by both (impulsivity). An ambitious study by Perry and Klerman (1980) compared 104 separate criteria, identified in the literature as discriminating features of borderlines, and provided empirical support for the *DSM-III* model.[2]

Research has suggested that the Gunderson model may be much more encompassing that the *DSM-III* BPD (e.g., Kroll, Sines, et al., 1981). In contrast, Nelson et al. (1985) found a slightly higher prevalence of *DSM-III* than Gunderson borderlines and poor correspondence between the two systems (52.2%). To further complicate matters, Nelson et al. (1985) found substantial agreement between Kernberg structural criteria (Kernberg, 1979) and *DSM-III*. One possible explanation is that the structural conceptualization (e.g., primitive ego defenses) provided by Kernberg does not require substantial evidence of impairment, as is the case with Gunderson. In support of this perspective, Koenigsberg, Kernberg, and Schomer (1983) found a high level of agreement between the two systems for inpatients; the level was substantially diminished in outpatients. This body of research will be examined more closely within the context of construct validity.

The remainder of this chapter is devoted to a review of Gunderson's (1982) Diagnostic Interview for Borderlines (DIB). In understanding the DIB, however, psychologists must also appreciate its place in the enduring controversies over borderline as a personality organization and a disorder.

Description and Development

The DIB comprises 123 items for assessing clinical characteristics of borderlines, in addition to symptoms chiefly associated with psychotic and affective syndromes. The time of administration is approximately 1 hour, although this may vary substantially across patients (50 – 90 minutes). Items are composed of (a) structured questions, (b) tables of information to be completed from multiple sources, and (c) clinical observations.

The items/ratings are organized into 29 "statements" or criteria that relate specifically to borderlines (see Table 10.1). The 29 criteria are subsequently categorized into five "sections" or scales.

The DIB is a semistructured diagnostic interview. Standard questions are presented verbatim to each interviewee. These inquiries are followed by unstructured questions, created by the clinician, for the clarification of individual ratings (e.g., frequency, duration, and circumstances) for a particular patient. Clinical data from other sources are also integrated into specific ratings; however, no item is scored as "present" without some confirmation from the patient.

The purpose of the DIB (Kolb & Gunderson, 1980) is to assess comprehensively five general dimensions of borderline functioning: Social adaptation, Impulsive action patterns, Affects, Psychosis, and Interpersonal relations. The *Social adaptation* dimension combines an instability at work or school with a substantial and socially appropriate involvement with others. The *Impulse action patterns* dimension consists of potentially self-destructive behavior (e.g., suicide attempts, self-mutilation, and drug abuse) and behavior that does not

---

[2]However, a number of criteria not included in these models (i.e., *DSM-III*, Kernberg, or Gunderson) were also seen as highly discriminating.

conform to social norms (sexual deviance and antisocial actions). The *Affects* dimension incorporates negative affect (dysphoria, anhedonia, anger, and depression) with demandingness and an absence of flat or elevated mood. The *Psychosis* dimension refers to transient psychotic experiences (derealization, depersonalization, paranoid experiences) in the absence of prolonged psychotic symptoms such as hallucinations and delusions. The *Interpersonal relations* dimension is characterized by unstable and dependent roles, an active avoidance of isolation, and several facets of impaired functioning (e.g., devaluation, manipulation, and splitting). In discriminating borderline patients from others, Gunderson and Kolb (1978) believed that components of these dimensions constituted important criteria. More specifically, they identified seven cardinal features: low achievement, impulsivity, manipulative suicide, heightened affectivity, mild psychotic experiences, high socialization, and disturbed close relationships.

Table 10.1
Organization of the Diagnostic Interview for Borderlines (DIB)

	Composition		Reliability (ICC)	
Section	**Statements**	**Ratings**	**Statements**	**Ratings**
Social adaptation	4	16	.79	.65
Impulse action patterns	5	12	.82	.64
Affects	5	37	.78	.61
Psychosis	8	24	.71	.69
Interpersonal relations	7	34	.71	.53

Note. The ICCs are the *M* intraclass coefficients reported by Gunderson, Kolb, and Austin (1981) in the development of the DIB.

The DIB is scored on a 3-point scale that consists primarily of the following metric: 0 for "no," 1 for "probable," and 2 for "yes" or "definite." In order to maximize the discrimination, two variations in the scoring occur (see Gunderson, Kolb, & Austin, 1981). First, symptoms of schizophrenia and mood disorders are given negative weights. Second, two cardinal features of borderlines (manipulative suicide attempts and dissociative experiences) are given greater weights, with a maximum rating of 4.

Ratings of individual items are synthesized into a global rating for the presence or absence of the 29 statements. Section totals involve the summing of these global ratings, with maximum scores ranging from 8 to 16. Finally, scores for the five sections are "scaled" so that each section is rated from 0 to 2. Based on Kolb and Gunderson (1980), any scaled score of 7 or above is used to designate BPD.

Gunderson et al. (1981) reported that the DIB was developed through 4 years of pilot testing and item refinement. The content and parameters of the DIB were based on a comprehensive review of the borderline literature by Gunderson and Singer (1975) and two longitudinal studies (Carpenter & Gunderson, 1977; Gunderson, Carpenter, & Strauss, 1975). According to Hurt,

Clarkin, Koenigsberg, Frances, and Nurnberg (1986), the first draft of the DIB was authored by Gunderson and Kolb in 1976. Descriptions of the item refinement and initial testing are not published. Preliminary evidence from training interviews (cited in Kolb & Gunderson, 1980) suggests adequate reliability for individual items (*M* ICC = .66) and descriptive statements (*M* ICC = .77).

Zanarini, Gunderson, Frankenburg, and Chauncey (1989) described briefly the Revised Diagnostic Interview for Borderlines (DIB-R) that was undertaken in the fall of 1982. Zanarini et al. reported that the DIB-R was revised over a 10-month period with the goal of improving its discriminant power. Further DIB-R modifications made in 1992 resulted in the most recent version (Gunderson & Zanarini, 1992). In addition to sociodemographic information, the DIB-R requires that the clinician address 106 individual ratings, 22 ratings of statements, and 8 ratings of sections (see Table 10.2).

Table 10.2
Organization of the Revised Diagnostic Interview for Borderlines (DIB-R)

Section	Composition	
	Statements	Ratings
Affect	5	19
Cognition	3	29
Impulse action patterns	5	17
Interpersonal relationships	9	41

Note. The reliability of the DIB-R has yet to be investigated.

The scoring system for the DIB-R remains essentially the same with two exceptions. First, the total DIB-R score is based on four sections, with Impulse action patterns and Interpersonal relationships given greater weights (0 – 3). Second, the cutting score for BPD has been made more stringent, with a total score of 8 or higher necessary for the diagnosis. In addition, the time framework for applying these scores has been standardized in the DIB-R to be based on the last 24 months.

The DIB-R differs substantially from the original DIB in its structure and organization. First and foremost, the organization of sections has been fundamentally changed, with the deletion of the Social adaptation section and broadening of the earlier psychosis into a *Cognition* section that includes nonpsychotic but disturbed thinking. Of the remaining sections, *Affect* concentrates on negative affect entailing chronic anxiety, in addition to other dysphoric states, and transfers demandingness to "interpersonal relationships." *Impulse action patterns* remains close to the original version; "other impulsive patterns" was substituted for antisocial behavior, with a somewhat broader scope than in the original. *Interpersonal relationships* was recast with statements that addressed an intolerance of being alone; fears of abandonment, engulfment, and annihilation; counterdependency; and problems in psychiatric treatment (i.e., regression, object of countertransference, "special relationship" with therapist). In addition, the revised section considered problems associated with close relationships: (a) instability and conflict; (b) dependency or masochism; (c) devaluation, manipulation, or sadism; and (d) demandingness or entitlement.

I have gone to some pains to describe the DIB and DIB-R separately because of the fundamental differences between the two measures. No studies have been published on the equivalence of the DIB and DIB-R. In their absence, we must assume that these are two different but related measures. Given the appreciable differences in time framework, individual ratings, summary statements, composite ratings, and total cutting score, it would be improper to attempt to generalize from the DIB to the DIB-R. At present, nearly all the research has focused on the DIB.

I understand that many researchers employ the DIB-R rather than the DIB. While there is a natural tendency to employ the most up-to-date version of any structured interview, both researchers and clinicians should carefully weigh the theoretical differences and consider the respective validation of the DIB and DIB-R in making their decisions.

Reliability of the DIB

Research on the DIB has concentrated primarily on establishing its interrater reliability. Comparatively less attention has been paid to the internal consistency of the five scales and to the test-retest reliability. Table 10.3 summarizes the available reliability studies, which we will review in detail.

Gunderson et al. (1981) reported the first interrater reliability study of the DIB, which was based on the independent ratings of two highly experienced psychiatrists (Gunderson and Kolb) who were instrumental in the development of the DIB. They examined the consistency of their ratings for 70 inpatients and found excellent agreement across items, statements, and overall ratings. Subsequent studies have not achieved these reliability coefficients; possibly the sophistication and implicit scoring conventions of Gunderson and Kolb do not generalize to other clinicians in other settings.

An early study of DIB interrater reliability yielded moderate results. Kroll, Pyle, Zander, Martin, et al. (1981) examined levels of agreement for 30 consecutive psychiatric admissions. They found moderate agreement (median κ = .74) across three interviewers.

Several more-recent studies have confirmed the DIB's moderate to good reliability. Frances, Clarkin, Gilmore, Hurt, and Brown (1984) employed weighted kappas to measure reliability between clinicians for 76 outpatients, including 26 borderlines. Reliabilities for items and statements were unreported but were described as "acceptable." For diagnosis, the weighted kappa was .78 and represented a marginal improvement over clinical diagnosis (unweighted κ = .72). Several of these investigators were involved in a subsequent study (Hurt, Clarkin, Koenigsberg, Frances, & Nurnberg, 1986) that combined inpatients and outpatients.[3] Overall reliability appeared to be good (κs $\geq$ .75), but is not

---

[3] Although not stated explicitly, the 76 inpatients reported in this study appear to be the same patients reported previously in Frances et al. (1984).

reported in detail. McManus, Lerner, Robbins, and Barbour (1984) evaluated the interrater reliability of the DIB with 48 adolescents in a university hospital and found acceptable reliability estimates. The range of reliabilities obtained for the DIB scales is .74 to .94, with 26 of the 29 statements achieving adequate reliability ($r \geq .60$).[4] Some differences were observed among the three raters who achieved moderate to high reliabilities (range = .72 – .85). Derksen (1990) cited an earlier Dutch study (van de Loo, Derksen, Dassel, & Becking, 1987) in which two psychologists assessed interrater reliability for 20 eating-disordered female patients. Although no reliability estimates were reported, perfect agreement was achieved with respect to DIB scores. Finally, Kavoussi, Coccaro, Klar, Berstein, and Siever (1990) found a moderately high agreement ($\kappa = .79$) for 56 personality disordered VA patients.

Table 10.3
Reliability Studies of the Diagnostic Interview for Borderlines (DIB)

Study	Agreement
Gunderson, Kolb, & Austin (1981) Interrater reliability study by two psychiatrists used 70 inpatients classified into one of four categories: borderline, schizophrenic, neurotic, or depressed disorders.	Interrater for DIB, ICC = .91; interrater sections, ICC = .92; interrater borderline items, ICC = .82
Kroll, Pyle, & Zander (1981) Interrater reliability study used 30 consecutive psychiatric inpatients with chronic schizophrenic and demented patients excluded. Three interviewers of varied backgrounds performed the evaluations.	Interrater for diagnosis, $\kappa = .74$
Cornell, Silk, Ludolph, & Lohr (1983) This study was a combination of interrater reliability ($n = 12$) and test-retest reliability ($n = 24$) at an average interval of 14 days; four experienced clinicians administered the DIB to 24 psychiatric inpatients who had at least one characteristic of borderlines.	Interrater for DIB, $r = .78$; interrater for sections, $r = .66$. Test-retest for DIB, $r = .71$; test-retest for sections, $r = .55$
McManus, Lerner, Robbins, & Barbour (1984) Interrater reliability study used 48 hospitalized adolescent inpatients, excluding those with neurological dysfunction. Patients were evaluated by pairs of experienced clinicians.	Interrater reliability, $\kappa = .72$

---

[4]Please note that this is a correction of a misprint (McManus et al., 1984, p. 687).

Table 10.3   (continued)
Reliability Studies of the Diagnostic Interview for
Borderlines (DIB)

Study	Agreement
Frances, Clarkin, Gilmore, Hurt, & Brown (1984) Interrater reliability study with three clinicians was conducted using 76 outpatients whose primary diagnosis was a personality disorder.	Interrater reliability, κ = .78[a]
Hurt, Clarkin, Koenigsberg, Frances, & Nurnberg (1986) Although the total sample consisted of 140 inpatients and outpatients, the investigators did not specify how many were used in the reliability study, but simply reported the threshold level (i.e., ≥ .75) of agreement.	Interrater reliability, κ ≥ .75
Kavoussi, Coccaro, Klar, Berstein, & Siever (1990) Interrater reliability study with two raters was conducted using 56 personality-disordered VA patients.	Interrater reliability, κ = .79

Note. κ = unweighted κs; r = Pearson's correlations; ICC = intraclass coefficients. Except where otherwise noted, median statistics are reported.
[a]The *M* weighted kappa; in comparison, the unweighted kappa for *DSM-III* borderline personality disorder was .72.

Hurt et al. (1986) examined the scale characteristics for the DIB, with rather disappointing results. Estimates of internal consistency were modest, with a range of .32 to .69 (median = .53). Both inter-item (.04 – .36) and item-scale (.09 – .60) correlations evidence marked variability. Of the five scales, Social adaptation appears to have very poor homogeneity. Based on these findings, clinicians must be very circumspect in making any scale interpretations.

Dewey, Silk, Ludolph, and Lohr (1983) employed four experienced clinicians in a test-retest reliability study of the DIB. They evaluated 24 newly admitted inpatients, 23 of whom had Axis I disorders. Personality disorders were poorly represented in the study (i.e., eight borderline, two dependent, and two histrionic personality disorders). Patients were retested by clinicians, unaware of previous results, after an average interval of 14 days. Importantly, the investigators augmented the DIB by the adoption of additional scoring conventions designed to improve its reliability. Results remained moderately stable across interviewers (median r = .66) and time (median r = .55). Agreement on diagnosis was satisfactory for the test-retest component (κ = .71). However, generalizability of the results is constrained by (a) the sample characteristics, and (b) the augmented scoring.

Taken together, the studies provide evidence of moderate reliability for the DIB. Most studies suggest high concordance rates for BPD (> 80%), although studies have typically preselected patients to represent only a few diagnoses. By narrowing the number of diagnoses, the levels of agreement may be inflated. Only one study addressed the temporal stability of diagnosis; it yielded modest results. While DIB reliability is adequate for clinical practice, further refinements are needed in scale development and replicability of results.

Validation of the DIB

The primary emphasis has been on comparing the DIB to clinical diagnosis as part of a bootstrapping operation. Comparatively less attention has been paid to concurrent validity through comparison with other psychological measures or longitudinal dimensions (i.e., course of the disorder and treatment outcome) of DIB-diagnosed borderlines. In general, evidence of construct validity through factor-analytic and cluster-analytic techniques has rarely been investigated for the DIB.

The original validity study by Gunderson and Kolb (1978) sought to discriminate 31 borderline from 22 schizophrenic and 11 neurotically depressed inpatients. A stepwise discriminant analysis was applied to the five scales and 29 statements.[5] Employing four scales (Psychosis excluded), the discriminant model accurately classified 85.0% of patients as borderline or nonborderline. In comparison to clinical diagnosis, the sensitivity was 75.9%, with specificity unreported.

Soloff and Ulrich (1981) attempted a replication of the Gunderson and Kolb study. They followed the same inclusion criteria as the earlier study, except that patients were not always interviewed in their first week of hospitalization. The study was composed of 23 borderline, 22 schizophrenic, and 20 depressed patients. They largely corroborated the findings of Gunderson and Kolb, with significant differences between borderlines and the other two groups on 12 of 29 statements. The most pronounced differences were established for Impulsive Actions and Interpersonal Relations.

Gunderson and his colleagues conducted two additional studies of the DIB (Kolb & Gunderson, 1980; Gunderson et al., 1981). Kolb and Gunderson (1980) examined differences on the DIB between 32 BPD patients and a comparison group of 38 inpatients of whom the majority were schizophrenic. They found that a cutting score ≥ 7 produced a sensitivity of .73 and a specificity of .81. Gunderson et al. (1981) investigated the underlying factor structure of the DIB as evidence of its construct validity.[6] Preliminary support was found for three of the five sections (i.e., Social Adaptation, Impulse/Action, and Interpersonal Relations).

---

[5]The sample size ($N = 62$) is insufficient to warrant a discriminant model on the statements.

[6]This factor solution is likely to be unstable, given the small sample ($N = 71$) and substantial number of statements ($N = 29$).

Criterion–Related Validity With Clinical Diagnosis

Koenigsberg et al. (1983) compared DIB diagnosis to clinical diagnosis based on the *DSM-II* by clinicians trained in the Kernberg (1975) structural model of borderlines. In a study of 74 outpatients and 62 inpatients, they established a sensitivity of .58 and a specificity of .88. Interestingly, the *DSM-II*/Kernberg interviews yielded substantially more BPDs in the outpatient population. The current relevance of this study is clearly limited by the use of *DSM-II* and by the obvious focus on the Kernberg perspective of borderlines.

Kroll, Sines, et al. (1981) evaluated the criterion-related validity of the DIB by comparing its results to *DSM-III* criteria, the Spitzer checklist (Spitzer et al., 1979), and the MMPI. In a study of 117 consecutive inpatient admissions, they found that the DIB borderlines (scaled score ≥ 7) was more encompassing than either the *DSM-III* or Spitzer checklist. More specifically, the DIB diagnosed borderlines approximately twice as often, although most patients diagnosed as borderline by the *DSM-III* (80.0%) and the Spitzer checklist (72.7%) were also diagnosed on the DIB. The MMPI profile most closely identified with DIB borderlines was an 8-4-2 profile (28.5%); previous research had associated this profile with several other *DSM-II* disorders.

Nelson et al. (1985) followed the same basic design of Kroll, Sines, et al. (1981), except they omitted the MMPI. In a study of 51 inpatients, their results suggested a moderate correspondence between *DSM-III* and DIB diagnoses, with a sensitivity of .65 and a specificity of .90.[7] Unlike Kroll, Sines, et al., however, Nelson et al. found the prevalence rate for DIB diagnosis to be *lower* than that for *DSM-III* (29.4% vs. 39.2%).

McManus et al. (1984) compared DIB and *DSM-III* diagnoses of BPD. In a study of 48 adolescent inpatients, including 12 borderlines, they established the sensitivity of the DIB at 75.0% and the specificity at 88.9%. Interestingly, they found that different scale scores contributed to the discrimination between borderlines and other specific disorders. For example, Affect, Impulse, and Interpersonal relations scales differentiated major affective disorders from BPD, while only the Interpersonal relations scale separated schizophrenia from DIB. This finding of the McManus study may offer an important insight into variable results in criterion-related validity studies: the proportion of diagnostic groups represented in specific studies may determine the concordance between DIB and *DSM-III*.

Frances et al. (1984), Hurt, Hyler, Frances, Clarkin, and Brent (1984), and Hurt et al. (1986) conducted three related studies of the DIB and *DSM-III* at the Payne Whitney Clinic. Based on 76 outpatients, Frances et al. reported a sensitivity of .73 and a specificity of .94. One advantage of this study was the inclusion of other Axis II disorders, including substantial numbers of histrionic, avoidant, and dependent disorders. Consistent with McManus et al., they found that the Social Adaptation scale was ineffective at discriminating between criterion groups. The Hurt et al. (1984) study examined 40 additional outpatients with DIB diagnosis supplemented by the *DSM-III* and the Personality Diagnostic Questionnaire (PDQ; Hyler & Reider, 1987). They found lower sensitivity (.63)

---

[7]Agreement between the Spitzer checklist and the DIB was very similar.

and specificity (.62) when the DIB was compared to the *DSM-III*. Though data were not reported in detail, the DIB appeared to have a close correspondence with the PDQ. In the third study, Hurt et al. (1986) combined the data from Frances et al. (1984) with data from 64 additional inpatients. They reported on the combined samples a sensitivity of .75 and a specificity of .78.

Barrash, Kroll, Carey, and Sines (1983) examined DIB and *DSM-III* diagnosis of BPD. They established a sensitivity rate of .72 and a specificity of .85.[8] Through the application of cluster analysis, two clusters of BPD emerged. Cluster 1 borderlines (compared to Cluster 2 and nonborderline patients) were more socially isolated, more unstable in their work histories, less appropriate in appearance, and less disturbed in interpersonal relationships. In contrast, Cluster 2 borderlines were more social, more intolerant of being alone, more generally impulsive, and more involved in intense but unstable relationships. Both clusters were characterized by self-mutilation, manipulative suicide gestures, splitting, and regression in treatment. Use of these clusters improved the identification of *DSM-III* diagnosed borderlines.

Bateman (1989) explored the relationship between the DIB and ICD diagnoses based on Present State Examination results for 42 inpatients. The 12 patients diagnosed as borderline on the DIB were given an assortment of diagnoses on the ICD-9 and a range of elevations on PSE syndromes. Interpretation of these negative findings must be tempered by noting the substantial differences in diagnostic systems and the lack of PSE syndromes that correspond to the cardinal features of BPD.

Criterion–Related Validity With Psychological Measures

Singer and Larson (1981) examined Rorschach protocols for 114 patients including 25 BPDs. Employing a specialized scoring system with 30 subscores on ego functioning, they were able to identify eight variables as part of a discriminant function which enabled the researchers to classify 80% of the borderlines and approximately two-thirds of those with schizophrenic disorders. While the study documents cognitive problems in borderlines, it offers little direct evidence regarding the diagnostic validity of the DIB or related measures.

Swartz, Blazer, George, and Winfield (1990) developed from the DIS a borderline index consisting of 24 borderline symptoms (see Chapter 3). As a measure of concurrent validity this index was compared to the DIB. Using a cutting score of ≥ 11, the two measures evidenced a high convergence (> 80%) and a moderate coefficient of agreement ($\kappa = .67$) for 79 psychiatric patients.

Kavoussi et al. (1990) compared the DIB to two other diagnostic interviews: the Structured Interview for Personality Disorders (SIPD; Pfohl, Stangl, & Zimmerman, 1982) and the Schedule for Interviewing Borderlines (SIB; Baron, 1980). In a study of 56 personality-disordered patients, Kavoussi et al. found only modest correspondence among the three measures. In establishing categorical diagnosis, the DIB showed a modest association with the SIPD ($\kappa = .42$) and poor

---

[8]As in their earlier study (Kroll, Sines, et al., 1981), they found that the DIB diagnosed BPD more than twice as often as did the *DSM-III*.

association with the SIB (κ = .18). From a dimensional perspective, moderate correlations (.49 – .65) were found for the severity of borderline symptoms. Kavoussi et al. recommended a lower cutting score for the DIB ($\geq$ 6) to increase its concordance with the other borderline measures.

Angus and Marziali (1988) compared the DIB to the PDE (see Chapter 7) and the PDQ in a small sample of 22 outpatients. They found very poor diagnostic concordance among the three measures. The kappa coefficient between the DIB and the PDE was .08; between the DIB and the PDQ, –.33.

Two studies (Derksen, 1990; Kullgren & Armelius, 1990) have examined the convergent validity of the DIB with the Structural Interview (SI) by Kernberg (1981). The term "structural" here refers to personality structure (not structured interview), which is assessed by the SI through a psychoanalytically oriented interview evaluating identity diffusion and primitive defense mechanisms found in borderlines (see Derksen, 1990). Derksen (1990) administered the DIB and SI to 20 eating-disordered patients and 43 patients with Axis II disorders. The level of agreement between the two measures was relatively modest (62.5%) and suggested that some persons may have borderline organization on the SI without borderline behavior on the DIB. Kullgren and Armelius (1990) examined 44 psychiatric inpatients on the SI and DIB. They found that 24 subjects with borderline organization on the SI had higher DIB scores than those with psychotic, but not neurotic personality organization. Unexpectedly, the SI scores for the borderline organization (*M* = 5.7, *SD* = 1.9) would suggest that the majority would not meet the DIB cutting score ($\geq$ 7) for borderlines.

Segal, Westen, Lohr, Silk, and Cohen (1992) employed an experimental projective technique based on patient-created stories for the WAIS-R Picture Arrangement subtest to study differences among borderline, borderline/depressed, and depressed patients, and normal controls drawn from hospital units and the community. Small but statistically significant differences were found that were consistent with hypotheses: borderline patients had less capacity for emotional investment and a more malevolent world view. While theoretically interesting, the study does not really contribute directly to DIB construct validity.

In general, the criterion-related validity of the DIB has received only modest support, partly due to heterogeneity on the borderline construct itself. At best, coefficients of agreement fall in the moderate range. I find it encouraging, however, that despite only modest diagnostic agreement, dimensional scores appear to demonstrate moderate degrees of association (see Kavoussi et al., 1990). As noted in the introduction, the controversy continues to simmer on the nature of BPD itself. Not until this controversy is resolved are we likely to see high levels of agreement among any measures of BPD.

Outcome Studies

An important dimension to diagnostic validity is the establishment of outcome criteria[9] for specific disorders. Pope, Jonas, Hudson, Cohen, and Gunderson (1983) examined 33 BPD patients who received a score of at least 6

---

[9]The other side of outcome criteria, namely antecedent conditions, has rarely been examined for DIB-diagnosed BPD (e.g., see Dahl & Bordahl, 1993).

on the DIB, based on chart diagnosis and follow-up interviews, 4 to 7 years later. Complicating the interpretation of their findings was the fact that most patients qualified for at least two diagnoses in addition to BPD. Of clinical interest, the patients with BPD and a major mood disorder appeared to have marginally better outcomes (global rating of 1.86) than BPD patients without the affective component (global rating of 1.27).[10] Moreover, BPD patients without mood disorders had very poor response to medication. Overall, few BPD patients were performing adequately in social relations and occupational functioning at follow-up. With respect to outcome criteria, the diagnosis of BPD remained stable for approximately two-thirds of the sample, although this finding is obscured by the fact that most also qualified for other personality disorders. In summary, the Pope et al. (1983) study offers only equivocal evidence of BPD as a chronic and debilitating disorder. Conclusions are hampered by the existence of multiple disorders and substantial changes in these disorders during the follow-up period.

Silk, Lohr, Ogata, and Westen (1990), in line with the Pope et al. study, followed nine borderline patients (interval from 1 – 3.5 years) with previous but not current depression. They found significant improvement on the DIB, particularly with respect to affect and psychosis, although most continued to meet *DSM-III* BPD diagnosis. Without comparison groups of never-depressed and still-depressed borderlines, these results are difficult to interpret.

Soloff, George, Cornelius, Nathan, and Schulz (1991) studied differences in pharmacologic responses for BPD, schizotypal personality disorder (SPD), and the combined BPD/SPD. The diagnosis of BPD was established with the DIB (≥ 7). Of 85 consecutive admissions, 34 were BPD only and 50 were BPD/SPD.[11] Drug trials (i.e., haloperidol, amitriptyline, and placebo) lasted 5 weeks. As expected, BPD/SPD patients had a greater decrease in symptoms than BPD patients when treated with haloperidol. However, the BPD patients also evidenced considerable improvement. Interestingly, both groups also had significant improvement in their clinical status when treated with an antidepressant. While such research suggests the treatment potential for BPD and its variants, this study did not establish specific treatment effects for BPD alone.

Kelly et al. (1992), in a double-blind pharmacological study of 97 DIB-diagnosed borderlines, found that nearly half (46.4%) dropped out of treatment before the 22-week program was completed. Anger as measured by the DIB, impulsiveness, lack of improvement, and substance abuse appeared to be linked to attrition. The study is useful in delineating elements of BPD that complicate treatment compliance, including components of the DIB. Links, Steiner, Boiago, and Irwin (1990) also experienced high rates of noncompliance. Only 17 of 43 DIB borderline patients agreed to participate in a drug treatment study, and 7 of these 17 did not complete the treatment protocol. Predictably, the marked instability of borderlines is reflected in their treatment compliance.

---

[10]Worthy of further investigation is a finding by Westen et al. (1992) that the depressive experiences of borderlines are qualitatively different from those of depressed patients.

[11]Only one patient qualified for SPD alone; inexplicably, this patient was combined with the BPD/SPD.

Validation of the DIB-R

Zanarini et al. (1989) compared 95 BPD patients with 142 patients having other personality disorders. The sample was drawn from a combination of outpatients and inpatients of average to above-average intelligence and without a major psychotic or organic disorder. They found that a cutting score of ≥ 8 had a sensitivity of .82 and a specificity of .80 when compared to clinical diagnosis. One worrisome observation is that the modal score for other personality disorders was very close to the cutting score (i.e., 35% had a score of 7). Surprisingly, the DIB-R tended to misclassify a relatively high percentage of personality disorders from the anxious cluster (27%), which share few symptoms with BPD. As noted by the authors, the diagnostic validity of the DIB-R compares favorably with that of other measures in current use.

Zanarini, Gunderson, and Frankenburg (1989), in a further analysis of the Zanarini et al. (1989) study, compared the comorbidity of borderlines, as evaluated by the DIB-R, with other personality disorders, as measured by the DIPD. They found that dysthymia was common among the patients studied and that substance abuse was common among BPD and APD patients. Their results do little, however, to elucidate the complex comorbidity problems with borderline patients.

Clinical Applications

The DIB and DIB-R are best conceptualized as two distinct although related measures of BPD. Fundamental differences in questions, time framework, and scoring argue against treating the DIB-R as simply an extension of the DIB. Of course, a systematic study of their comparability is clearly needed.

The great bulk of the research addresses the DIB, which is, therefore, likely to be the measure of choice in the clinical investigation of borderlines. Whether the Gunderson and Singer (1975) model of borderlines is "correct" remains unresolved. However, the DIB allows the treating mental health professional to make explicit statements about patients' clinical characteristics vis-a-vis this model. Moreover, the practitioner may take some comfort in the fact that these clinical judgments are generally consistent across raters. From this vantage point, perhaps the greatest advantage of the DIB, and presumably the DIB-R, is its ability to offer clear statements that are driven from a clear theoretical perspective.

Global judgments attempting to integrate these 29 statements appear to be ineffective, since the five "scales" or sections evidence only modest internal consistency (Hurt et al., 1986). In addition, cluster-analytic and factor-analytic techniques have not been thoroughly explored with the DIB, leaving the relationship between clinical items, statements, and sections largely untested. I would therefore recommend that the DIB be employed as primarily a descriptive measure, with interpretations based on the 29 statements.

The DIB should not be employed as a substitute for BPD diagnoses. Diagnostically, very high scores on the DIB (≥ 8) are most often found with borderlines, although cases have been reported in which nonborderlines received a score of 10, the highest score (see McManus et al., 1984). Conversely, substantial numbers of BPD subjects score in the middle range (4–6) on the DIB. Although not a substitute for diagnosis, the DIB provides important corroborative data.

The recent adoption of *DSM-IV* is likely to have little effect on the clinical usefulness of the DIB and the DIB-R. Indeed, the one or two substantive changes in the *DSM-IV* inclusion criteria would appear to increase the correspondence between *DSM-IV* and DIB. The addition of transient dissociative or paranoid symptoms appears bring *DSM* criteria into agreement with the psychotic section on the DIB. The effect of the second change (i.e., the redefinition of identity disturbance) appears to be less clear in its implications for DIB and DIB-R.

Borderline patients are often viewed as notoriously poor informants, with substantial numbers having a factitial component to their presentation (Pope et al., 1983) as well as other forms of deception (Ford, King, & Hollender, 1988). A potential problem with the DIB and DIB-R is that the face validity of the individual items, clustering of items, and unidimensional scoring (i.e., endorsements are almost invariably evidence of psychopathology) all increase the likelihood that BPD patients can distort their clinical presentation without detection. In clinical practice, psychologists may wish to employ psychological testing in addition to structured interviewing with borderline patients. For example, the Personality Assessment Inventory (PAI; Morey, 1991b) has both a borderline scale and validity scales.

The advantages of the DIB are summarized in Table 10.4. As previously noted, these advantages include its strong conceptual model, comprehensive coverage of associated symptomatology, and satisfactory interrater reliability.

The DIB's exhaustive coverage is also a potential liability, since the 60 to 90 minutes for its administration may burden clinical resources. Psychologists primarily interested in diagnosis may wish to consider other structured interviews, such as the PDE and SIDP, which allow for differential diagnosis as well as multiple diagnoses. In contrast, the DIB is likely to be the assessment method of choice for those psychologists involved in psychotherapeutic interventions with borderlines from the Gunderson and Singer model.

Table 10.4
Advantages of the Diagnostic Interview for Borderlines (DIB) in the Assessment of Borderline Personality Disorder

1. Strong conceptual model

   The DIB and DIB-R were carefully built on the Gunderson and Singer (1975) model of BPD. This model has been tested and refined over the last decade; it represents the most enduring classification for the difficult and controversial diagnosis of BPD.

2. Comprehensive coverage of associated symptomatology

   The DIB provides an exhaustive coverage of symptoms that are associated with BPD. While rationalistically derived, its systematic review of BPD symptoms has substantial clinical value.

3. Adequate to good interrater reliability

   As noted in Table 10.3, the interrater reliability of the DIB has been demonstrated in many populations and clinical settings with generally satisfactory reliability estimates (i.e., $\geq .70$).

11

Psychopathy Checklist (PCL)

Overview

The related constructs of antisocial personality disorder (APD) and psychopathy have crucial ramifications for how psychologists evaluate and treat individuals who are in conflict with the law. As noted by Rogers and Dion (1991), mental health professionals have remained undecided in how to distinguish antisocial "behavior" (i.e., a choice of actions) from antisocial "personality" (i.e., a mental disorder embedded in childhood antecedents and characterological deficits). This indecision about what constitutes APD is clearly chronicled in successive versions of the *DSM*. In *DSM-II*, the emphasis was placed on characterological dimensions that reflected "grossly selfish, callous, irresponsible, impulsive, and unable to learn from experience and punishment" (APA, 1968, p. 43), with no specification of criminal actions. In *DSM-III*, the focus was centered on dysfunctional behavior that indicated a lack of socialization and achievement, both as a child and as an adult, and a pervasive willingness to violate the rights of others. In *DSM-III-R*, the attention was refocused on violent criminal acts, particularly those which emerged prior to adulthood. In the development of *DSM-IV*, three divergent models (*DSM-III-R*, ICD-10, and psychopathic personality disorder) were debated vigorously (Hare, Hart, & Harpur, 1991) before the American Psychiatric Association settled on a similar though simplified version of *DSM-III-R*.[1]

Psychologists are confronted with a bewildering array of symptoms that have been associated with the diagnosis of APD. As outlined in Chapter 1, Rogers and his colleagues (Rogers, Dion, & Lynett, 1992; Rogers, Duncan, Lynett, & Sewell, in press) established, through prototypical analysis, broad dimensions of APD. In the Rogers et al. (in press) study, four distinct factors emerged: (a) *unstable self-image, unstable relationships, and irresponsibility;* (b) *manipulation and lack of guilt;* (c) *aggressive behavior;* and (d) *nonviolent delinquency.* While relying on the *DSM-IV* for APD diagnosis, psychologists may find these dimensions helpful in the conceptualization of what constitutes APD.

---

[1]Although field trials were supposed to play a major role in establishing the optimal criteria for APD (Widiger, Frances, Pincus, Davis, & First, 1991), political and nonempirical considerations appear to have won out (see Hare & Hart, in press; Widiger & Corbitt, 1993, in press).

Hare (1980, 1985a) initiated his own efforts to assess psychopathy which were relatively independent of the *DSM* versions. His concept of psychopathy (Hart, Hare, & Harpur, 1992) is more encompassing than that found in recent versions of APD because of its inclusion of affective and interpersonal dimensions. According to Hare and Hart (1993), psychopathy is defined as "a cluster of personality traits and socially deviant behaviors: a glib and superficial charm; egocentricity; selfishness; lack of empathy, guilt, and remorse; deceitfulness and manipulativeness; lack of enduring attachments to people, principles, or goals; impulsive and irresponsible behavior; and a tendency to violate explicit social norms" (p. 104). Hare's work resulted in the development of the Psychopathy Checklist (PCL).

Description

The Psychopathy Checklist is presently available in three closely related versions: the original 22-item PCL, a revised 20-item version (PCL-R), and a briefer 12-item version (known as the PCL-Screening Version or PCL-SV[2]). This chapter will focus primarily on the PCL-R because of its extensive validation and its commercial availability.

The PCL-R is composed of a 16-page Interview and Information Schedule and a 2-page answer sheet. The Interview and Information Schedule is organized into 10 sections: School Adjustment, Work History, Career Goals, Finances, Health, Family Life, Sex/Relationships, Drug Use, Childhood/Adolescent Antisocial Behavior, and Adult Antisocial Behavior. Unlike most semistructured interviews, these sections and their concomitant questions are not explicitly linked to specific ratings. Instead, psychologists utilize responses and collateral information to address multiple PCL-R ratings.

The PCL-R Interview and Information Schedule is organized into (a) standard questions (enumerated) which are asked of all respondents and (b) optional probes (bracketed) which are asked when more detailed information is required. In addition, several branching questions are asked, depending on responses to earlier questions; branching questions are identified by instructions to the interviewer which are presented in capital letters (e.g., IF NO, ASK). Although the Interview and Information Schedule provides very limited space for recording responses, all ratings are made on a separate answer sheet. Psychologists may wish to develop their own system for recording patient responses.

Responses to the Interview and Information Schedule are scored on the answer sheet, which includes a list of the criteria and the possible ratings. The 20 items are rated on a 3-point rating with the general criteria of 0 for "no," 1 for "maybe/in some respects," and 2 for "yes." Unfortunately, the actual criteria for rating items are not included on the form. Rather, psychologists must consult a third source, the PCL-R Rating Booklet, in order to make the necessary ratings.[3] In addition to space for the individual ratings, the answer sheet provides tables for prorating scores when individual ratings are omitted and percentile ranks for male inmates and forensic patients.

---

[2]The PCL-SV was originally described as the PCL-Clinical Version (PCL-CV).

[3]An unexplored issue is the number of administrative and interpretative errors that occur from this unnecessarily complicated organization.

The individual ratings are summed into two factor scores. The PCL-R test manual (Hare, 1991) does not provide any extensive description about how psychologists should make differential use of factor scores in their clinical use of the PCL-R. According to Hart et al. (1992), high scores on Factor 1 should be interpreted as reflecting interpersonal and affective characteristics of psychopathy that are linked to narcissistic and exploitative dimensions. In contrast, high scores on Factor 2 are indicative of criminal and impulsive behaviors and are associated with APD diagnosis.

The PCL-R also yields an overall or global score, intended as "a dimensional score that represents the extent to which a given individual is judged to match the 'prototypical psychopath'" (Hare, 1991, p. 17). In addition, a cutting score of ≥ 30 is provided which has a sensitivity of .72 and specificity of .93 when employed with white male inmates (Hare, 1985a).

Hare (1991) warned against problems in using cutting scores based on the standard error of measurement (SE_M). The SE_M for the PCL-R total score was 3.25. If a liberal standard (1 SE_M) were employed, then a cutting score of ≥ 33 should be used. If a conservative standard (2 SE_M) were employed, then a cutting score of ≥ 37 should be used. Similar adjustments should be made for determination of nonpsychopathic individuals. If a conservative standard (based on 2 SE_M) were fully implemented, then the cutting scores would be 0–23 for nonpsychopathic, 24–36 for indeterminate, and 37–40 for psychopathic. Of course, a problem with this conservative categorization is that most psychopaths would be missed.

Rationale and Development

Hare and Cox (1978) originally devised a series of 16 ratings that were derived from Cleckley's (1976) conceptualization of psychopathy. These global ratings were organized on a 7-point Likert scale and required that interviewers were highly versed in Cleckley's theory and sophisticated in their ability to interview inmates and integrate relevant data. This approach evidenced considerable promise as a reliable assessment method. For example, Hare (1985a) established high interrater reliability (.90) using 229 inmates.

Several problems were observed, however, with this "global ratings" approach. First, as previously noted, interviewers were required to have sophisticated training. Second, the rating items varied in the accessibility of required information and in the range of resulting scores. Third, the global ratings approach provided only partial standardization of criterion variance and offered little assistance with information variance. For these reasons, Hare (1980) decided to develop a more criterion-based checklist approach.

The first step in the development of the PCL was the generation of characteristics that would likely differentiate between psychopathic and nonpsychopathic inmates (Hart et al., 1992). Based on literature reviews and practical experience with criminals, the Hart team constructed a list of over 100 characteristics. Although specific details are not readily available, Hart et al. (1992) have described the general process of item selection and refinement. Items were selected which appeared to discriminate between psychopaths and nonpsychopaths and which met the following conditions: they were (a) nonoverlapping, (b) sufficiently correlated with global ratings, (c) not extreme in base rates, and (d) generally reliable. According to Hare (1985b), a series of analyses was carried out to refine these items and create the PCL.

The original PCL was composed of 22 items that reflected interpersonal, affective, and behavioral indicators of psychopathy. As described by Hare (1991, p. 1), the PCL/PCL-R was intended to assess "a widely understood clinical conception of psychopathy, perhaps most clearly exemplified by Cleckley's (1976) *Mask of Sanity.*" Although originally based on Cleckley's conceptualization, the resulting PCL and PCL-R actually deviated significantly from its own theoretical underpinnings. Table 11.1 summarizes the differences between Cleckley's (1976) formulation and Hare's interpretations and refinements on the PCL and PCL-R.

Table 11.1 succinctly illustrates the fundamental differences between the Cleckley and Hare conceptualizations of psychopathy. Of the 16 Cleckley criteria, only four characteristics (untruthfulness, remorse, affect, and planning) are closely paralleled by the PCL/PCL-R. Three other characteristics (charm, sex, and egocentricity) share key elements.[4] The remaining nine characteristics are not represented on the PCL/PCL-R. Likewise, the majority of the PCL characteristics (68.2%) do not correspond to Cleckley's model.

Hare (1991) reported that other theoretical contributions to the PCL/PCL-R include the work by W. M. McCord and J. McCord (1964), Craft (1965), Karpman (1961) and Buss (1966). These studies focus on affective, impulsive, dishonest, and antisocial aspects of psychopathy. He also presented evidence that the PCL criteria were similar to those employed clinically by Canadian psychiatrists (Gray & Hutchinson, 1964) and British physicians (Davies & Feldman, 1981).[5]

Hare (1985b) described the modifications made in the PCL to create the revised 20-item version, the PCL-R. One PCL item (concerning alcohol and drug use) was dropped because of difficulty in scoring, and a second item (previous diagnosis as psychopath) was deleted because of its redundancy with the PCL itself. The PCL-R manual (Hare, 1985b) provides detailed descriptions of each PCL-R item and its scoring. The more recent PCL-R manual (Hare, 1991) corresponds closely to the 1985 manual in its description regarding 11 items. However, the remaining 9 items evidence small but observable changes in the wording and the resulting criteria. Given the fact that these descriptions constitute the scoring criteria itself, the lack of data on the comparability of these two versions is a rather serious oversight. In other words, does the validity data on the 1985 version generalize to the 1991 version?

---

[4]Please note, however, that egocentricity was eliminated in the PCL-R version.

[5]Following Hare's (1991, p. 41) own description, however, the PCL-R appears to be consistent with only five characteristics from the Canadian study and six from the British study.

Table 11.1

Similarities and Differences between Cleckley's Formulation of Psychopathy and Hare's PCL/PCL-R

Similar constructs

Cleckley	PCL	PCL-R
Superficial charm and good intelligence	Glibness/superficial charm	Glibness/superficial charm
Untruthfulness and insincerity	Pathological lying and deception	Pathological lying
Lack of remorse or shame	Lack of remorse or guilt	Lack of remorse or guilt
General poverty of major affective reactions	Lack of affect and emotional depth	Shallow affect
Sex life impersonal, trivial, and poorly integrated	Promiscuous sexual relations	Promiscuous sexual behavior
Failure to follow any life plan	Lack of realistic, long-term plans	Lack of realistic, long-term plans
Pathological egocentricity and incapacity for love	Egocentricity/grandiose sense of self worth	Grandiose sense of self worth

Dissimilar constructs

Cleckley	Hare
Absence of delusions/irrational thinking	Previous diagnosis of psychopath[a]
Absence of nervousness and psychoneurotic manifestations	Proneness to boredom/low frustration tolerance[b]
Unreliability	Conning/lack of sincerity[b]
Inadequately motivated antisocial behavior	Callousness/lack of empathy
Poor judgment/failure to learn by experience	Parasitic lifestyle
Specific loss of insight	Early behavior problems[b]
Unresponsiveness in general interpersonal relations	Short temper/poor behavioral controls[b]
Fantastic and uninviting behavior with drink and sometimes without	Impulsivity
Suicide rarely carried out	Irresponsible as a parent[b]
	Frequent marital problems[b]
	Juvenile delinquency
	Poor probation or parole risk[b]
	Failure to accept responsibility for own actions
	Many types of offense[b]
	Drug or alcohol abuse not direct cause of antisocial behavior[a]

Note. Cleckley = Cleckley's (1976) criteria; PCL = Psychopathy Checklist; PCL-R = Psychopathy Checklist–Revised.
[a]Deleted in the PCL-R. [b]Modified in the PCL-R.

Validation of the PCL-R

Reliability

I have divided this section into original studies (i.e., research reported by Hare, 1991 in the validation of the PCL-R) and supplementary studies (i.e., subsequent research on the PCL-R). Both sets of studies will be examined with reference to interrater and test-retest reliabilities.

Original Studies. Hare (1991) summarized the interrater reliability regarding the total PCL-R scores for four inmate and two forensic-psychiatric samples. As presented in Table 11.2, the overall ICCs were relatively high across four inmate samples (range = .78 – .89, median = .84). Moreover, the sole forensic study appeared to have excellent interrater reliability, with an ICC of .91.[6] In addition, the PCL-R appears to have excellent internal consistency, with all studies reporting alpha coefficients above .80.

The interrater reliabilities for the individual items, combined across these studies, ranged substantially from a relatively modest .42 to an excellent .86. The median interrater reliability for individual items of .59 is relatively good when compared to that of other structured interviews.

Test-retest reliability has not been thoroughly addressed in studies of the PCL-R. Cacciola, Rutherford, and Alterman (1990) performed a test-retest reliability study using 10 male opiate addicts in outpatient treatment. This preliminary study, with an interval of 1 month, produced promising results with an r of .94. Drawing on PCL data to address the PCL-R, Hare (1991) and Schroeder, Schroeder, and Hare (1983) examined the stability of ratings on the earlier PCL. Schroeder et al. established excellent test-retest reliabilities. Although their description is rather elliptical, it would appear that they compared the same rater across the two occasions, which would likely inflate the reliability estimates. Given this methodological constraint and the meager sample of Cacciola et al. (1990), we have little data on the stability of PCL-R ratings.

Supplementary Studies. Cooney, Kadden, and Litt (1990) administered a slightly shortened 19-item version of the PCL to 79 male and 39 female inpatient alcoholics. Ratings were rendered independently by primary clinicians and occupational therapists. Unlike those of the original studies, these interrater reliabilities were exceptionally poor, with an overall ICC of –.12. Although Cooney et al. explained this difference by asserting that the occupational therapists had limited knowledge of the patient, this explanation appears to be unsatisfactory based on two factors: (a) occupational therapists conducted individual PCL interviews, and (b) the PCL and PCL-R are designed for use by mental health professionals who are unfamiliar with patients.

Hart, Forth, and Hare (1991) reported a further analysis of reliability data presented in the original studies. Two raters had independently administered the PCL-R to 119 male inmates, which yielded an excellent overall estimate of interrater reliability (ICC = .87). Importantly, the researchers found that Factor 1 of

---

[6]The data on a possible second study reported by Hare (1991) appear to be inconsistent: on page 33, unpublished data by Wong are stated as having only one rater; on page 35, interrater reliability data are recorded for the same study.

the PCL-R had a significantly lower ICC (i.e., .75) that did Factor 2 (i.e., .92). Additionally, the level of agreement on psychopathy, using a cutting score of > 30, was relatively modest, with a kappa of .54.

Gacono and Hutton (in press) reported that psychologists were able to achieve high reliabilities after completing a training program (i.e., workshops, practice cases, and videotapes). They reported only the reliability for the total score (median r = .98). These data suggest that extended training may result in nearly perfect agreement for interrater reliability.

Table 11.2
A Distillation of Hare's Interrater Reliabilities for the PCL-R

Study	Sample	ICC	α
Hare studies[a]	176 male inmates	.78	.86
Hare studies[a]	37 male inmates	.89	.88
Kosson, Smith, & Newman (1990)	72 male inmates	.80	.87
Cote & Hodgins (1989)[b]	70 French-speaking inmates	.87	.89
Johnson (1990)[b]	60 male inmates	–	.91
Hart & Hare (1989)	80 pretrial forensic inpatients	.91	.85
Rice, Harris, & Quinsey (1990)	20 male forensic inpatients	–	.89
Hare studies[a]	64 male forensic outpatients	–	.83

Note. All studies with independent PCL-Rs by two or more raters are included (Hare, 1991). Interestingly, interrater reliabilities were not reported for several of these studies.
[a]Hare (1991) did not specify which studies were used for these reliability coefficients.
[b]Unpublished data reported in Hare (1991).

Alterman, Cacciola, and Rutherford (1993) trained and "pilot-tested" two psychologists and two B.A.-level research assistants on 10 videotaped PCL-R interviews with substance abuse patients. They achieved an overall interrater reliability estimate of .84 for the 10 videotapes. A test-retest design was employed with an additional 88 substance abuse patients, who were evaluated by a second interviewer at an interval of approximately 1 month. To increase the sophistication of the study, some raters were given additional information (clinical chart and criminal records) to test their respective effects on reliability. Additional information appeared to have a slightly positive effect, increasing correlations from .85 to .89. However, the PCL-R scores appeared to be reliable for both Factors (F_1 = .71, F_2 = .79) when based on PCL-R interviews alone. This research is important as the first major PCL-R test-retest reliability study. Not only did the Alterman et al. (1993) study yield very satisfactory results, it also suggested that interviewers with less-than-optimal data could still achieve reasonably consistent findings.

In summary, reliability studies, with the exception of Cooney et al. (1990), have demonstrated excellent interrater reliability for PCL-R total and factor scores. Reliability of individual items has fared less well, although 10 of the 20 items had moderately high ICCs of .60 or higher. Test-retest reliability has been examined only recently (Alterman et al., 1993), but has yielded very promising results. Finally, measures of internal consistency have been uniformly high.

Validity

Extensive research exists on the validity of the PCL-R. Investigators have probed and evaluated its factor structure, concurrent validity, predictive validity, and convergent validity. I will examine each component of the PCL-R validation separately. I will then briefly summarize validity data on the alternate versions (i.e., PCL and PCL-SV).

Factor Structure. The establishment of the PCL-R's underlying dimensions appears central to its validation. If its factor structure is either unstable or poorly formed, then the ability to utilize these factors in clinical practice is severely eroded. Hare (1991) performed an analysis of congruence coefficients for four separate factor analyses rotated to oblique solutions. Of the 17 items that loaded on the two factors, 10 items were completely replicated across the four studies. Of the remaining 7 items, 5 were consistent across three of the four studies. These data strongly support a very stable two-factor solution. Although Hare et al. (1990) and Hare (1991) did not report the variance accounted for by each factor, earlier estimates by Harpur, Hare, and Hakstian (1989) suggested that the first factor accounted for 29% to 34% of the variance.

Hare (1991) described the two factors. Factor 1 is characterized as "selfish, callous, and remorseless use of others" (p. 38), and Factor 2 is depicted as "chronically unstable and antisocial lifestyle; social deviance" (p. 38). Rogers and Bagby (in press) have taken issue with these descriptions. They argue that Factor 1 has the highest loadings on interpersonal components of psychopathy that were overlooked by Hare (1991): glibness/superficial charm (.86) and grandiose sense of self-worth (.76). They further argue that Hare's Factor 2 misses important problems in the self-modulation of behavior, as observed in impulsivity (.66), poor behavioral controls (.44), and need for stimulation (.56).

In summary, the empirical data have convincingly established two strong, replicable dimensions of psychopathy. At question, however, is the best conceptualization of these factors. In subsequent sections, these dimensions will be discussed with reference to their concurrent and predictive validity.

Concurrent Validity. A substantial body of research has compared the PCL-R to ratings of psychopathy and to the APD diagnosis. Hare (1991) reported two studies of the PCL-R that compared its scores to the previously described global ratings of psychopathy. Both studies evidenced strong correlations with the PCL-R total score (i.e., .87 and .90) and factor scores (.70 – .87, median = .79). Despite its divergence from Cleckley's conceptualization, the PCL-R appears to be closely related to notions of psychopathy found in clinical practice.

The PCL-R appears to be moderately correlated with *DSM-III* APD diagnosis (see Hare, 1991); studies established comparable correlations with total scores for White (*r*s = .45 and .63) and African-American (*r* = .58) offenders. Hare (1991) reported only a single PCL-R/*DSM-III-R* study, again with a moderate correlation (*r* = .54). One consistent finding across both *DSM-III* and *DSM-III-R* is that the APD diagnosis is more strongly correlated with Factor 2 (median *r* = .59) than with Factor 1 (median *r* = .36).

Hare (1991) provided a cogent discussion of the asymmetrical relationship between PCL-R and APD. Because APD diagnosis (prevalence of 50% to 80%) is much more common than PCL-R psychopathy (prevalence of 20% to 30%) in correctional populations, most individuals with psychopathy also qualify for APD. In contrast, less than one-third of offenders with APD warrant the psychopathy designation.

Predictive Validity. An important feature of the PCL-R is the body of well-designed studies to examine its predictive validity. These studies have focused exclusively on its correctional/forensic application as it relates to two predictions: (a) future violent and criminal behavior, and (b) treatment response. The PCL/PCL-R studies which relate to criminal behavior are summarized in Table 11.3.

Hare (1991) summarized three PCL and one PCL-R study that examined the ability of parolees to adapt successfully to the community. Wong (1984), in a technical report cited by Hare (1991), found a low but positive correlation ($r = .30$) between the total PCL score and future criminal behavior. This finding is corroborated by Hart, Kropp, and Hare (1988; $r = .33$) and Serin (1991; $r = .31$). Use of simple cutting scores performed surprising well, with sensitivity ranging from .65 to .85 and specificity from .62 to .93. As observed in Table 11.3, these data apply only to released male inmates. In addition, the cutting scores remain relatively stable when PCL scores are prorated (i.e., 31 for Hart et al., 1988; 28 for Serin, 1991).

Table 11.3
Predictive Validity Studies of Criminal Behavior With the PCL and PCL-R

Study	Sample	Version	Cutting	Sens	Spec	Total r
Wong (1984)	315 M/C	PCL	–	–	–	.30
Hart, Kropp, & Hare (1988)	231 M/C	PCL	>34	65	.76	.33
Serin, Peters, & Barabaree (1990)	93 M/C	PCL	>31	.67	.93	–
Serin (1991)	81 M/C	PCL-R	>28[a]	.85	.62	.31
Harris, Rice, & Cormier (1991)	166 M/FP	PCL-R	>25	.77	.79	.42
Rice, Harris, & Quinsey (1990)	54 M/FP	PCL-R	–	–	–	.35
Heilbrun, Gustaffson, Hart, & Hare (1992)	208 FP	PCL-R	–	–	–	.16

Note. Cutting = cutting score (scores above the cutting score are designated as "psychopathic"); Sens = sensitivity (i.e., proportion of psychopaths who commit further criminal acts); Spec = specificity (i.e., proportion of nonpsychopaths who do not commit future criminal acts); Total r = correlation of total score with criminal offenses; M/C = male correctional subjects; M/FP = male forensic psychiatric patients.
[a]Nonpsychopaths were designated as those with PCL-R scores less than 18.

Two studies (Harris, Rice, & Cormier, 1991; Rice, Harris, & Quinsey, 1990) have investigated the use of the PCL-R ratings in predicting future criminal behavior in forensic patients, based on record review alone and not on PCL-R interviews.[7] These results are similar to those found with male inmates, except that a much lower cutting score (i.e., > 25) proved useful. In contrast, Heilbrun, Gustaffson, Hart, and Hare (1992), in an unpublished study cited by Hare and Hart (1993), found only a very modest correlation ($r = .16$) between the PCL-R total score and violent recidivism.

Simourd, Bonta, Andrews, and Hoge (1990) performed a meta-analysis for studies of the PCL/PCL-R, the So scale of the CPI, and the *Pd* scale of the MMPI. They found relatively modest effect sizes for the PCL/PCL-R, with a mean of .28. One difficulty in interpreting these results is the combination of external criteria (reincarceration, parole violation, and violent offense). However, when calculated for violent offense, the most common criterion, the effect sizes remain low (.25). One important consideration in understanding these results is that the comparisons are made within offender groups; higher effect sizes would be expected if offender groups were compared to nonoffender groups. Simourd et al. concluded that the PCL/PCL-R and the So scale were comparable and that both were superior to the MMPI *Pd* scale.

Psychopaths have often been viewed as less treatable than other offenders, although the empirical literature is far from conclusive (Wong & Elek, 1989). Ogloff, Wong, and Greenwood (1990) studied the treatability of 21 psychopaths (PCL-R > 26), 12 nonpsychopaths (PCL-R < 18), and 47 "mixed" offenders (PCL-R > 17 < 27). In a predictive study, they found that psychopathic inmates were less motivated and showed less improvement than either of the other two groups. Interestingly, the nonpsychopathic and mixed groups had comparable scores on all indices.

Convergent Validity. Studies of convergent validity form two general categories. First, a large body of research exists on the PCL/PCL-R and its relationship to current aggression, antisocial behavior, and rule-breaking. Second, a much smaller literature has examined the PCL-R in relationship to inventories and self-report measures which evaluate constructs similar to psychopathy.

Hare (1991) and Hare and Hart (1993) provide comprehensive reviews of the relationship between the PCL-R and violent and criminal behavior. They provide a summary of nine PCL/PCL-R studies which clearly demonstrate that psychopaths commit more criminal offenses, commit more violent offenses, and pose greater management problems in correctional settings. Very recent research with sex offenders (Miller, Geddings, Levenston, & Patrick, 1994) has continued to corroborate these findings. Although some differences occurred in cutting scores, psychologists can feel comfortable in utilizing the PCL-R in risk assessment of correctional referrals. The next logical step would be a meta-analysis of these studies to establish effect sizes and optimal cutting scores.

An important issue is whether the association found between psychopathy and crime might not be mediated by other coexisting disorders. Towards this

---

[7]Wong (1988) reported that reliable ratings ($r = .74$) can be achieved on file information alone with a moderate agreement in levels of psychopathy ($\kappa = .63$) between file information and the more typical interview-plus-file information.

end, Heilbrun et al. (1992) examined the relationship of schizophrenia to PCL-R ratings and found virtually no relationship ($r = .06$). Research (see Hare, 1991) on the PCL/PCL-R has postulated that psychopaths would experience less anxiety on the State-Trait Anxiety Inventory (STAI) than would their nonpsychopathic counterparts; this hypothesis is partially confirmed for Factor 1 (median r with the STAI of $-.23$) but not Factor 2 (median r with the STAI of .16). Studies have also been conducted on substance abuse (Smith & Newman, 1990; Hart & Hare, 1989; Hemphill, Hart, & Hare, 1990[8]), which appears to have virtually no relationship to PCL-R Factor 1 ($rs = .05 - .15$) and a modest relationship to Factor 2 ($rs = .26 - .40$). Although studies of criminal behavior with psychopaths, psychopaths/substance abusers, nonpsychopaths/substance abusers, nonpsychopathics/nonsubstance abusers would be instructive,[9] the existing data suggest that psychopathy as a construct is relatively independent of substance abuse disorders.

Several studies have investigated convergent validity by correlating PCL/PCL-R scores with multiscale inventories. For example, Hare (1985b) found modest correlations between MMPI scales 4 ($r = .36$) and 9 ($r = .27$) and the PCL, but no other correlations with clinical scales ($rs < .15$) except scale 5 ($r = -.30$). Hart, Forth, and Hare (1991) found modest correlations between the PCL-R and the MCMI-II antisocial scale ($r = .45$) and aggressive-sadistic scale ($r = .36$), although the interpretation of these results is obtenerated by similar correlations (i.e., $rs > .30$) on five additional scales: narcissism, paranoia, drug dependence, thought disorder, and delusional disorder.

Gacono and Meloy (1991) compared Rorschach variables for 22 psychopaths (i.e., scores ≥ 30) and 21 nonpsychopaths (< 30). Across 25 Rorschach scores, they found differences on three variables. These data were interpreted in light of object relations theory to indicate lack of attachment and anxiety in severe psychopaths. While theoretically interesting, the study does not address directly the diagnostic validity of PCL-R classifications.

Alternative Versions. Two alternative versions of the PCL-R are the original PCL and the PCL-SV. The original PCL has been previously described and correlates highly ($r = .88$) with the PCL-R. Given the extensive research available on the PCL-R and the administrative problems associated with the two deleted PCL items, there appears to be little justification for administering the original PCL. Therefore, this section will devote its space to a discussion of the abbreviated PCL-SV.

Hart et al. (1991, in press) developed the PCL-SV to meet the following requirements: (a) to be conceptually and empirically related to the PCL-R, (b) to be suitable for clinical and forensic populations, and (c) to evidence good reliability and validity. Previous experience with a six-item version suggested that good reliability could be achieved on a briefer measure. Hart et al. selected six

---

[8]The Hemphill et al. presentation was summarized in Hare and Hart (1993).

[9]The empirical question is whether correlations between criminal behavior and psychopathy might be explainable in terms of substance abuse/recidivism. Given the modest correlations and the documented role of substance abuse with future criminal behavior (e.g., Holcomb & Ahr, 1988), chronic substance abuse might represent an important causal factor in repeated criminal behavior.

items each for Factors 1 and 2 of the PCL-R. In addition, they altered the descriptions of the last two items (adolescent and adult antisocial behavior) so that they would be more applicable than the PCL-R to nonforensic clinical populations (Hare, Cox, & Hart, in press). The cutting score for psychopathy was prorated from the PCL-R and set at ≥ 18.

Hart et al. (1991) examined the interrater reliability of the PCL-SV on six separate samples (two inmate, two forensic psychiatric, one nonforensic psychiatric, and one university sample). The resulting ICCs ranged from moderate to high (.67 – .92) with a median of .82. Factors 1 and 2 had comparable reliabilities (median ICCs = .77 and .81, respectively). Moreover, Hart and Hare (1994) computed an ICC of .96 for averaged ratings on 12 offenders and 12 controls.

The PCL-SV was highly correlated with the PCL-R (median r = .80) and moderately correlated with APD diagnosis (median r = .64). As a stringent test of convergent validity, the PCL-SV was administered to 27 nonpsychotic inpatients with independent evaluations of Axis II disorders on the PDE. The PCL-SV was highly correlated with the PDE Antisocial Scale (r = .83) but also manifested moderate correlations (≥ .60) with Borderline, Histrionic, Narcissistic, and Sadistic. Given the inpatient status of the sample, the multiplicity of Axis II disorders is not surprising. Interestingly, the PCL-SV appeared to be more highly correlated with the MCMI-II antisocial scale (i.e., .68) than did the PCL-R (.45).

Hare et al. (1991), based on the psychometric strengths of the PCL-SV, recommended a slightly modified version as an alternative to the *DSM-IV* APD diagnosis. Although not incorporated into *DSM-IV*, the advantages of the PCL-SV are twofold: (a) it is intended for general clinical use, and (b) it has the psychometric rigor of the PCL-R but is more streamlined.

Clinical Applications

The great bulk of the PCL and PCL-R studies involve their validation with White male correctional subjects. For this population, the PCL-R offers incremental validity (see Hare, 1991) for making accurate risk assessments. These risk assessments are best utilized with (a) institutional placement decisions in corrections (e.g., level of security and treatment needs), (b) parole and conditional release decisions, and (c) hearings on community placement of forensic patients. In these cases with White male inmates, the PCL-R should definitely be employed as a critical and unequalled measure in determining their specific risk assessments. For other decisions within the forensic system, psychologists are likely to be much more circumspect on the direct relevance of PCL-R data.

Rogers and Ornduff (in press) recommend that mental health experts may have the strongest case in risk assessment when male correctional evaluatees have very high scores on the PCL-R and clearly exceed the minimum criteria for APD. Such high scores circumvent the earlier-noted concerns regarding the SE_M and increase the sensitivity of predictions. Conversely, very low scores (< 18) combined with the relative absence of APD symptoms may provide encouraging evidence regarding treatability and lower risk of recidivism. Psychologists who employ these predictive data must be equally willing to provide both positive as well as negative opinions or run the very real risk of being labeled as biased.

The PCL-R is a polythetic model, with more than 15,000 possible variations of psychopathy (i.e., different combinations of symptom scores $\geq$ 30). Whether every score of 30 or above presents the same risk has yet to be empirically assessed. However, criteria of Factor 1 appear to have generally low correlations (< .20) with future criminal behavior, compared to criteria of Factor 2 (> .30) (see Hare, 1991). This observation would suggest that PCL-R psychopath designations based primarily on Factor 1 items may pose less of a risk than individuals with similar designations based largely on Factor 2 items. I would recommend that psychologists be more cautious in making predictive statements when scores are predominantly composed of Factor 1 items.

I would also recommend, consistent with the SE_M discussion in the *Description* section of this chapter, that a minimum cutting score of $\geq$ 33 be employed in making predictive statements regarding recidivism. I am aware that others would take issue with this conservative approach; for example, Gacono and Hutton (in press) suggest that total scores of 28 and 29 be labeled as "high moderate," 30 to 32 as "low severe," and 33 and above as "severe." I believe that such a classification, at the present time, is an overrefinement of PCL-R interpretation. First, the available predictive literature is based on cutting scores which do not allow for such specific probabilities. Even when high scores are achieved, a substantial minority of false-positives occur. Second, referral sources are unlikely to understand these distinctions and may treat a "high moderate" score on psychopathy in a similar fashion as a "severe" score.

Available research data would suggest that the PCL-R may be used descriptively (but *not* predictively) with African-American samples. Kosson, Smith, and Newman (1990) demonstrated that both White and African-American samples manifest similar differences in prior criminal behavior between psychopaths and nonpsychopaths. Normative data on female offenders suggest somewhat lower scores (Hare, 1991). At present, data are insufficient to recommend use of the PCL-R with female populations.

Relatively little information is available on the usefulness of the PCL-R with adolescent offenders. Forth, Hart, and Hare (1990) administered an 18-item PCL-R version to 75 youthful offenders and were able to achieve a high level of interrater reliability (ICC = .88). The PCL-R scores ($\geq$ 30) were correlated with conduct disorder symptoms (r = .64), institutional problems (r = .46), and prediction of postrelease violent offenses (r = .26). Psychologists may well feel conflicted on whether to use the PCL-R with male adolescent offenders. On one hand, the PCL-R has not been cross-validated for this or any other adolescent population. On the other, the lack of any other predictive measures of aggressive/criminal behavior forms a pragmatic argument for its cautious use.

The empirical data on the PCL-R are very limited with respect to treatability. The study by Ogloff et al. (1990) suggests that psychopaths are less motivated for, and are less likely to continue in, treatment. Please note that the study did not address treatment effectiveness. At present, we do not know whether the smaller percentage of psychopaths who do complete treatment garner positive effects from this treatment. Based on the incalculable social costs (e.g., police investigations, criminal courts, lengthy incarcerations, and damages to victims), I would argue against summarily dismissing treatment efforts with psychopaths, because even modestly successful programs may be cost-effective (see Rogers & Mitchell, 1991).

The PCL-SV has not been widely adopted in either clinical or forensic/correctional practices. Given the substantial samples of nonforensic patients and females, the PCL-SV would appear to be particularly useful for the evaluation of patients with antisocial histories. As with Axis II structured interviews, a screening measure like the PDQ-R may assist in identifying patients for whom the PCL-SV may be especially relevant. I would recommend the clinical adaptation of the PCL-SV which is currently available from its authors.

A potential problem with the PCL-R and PCL-SV is the possibility of creating halo effects. This problem is compounded by the extensive amount of description of each item, which unavoidably creates varying degrees of overlap. I have pilot-tested an alternative answer sheet for the PCL-SV that requires the psychologist to make particular ratings of each descriptor, as opposed to more global ratings. The advantage of rating each subcriterion individually is twofold: (a) the psychologist gathers more case-specific information, and (b) this more systematic process may help prevent the halo effect.

Some psychologists may be concerned about the atheoretical nature of the PCL-R and PCL-SV. Contributions from Cleckley and others would appear to account for only one-half of the PCL items. Other psychologists may view the lack of a coherent theory as a strength, in that interpretations are not forced or unduly influenced from a particular theoretical perspective. Certainly, the existence of two stable factors greatly increases the interpretability of the PCL-R and PCL-SV.

The advent of the *DSM-IV* is likely to have little affect on the clinical usefulness of the PCL-R and PCL-SV. First and foremost, the PCL versions do not rely upon the *DSM* for their validation. In other words, no attempt has been made to utilize the *DSM* as a gold standard. Second, the changes in *DSM-IV* diagnosis of APD have involved a reduction in and simplification of symptoms. The actual consequences of these changes to the prevalence of APD are not known. While the number of criteria has been reduced to seven, the *DSM-IV* has also reduced the minimum number of criteria needed to render the diagnosis.

In summary, the PCL-R and PCL-SV have considerable strengths in their ability to identify two critical dimensions of psychopathy and to relate these dimensions to violent and criminal behavior. Certainly, the PCL-R is highly reliable with evidence of short-term stability. These and other advantages are summarized in Table 11.4.

The primary limitations of the PCL-R are (a) the relative absence of studies on its generalizability beyond correctional facilities and maximum security forensic hospitals, and (b) the paucity of research on adolescents, minorities, and women. Other limitations include the dearth of specific studies on the polythetic model and the PCL-R's vulnerability to halo effects, given the global nature of its ratings. These limitations do not detract, however, from its careful applications to white male offender and forensic populations.

Table 11.4
Advantages and Limitations in Using the PCL-R and PCL-SV

Advantages

1. The PCL-R is the best-validated and most reliable clinical method for determining risk assessment in White male offenders.

2. For male forensic patients placed in maximum security hospitals, the PCL-R offers useful data for risk assessment when released into the community.

3 The PCL-R and PCL-SV provide a replicated and stable two-factor solution that allows psychologists to describe two broad dimensions of psychopathy.

4. Because of their nonspecific interview format and insistence on collateral data, the PCL-R and PCL-SV are probably much harder to foil than are APD sections of other structured interviews.

Limitations

1. Psychologists are likely to be tempted to apply the previously described risk assessment beyond these parameters.

2. Nearly all the predictive studies were conducted on subjects within the Canadian criminal justice system. Although the Canadian and American systems are similar, the generalizability of these findings to the American system has not been formally investigated.

3. Variations in cutting scores and different combinations of endorsed PCL-R items are likely to affect interpretation, although little data exist on this critical point.

12

Structured Interview of Reported Symptoms (SIRS)

An important dimension of psychological assessment is the ascertainment of response styles. While traditionally clinicians have assumed that patients are honest and self-disclosing, the increasing complexity of mental health service delivery and competing interests among persons, agencies, and government militate against this forthrightness (Rogers & Cavanaugh, 1983). Despite the reliance on self-report measures such as the MMPI and MMPI-2 (see Rogers, 1984; Schretlen, 1988), psychologists and other mental health professionals have more recently considered the use of structured interviews in determining response styles (Rogers, 1987, 1988), particularly in the assessment of malingering. This chapter focuses on the Structured Interview of Reported Symptoms as a standardized, interview-based measure of malingering and related response styles.

Overview

Description

The Structured Interview of Reported Symptoms (SIRS) was developed by Rogers and his colleagues (Rogers, 1992; Rogers, Bagby, & Dickens, 1992) to assess different response styles, particularly the feigning of mental disorders. The SIRS is composed of 172 items that are organized into eight primary and five supplementary scales. Scales are designated as "primary" if their cutting scores consistently differentiate feigners from clinical and community samples.[1] Three primary scales examine very unusual symptom presentation (Rare Symptoms [RS], Symptom Combinations [SC], and Improbable and Absurd Symptoms [IA]); four scales address the range and severity of symptom endorsements (Blatant Symptoms [BL], Subtle Symptoms [SU], Selectivity and Symptoms [SEL], and Severity of Symptoms [SEV]); and the remaining scale inspects differences between self-report and observation (Reported vs. Observed Symptoms [RO]). Some individuals feigning mental disorders focus mostly on the range and severity of symptoms (i.e., BL, SU, SEL, and SEV), while others manifest elevations on nearly all scales.

---

[1] Statistically significant differences were also found for supplementary scales (e.g., see Rogers, Gillis, Dickens, & Bagby, 1991). However, the overlap of distributions reduced the effectiveness of their cutting scores.

The format of the SIRS is structured rather than semistructured. In other words, psychologists are disallowed from asking their own unstructured questions during the formal administration of the SIRS. Once the SIRS is completed, they are permitted to ask for amplification of key questions. One valuable use of this postinquiry phase is to solicit examples, particularly of item endorsements reflecting very unusual symptom presentation (e.g., for neologisms, "What words have you invented?"). The rationale for making the SIRS a structured interview is to minimize the possibility of interactional factors influencing either (a) the types of unstructured questions employed, or (b) the nonstandardized interpretation of responses to these questions. In addition, a less structured format might occasionally allow a clinician to express implicitly or explicitly his/her perceptions of the patient's credibility, thereby negatively affecting rapport and influencing subsequent responses to the SIRS.

SIRS items are scored on a 3-point scale, with 0 reserved for "no" or nondeviant responses and 1 and 2 for increasing gradations of endorsement (Rogers, Bagby, et al., 1992). Different criteria are employed for scoring 1 and 2, based on the type of questions involved. For detailed inquiries, the scoring reflects severity: 1 is used for "a major problem," and 2 for "an unbearable problem." For general inquiries, the scoring reflects the level of certainty: 1 represents a qualified endorsement, and 2 an unambiguous endorsement.

The chief purpose of SIRS scales is the accurate classification of feigning and bona fide patients. Guidelines are offered for the further specification of feigning into malingering and factitious disorders.[2] In addition to the *DSM-III-R* and *DSM-IV* definitions of malingering, the SIRS manual offers an empirically derived model for the classification of malingering. Rogers (1990a, 1990b) proposed criteria for the overall classification of malingering that were cross-validated with both test and interview data. SIRS data are integrated into these criteria in making classifications of malingering. Beyond malingering and factitious disorders, the SIRS offers descriptive information on defensive and inconsistent responding.

Rationale

A structured interview was chosen over self-report inventories for several reasons (Rogers, Bagby, et al., 1992). First, in the absence of a gold standard, psychologists most often rely on clinical interviews in making their determinations of malingering and factitial disorders. The development of a structured interview would likely enhance this form of assessment. Moreover, research data (Tesser & Paulhus, 1983; Tetlock & Manstead, 1985) have clearly shown that persons may respond differently to self-report measures than to interview methods. To assume facilely that faked test results reflect a pervasive pattern of feigning is not empirically supported.

A second and closely related reason for developing a structured interview stems from the importance of the decisions related to response style and the concomitant need for a multimethod approach. Since the determination of feigning is likely to have far-reaching social consequences that often include the cessation

---

[2] See Rogers, Bagby, and Rector (1989) for a discussion of diagnostic and conceptual problems inherent in factitious disorders with psychological symptoms.

of mental health services, psychologists should render their decisions on multiple sources of data, including interview and psychometric data (Rogers, 1990a).

Development

Rogers (1984) conducted a comprehensive review of existing research and case studies on malingering, with an overriding goal of determining potential strategies for the identification of malingerers. This review yielded a total of 22 strategies, of which 15 were selected for further investigation with the SIRS. On a rational basis, a total of 330 items were generated to test in a preliminary manner these 15 strategies. These items were refined and tested on several inpatient samples to examine their fluency and transparency (i.e., ease with which they were recognized as bogus symptoms; Rogers & Resnick, 1988).

SIRS items were refined by the use of eight experts, who rendered independent judgments regarding the malingering strategies. Items on which general agreement was achieved were combined into scales consistent with each strategy. In addition, scale homogeneity was enhanced by dropping items that had very low item-to-scale correlations. The internal consistency of the scales was then evaluated by computing alpha coefficients based on data from three separate studies. The alpha coefficients ranged from .66 to .92.

Validation of the SIRS

Research on the SIRS validation will be summarized in three sections: reliability, validity, and generalizability. Each section will be described separately below.

Reliability

Research on an early version of the SIRS (Rogers, 1988, p. 266) suggested that good reliabilities (i.e., $rs > .80$) might be achievable. With the final version of the SIRS, Rogers, Bagby, et al. (1992) conducted two small studies of interrater reliability which yielded very positive results. Inpatient subjects were employed in both studies, since those who are seriously mentally ill are likely to provide the greatest challenge for reliability because of their idiosyncratic responses. Across the two studies, interrater reliabilities remained uniformly high (.89 – 1.00). Median reliabilities of .96 and 1.00 were reported.

Rogers, Bagby, et al. (1992) examined the reliability of individual scores through standard errors of measurement (SE_M). As expected, they found relatively low SE_Ms for patient and community samples responding honestly (1.51 and 1.19, respectively). In comparison, malingerers and simulators evidenced higher variability (2.64 and 2.38, respectively) as predicted, given their less consistent presentations.

Linblad (1993) trained five undergraduate research assistants in the administration of the SIRS. Interestingly, these assistants had no prior clinical training and were kept blind to the purpose of the SIRS and the goals of the research. Six patients were interviewed and independently rated by the five research assistants. Interrater reliability coefficients were uniformly high, with a median of .95 (averages across scales = .87 – .97).[3]

---

[3]Linblad reported reliabilities for six of the eight primary scales employed in his study.

Overall, these reliability studies indicate a high level of interrater reliability, even when used by nonprofessionals who are blind to the purpose of the SIRS. Psychologists can take comfort that high levels of reliability can be achieved with only a modest level of training and supervision in the SIRS.

Validity

Overview. Rogers, Harrell, and Liff (1993) described the three research models for the validation of tests of malingering: simulation, known-groups, and differential prevalence designs. Knowledge of these research models is a necessary prerequisite to understanding the SIRS's validation. As an introduction to this section, each is briefly defined:

1. *Simulation research* involves the use of "simulators," persons who are given experimental instructions to feign mental illness. They are subsequently compared to clinical samples and normal controls. As an analogue model, simulation research has the notable advantage of well-controlled experimental manipulation, but has serious limitations in generalizability.

2. *Known-groups design* entails the use of actual malingerers, independently classified by mental health professionals, who are compared to clinical and nonclinical samples. This model is constrained by problems in the identification of malingerers but is clearly generalizable to real-world settings.

3. *Differential prevalence design* assumes different rates of malingering based on referral issues and settings. Unfortunately, even when differential rates are found in the predicted directions, researchers have no way of knowing (a) whether these prevalence rates are accurate, or more importantly, (b) whether deviant scores truly represent malingering.

Rogers, Bagby, et al. (1992) has argued that for malingering measures to be accepted as valid, they must be cross-validated with both simulation research (maximizing the experimental design) and known-groups research (maximizing the generalizability).

Simulation Research by the Original Investigators. Rogers and his colleagues conducted a series of four studies (Rogers, Gillis, & Bagby, 1990; Rogers, Gillis, Bagby, & Monteiro, 1991; Rogers, Gillis, Dickens, & Bagby, 1991; Rogers, Kropp, & Bagby, 1993) that included a simulation design. In each study, subjects were given specific instructions to feign a mental illness and were offered an incentive (financial or course credit) for providing a convincing performance.

The studies varied with respect to setting and use of experimental instructions. Rogers, Gillis, and Bagby (1990) and Rogers, Kropp, and Bagby (1993) employed correctional subjects with prior experiences in psychological assessment and intervention to serve as simulators and controls. Rogers, Gillis, Bagby, et al. (1991) utilized college students in this regard, while Rogers, Gillis, Dickens, et al. (1991) used community subjects. The experimental instructions stated goals that ranged from avoiding placement in a more restrictive correctional institution to seeking voluntary hospitalization. In addition, two studies (Rogers, Gillis, Bagby, et al., 1991; Rogers, Kropp, et al., 1993) provided subgroups of simulators with coaching on the specific disorders being feigned or detection strategies built into the SIRS.

The combined samples for the four simulation studies were composed of 75 bona fide patients (35 outpatients and 40 inpatients), 170 simulators (70 from corrections, 40 from the community, and 60 from a university), and 97 controls (26 from corrections, 41 from the community, and 30 from a university). For each study, the primary scales evidenced highly significant differences for simulators in comparison to clinical and nonclinical samples.[4]

Rogers, Bagby, et al. (1992) combined the simulation studies described above and added 25 subjects to the clinical group in order to increase the inpatient representation. They performed a two-stage discriminant analysis to test overall differences in SIRS primary scales. To make the discriminant model more rigorous, they excluded nonclinical controls from the analysis. With both simulators and bona fide patients randomly divided into calibration (i.e., first) and cross-validation (i.e., second) samples, the discrimination function accurately classified 89.8% of the calibration and 88.3% of the cross validation samples.[5]

Taken together, the studies indicate highly consistent differences between simulators and others (clinical and nonclinical groups) on the SIRS primary scales. These differences appear to stand regardless of the sample (clinical, community, college, or corrections), the specific disorder feigned, and the presence or absence of coaching. The next step is to examine whether simulation research yielded convergent data with known-groups design.

Known-Groups Research by the Original Investigators. Samples of actual malingerers are difficult to establish. Rogers, Gillis, Dickens, et al. (1991), through systematic investigations of forensic inpatients, were able to identify 26 suspected malingerers who were independently classified by the assessment teams. Their primary SIRS scales were consistently elevated to comparable levels of simulators. Moreover, these suspected malingerers had significantly higher scores than clinical and nonclinical groups under standard instructions.

Rogers, Bagby, et al. (1992) combined the 26 suspected malingerers from Rogers, Gillis, Dickens, et al. (1991) with an additional 10 suspected malingerers to test for overall differences on the SIRS. The overall classification rate for a single-stage discriminant analysis was 94.3%; that included 97.5% of the clinical groups and 84.6% of the suspected malingerers. Results of the discriminant analysis with suspected malingerers were generally comparable to results with the simulators when contrasted to the same clinical samples.

Validation by Other Investigators. Connell (1991) tested the SIRS with 60 offenders (30 simulators and 30 honest responders) who were compared to 30 psychotic inpatients with highly significant differences on the primary scales. Unfortunately, he conducted a discriminant analysis on all three groups, rather than attempting to distinguish simulators from offender and patient samples.[6] In spite of this serious limitation, the discriminant analysis identified

---

[4]The sole exception was the SEL scale in the Rogers, Gillis, Dickins, and Bagby (1991) study.

[5]Although some fluctuations were observed in the classification of simulators and patients across the two studies, the purpose of the discriminant analysis, to provide evidence of construct validity, was still achieved. Issues of classification rates are addressed in the section on Clinical Applications.

[6]The purpose of the SIRS is to detect feigners, not to differentiate between offender and patient groups responding honestly.

23 of 30 simulators and 57 of 60 honest responders, for an overall classification rate of 88.9%.

Kropp (1992) addressed whether offenders with a high level of psychopathy as measured by the Psychopathy Checklist–Screening Version (PCL-SV; Hare, Cox, & Hart, 1989) would be more effective at feigning mental disorders than those with low PCL-SV scores. To this end, 100 male offenders were divided into groups of 50 high and 50 low psychopaths, who were randomly assigned to honest and malingering conditions. Results indicated that high levels of psychopathy did not generally improve the ability of the offenders to feign.[7] Highly significant differences were found in the predicted direction for all eight of the primary scales. Moreover, the SIRS appeared nonthreatening to simulators; approximately 90% of the feigning subjects believed that they had been successful at feigning mental illness.

Linblad (1993) conducted a within-subjects design using 66 participants recruited from correctional and forensic psychiatric settings. He compared three groups: (a) offenders without a mental health history, (b) forensic patients hospitalized with a primary diagnosis of a major mental illness, and (c) forensic patients hospitalized with a primary diagnosis of a personality disorder. Across samples, the results indicated highly significant differences on the primary scales, in the predicted direction. When the SIRS was combined with the MMPI-2, a very high rate of classification was achieved (95.5%). Experience as a psychiatric patient did not appear to improve simulators' ability to feign. In a finding similar to that of the Kropp study (1992), most simulators (77.6%) believed that they had successfully fooled both the SIRS and the MMPI-2.

Kurtz and Meyer (1994) tested the relative effectiveness of the SIRS, MMPI-2, and M Test (Beaber, Marston, Michelli, & Millws, 1985) in detecting coached inmates who feigned psychosis. They found that the SIRS (88.9%) was significantly more effective than the MMPI-2 (81.3%) or the M Test (< 75.0%). Indeed, the data for the MMPI-2 was particularly worrisome: a majority of the patients under the honest condition were misclassified as malingerers. Combining the SIRS with either the MMPI-2 or the M Test did not add to the incremental validity. The combined classification rates were nearly identical to the accuracy of the SIRS alone (i.e., 90.0% vs. 88.9%). These data suggest the superiority of the SIRS in the classification of malingerers in correctional settings.

Gothard (1993) performed an elaborate study of the SIRS with 60 offenders (30 simulators and 30 honest responders) who were compared to 48 patients referred for evaluations of their competency to stand trial. In addition, seven malingerers were independently identified and included as a known-groups component to the study. Like Kurtz and Meyer, Gothard established highly significant differences between honest responders (patients and controls) and feigners (simulators and malingerers) on each of the primary scales. With the use of three or more scales in the probable feigning range (established criterion by Rogers, Bagby, et al., 1992), the overall classification rate was 97%. The convergence between simulators and malingerers is very encouraging in this combination of

---

[7]Interestingly, when offenders under the honest condition were asked questions about whether they had malingered in the past, those with high psychopathy were more likely to acknowledge prior attempts.

simulation and known-groups design. Unlike earlier research, however, this study found that only a minority (24%) believed they had successfully fooled the SIRS.

Convergent Validity. Rogers, Gillis, Dickens, et al. (1991) established strong correlations between the SIRS and MMPI fake-bad indicators, with nearly all correlations (97.5%) at 60 or higher. Linblad (1993) found parallel differences between the SIRS and the MMPI-2, although he did not report any correlations between the two measures. Convergent results have also been reported (see Connell, 1991; Gothard, 1993; Kropp, 1992; Linblad, 1993; Rogers, Gillis, Dickens, et al., 1991) between the SIRS and the M Test (Beaber et al., 1985), a screening measure of feigned psychosis. Although many studies did not report correlations, parallel differences were consistently observed across criterion groups. Rogers, Bagby, et al. (1992) compiled data from earlier studies on 234 SIRS and M Tests. They found low to moderate correlations between SIRS primary scales and the M Test subscales: $M_{confusion}$, median $r = .51$; $M_{malingering}$, median $r = .26$; $M_{schizophrenia}$, median $r = .19$. These findings offer modest evidence of convergent validity.[8]

Rogers, Bagby, et al. (1992) performed two separate principal components analyses (PCA) with varimax rotation on feigners (simulators and malingerers) and honest responders (patients, offenders, and community and university subjects). With feigners, a single factor accounted for most of the variance (49.5%) and indicated one general dimension for the assessment of faked mental illness. The other two factors addressed defensiveness (16.8%) and dishonesty/inconsistency (10.5%). The factor analysis for honest responders was divided into non-bizarre faking (50.4%), bizarre faking (14.5%), and dishonesty/inconsistency (10.6%). Gothard (1993) performed a subsequent PCA with both feigners and honest responders. This PCA resulted in one general dimension of faking (approximately 63% of the variance) and a second factor possibly associated with defensiveness (approximately 8%). Overall, these results would suggest one general factor (50 – 60% of the variance) for feigning, with positive loadings from all the primary scales.[9]

Generalizability

An important element of scale validation is the generalizability of results across sociodemographic backgrounds, clinical status of patients, and the range of assessment settings. Rogers, Bagby, et al. (1992) examined the comparability of classification rules for 103 females and 299 males from the validation studies. Overall, the classification rates for nonclinical samples responding honestly remained similar. For the clinical samples, the Subtle Symptoms scale appeared to classify more female patients (15.8%) in the probable feigning category than male patients. Combined across honest responders, the specificity for individual primary scales in the probable feigning range remained identical for both genders at 97.6%. The sensitivity for individual primary scales was slightly higher for females (62.3%) than for males (56.3%).

---

[8]Only the first two subscales are supposed to be associated with malingering.

[9]The sole exception was found in the PCA of honest responders, in which the Improbable/Absurd scale loaded on the second factor (i.e., bizarre feigning dimension).

Two studies have examined the generalizability of the SIRS with minorities. Connell (1991) performed a MANOVA on 30 African-American and 60 White subjects and found no significant differences due to race. Gothard (1993) reported a very high classification rate in a diverse sample that included 31 African-Americans and 13 Hispanics in her study of feigning and competency to stand trial. The generalizability of the SIRS with other minority groups has not been investigated.

Rogers, Bagby, et al. (1992) investigated the comparative utility of the SIRS in correctional and noncorrectional settings. They found that the specificity rates remained similar (97.1% for correctional and 98.5% for noncorrectional settings) for individual primary scales. The sensitivity of individual scales was slightly higher for correctional (60.1%) and noncorrectional (53.9%) subjects.

The coaching of subjects has no effect on specificity of individual primary scales, but does cause a decrement in sensitivity from 65.2% to 49.1% of individual scales (see Rogers, Bagby, et al., 1992). Moreover, experience as a psychiatric patient does not appear to improve subjects' ability to elude detection (see Linblad, 1992). Finally, persons with APD (Rogers, Gillis, & Bagby, 1990) and high levels of psychopathy (Kropp, 1992) do not show increased likelihood of remaining undetected on the SIRS.

For the purposes of this chapter, I also scored unpublished pilot data on nine forensic experts (psychologists and psychiatrists) who attempted to feign mental disorders on the SIRS. In reviewing their protocols, five of the nine were designated as malingering (M number of primary scales in the probable feigning range was 3.8) and an additional three were placed in the indeterminate range. Only one expert (11.1%) was miscategorized on the SIRS as an "honest responder." These preliminary data suggest that the majority of highly experienced forensic experts will be correctly identified as feigning, although some are likely to be placed in the indeterminate range.[10]

Clinical Applications

Many psychologists discount the importance of malingering and related response styles in their assessment and facilely assume that (a) feigning is very rare, and/or (b) feigning is easily detectable because of its dramatic and highly atypical presentation. Neither of these assumptions is supported by the available data. A recent survey of 320 forensic experts (96% were psychologists) by Rogers, Sewell, and Goldstein (in press) estimated the prevalence of malingering to be 15.7% of forensic and 7.4% of nonforensic evaluations. While these estimates may be skewed for nonforensic assessments,[11] the problem of feigning is clearly not rare. Moreover, attempts by psychologists to detect feigning by

---

[10]Interestingly, the one expert who was miscategorized as an honest responder endorsed relatively few symptoms (bogus or bona fide). His case represents the nettling dilemma for many malingerers: If very few symptoms are feigned, then the likelihood of detection decreases dramatically. By the same token, if very few symptoms are feigned, then the likelihood of achieving an external goal (e.g., compensation) also decreases dramatically.

[11]Forensic experts, because of their expertise in complicated evaluations, may be referred a greater proportion of cases than other psychologists and psychiatrists where feigning is suspected.

employing their traditional assessment methods do not appear to be effective (see Rogers, Harrell, & Liff, 1993).

The assessment of malingering and related response styles is a critical determination with far-reaching ramifications. For bonafide patients, errors in classification may preclude the provision of mental health services and other benefits. For mental health services, those feigning mental illness utilize important resources. As noted in the SIRS manual, any conclusions regarding feigning must be based on a multi-source and multimethod approach. The SIRS may form an important component of this approach.

The validation of the SIRS has established it as a highly reliable measure that has been cross-validated on diverse populations. Because of its extensive validation, the SIRS should be employed in clinical and forensic cases where the possibility exists that some or all of the patient's presentation is feigned. Psychologists must be aware that substantial numbers of malingerers also have coexisting mental disorders. While the SIRS and other measures may assist psychologists in identifying response styles, the diagnostic task remains to establish which disorders are present with each patient.

A distinction has been made by the *DSM-III-R* and *DSM-IV* between factitious disorders and malingering: Factitious disorders are distinguished from malingering by motivation. Factitial patients are assumed to be motivated by desire to assume a "sick" role, while malingerers are apparently motivated by other external incentives. As observed by Rogers, Bagby, and Rector (1989), attempts to establish motivation are thwarted by the patient's obvious distortions and the competing theories for his/her feigning. More explicitly, if we cannot trust the patient's self-reporting, how can we rely on his/her account of motives? Conversely, should we willy-nilly assume, from the context of the evaluation, the patient's motivation? Following this argument, a *per saltum* inference that all patients in personal injury cases are motivated to feign by financial incentives is logically and empirically insupportable.

The clinical usefulness of the SIRS is unaffected by the *DSM-IV* revision. First, *DSM-IV* does not offer formal inclusion and exclusion criteria for malingering. Second, the indices provided by *DSM-IV* for malingering are identical to those presented in *DSM-III-R*. The criteria for factitious disorders have included minor changes in wording which do not appear to affect the diagnosis. A useful modification was made in subtyping factitious disorders which stresses in *DSM-IV* establishing the predominance of psychological or physical symptoms rather than attempting to rigidly dichotomize the two subtypes.

Preliminary data of the SIRS by Rogers, Bagby, and Vincent (in press) suggest substantial overlap between malingerers and patients with Factitious Disorders with Predominantly Psychological Signs and Symptoms (FDPS). They found (also see Rogers, Bagby, et al., 1992, p. 26), however, that some malingerers had marked elevations on primary scales that were not generally observed in factitial patients. For example, 50% of malingerers had Blatent Symptoms scores above 13, as compared to 12.5% of FDPS patients. Moreover, malingerers tended to be less consistent in their presentations, with 48.5% scoring higher than 6 on the Inconsistency scale, in contrast to 10.0% of FDPS patients. However, the real diagnostic task is to attempt to establish the patient's past and current relationships with doctors and health care systems. If the patient's admiration of and dependency on health care professionals can be firmly established, at least one important component of factitial disorders can be determined. The psychologist is then left to consider issues of secondary gain and other external benefits to the patient (e.g., disability insurance, removal of household responsibilities) while hospitalized.

The SIRS, as well as all other standardized measures of feigning, has limited usefulness in patients who are untestable. Fortunately, most of such cases are hospitalized and may be observed extensively to evaluate whether grossly disorganized speech or bizarre and highly regressed behavior (e.g., smearing and eating feces) are feigned or bona fide. Once patients are stabilized, the SIRS has an advantage over paper-and-pencil methods because the psychologist presents the questions and records the responses, thus minimizing administration problems. As a guideline for untestable patients, psychologists are instructed to discontinue testing if more than 15 minutes are spent on the first set of detailed inquiries. In this case, for whatever reason, the administration is obviously bogged down and unlikely to be following the standardized procedure.

The major advantages of the SIRS are summarized in Table 12.1. With respect to its validation, the SIRS is clearly superior to other specialized measures, such as the M Test (Beaber et al., 1985) and the SLAM test (Smith, 1990). The SIRS is highly reliable and clearly discriminates among criterion groups.

Psychologists often compare the efficacy of the SIRS to the validity scales of the MMPI and the MMPI-2. The SIRS has one major advantage over the MMPI/MMPI-2 in test validation and two advantages in clinical interpretation. The SIRS has been cross-validated with a known-groups design that employed suspected malingerers. In contrast, the MMPI (see Roman, Tuley, Villanueva, & Mitchell, 1990) and the MMPI-2 (see Lees-Haley, English, & Glenn, 1991) have only isolated studies of suspected malingerers that produced different results from MMPI/MMPI-2 simulation research.

The SIRS also has the advantage of establishing stable cutting scores that appear to be effective across a spectrum of feigned disorders and a diverse group of clinical and forensic settings. In comparison, the MMPI/MMPI-2 has been plagued with problems in establishing stable cutting scores. A meta-analytic study of the MMPI by Berry, Baer, and Harris (1991) found an extraordinary range of cutting scores. For example, optimal cutting scores for the F scale ranged from > 9 to > 34. Similarly, Rogers, Sewell, and Salekin (in press) reported in a meta-analytic study of the MMPI-2 a consistent lack of convergence in feigning studies. Again, cutting scores for F scale ranged widely from > 17 to > 30. With the SIRS, stable cutting scores greatly facilitate clinical interpretation.

A third advantage of the SIRS over the MMPI/MMPI-2 is that its interpretation is not confounded by alternative explanations. With the MMPI/MMPI-2, possible explanations for elevated fake-bad indicators include lack of reading comprehension, compromised attention, and severe mental illness. Because of its interview format, literacy problems are eliminated in the SIRS. Because of its relatively brief, interactive format, problems with attentionality are greatly reduced. Because of its systematic validation with inpatient and outpatient comparison samples, problems with misclassifying patients as feigners are minimized. In contrast, most of the fake-bad indicators of the MMPI/MMPI-2 were originally developed by distinguishing simulators from nonclinical controls (see Rogers, Sewell, et al., in press). Therefore, we should not be surprised about problems with these same scales in discriminating malingerers from psychiatric patients. As an illustration of this point, the recent research by Kurtz and Meyer (1994) found that the MMPI-2 had an unacceptably high false-positive rate of 60.0%.

Table 12.1
Advantages and Limitations of the Structured Interview of Reported Symptoms (SIRS)

Advantages

1. Interrater reliability

   Because of standardization, the SIRS is a highly reliable structured interview that produces virtually the same results when administered by mental health professionals or paraprofessionals with sufficient training.

2. Validation with simulation and known-groups design

   The SIRS is distinguished from other measures, such as the MMPI and MMPI-2, in providing scales that have been cross-validated by both analogue and known-groups designs. This approach combines the rigor of simulation studies with the clinical relevance of known-group research with suspected malingerers.

3. Stable cutting scores

   The SIRS cutting scores appear to be both stable and effective in classifying those persons feigning disorders.

4. Generalizable to minorities

   Although further studies are recommended, the SIRS has distinguished itself from other measures of malingering by its attention to minority status.

5. Specific information about individual patient's style of feigning

   An important feature of the SIRS, beyond the classification of feigning and honest responding, is its attention to the description of response styles. For example, treating psychologists may choose different interventions with patients who simply exaggerate the severity of their symptoms, as opposed to other patients who fabricate preposterous or incongruous symptoms.

Limitations

1. Neuropsychological impairment

   Although certain items were placed on the SIRS for the expressed purpose of evaluating feigned cognitive deficits, the SIRS has not been validated with those purporting severe intellectual or neuropsychological impairment.

2. Adolescent populations

   Adolescents have often evidenced atypical clinical presentations and responses to validity indicators on the MMPI (see Herkov, Archer, & Gordon, 1991). The usefulness of the SIRS with this population has yet to be fully investigated.

The purpose of this comparison is the delineation of the differences between the SIRS and the MMPI/MMPI-2 to rebut the frequent comment that the MMPI/MMPI-2 "covers the same ground" as the SIRS. Psychologists must decide which measures to employ to address the clinical needs of each individual case. As opposed to an either/or approach to the differences between the SIRS and the MMPI/MMPI-2, I would advocate the general employment of both as part of a multimethod assessment of possible feigning.

The testing of minorities is facilitated with the SIRS, since available research suggests that the SIRS is equally effective with both African-Americans and Whites. Psychologists, sensitive to ethnic and cultural issues, are likely to choose the SIRS as the only feigning measure to have addressed possible differences due to race.

The final advantage of the SIRS is its provision of specific information about response styles. As noted in Table 12.1, psychologists are able to describe characteristics of a particular patient's style of feigning. Knowing whether a patient in treatment is likely to be nonselective in symptom presentation, exaggerate the severity of genuine symptoms, or be inconsistent in self-reporting may assist the psychologist in assessment and subsequent interventions.

The presence of malingering does not preclude treatment, but may complicate the process of accurately assessing current diagnosis and treatment effectiveness. Whether the exaggeration of psychological problems represents a "cry for help" (i.e., strong motivation) or a breakdown/manipulation of the therapeutic relationship (i.e., low motivation) has not been explicated and likely varies from case to case. Unpublished data on the SIRS (Rogers, Bagby, & Prendergast, 1993) would suggest that a significant minority of chronic schizophrenic patients tend to be unreliable in their presentation and may dissimulate some of their symptoms. In spite of this, these patients continue to be involved in treatment. As a general guideline, I would recommend a frank but nonconfrontational discussion of the results and a sincere attempt to include the feigning patient in treatment decisions.

Two limitations of the SIRS are its circumscribed applications to cases of feigned cognitive deficits and adolescent populations. Rogers, Harrell, and Liff (1993) summarized the differences in feigning mental disorders versus intellectual and neuropsychological impairment. In the former case, the patient must fabricate or grossly exaggerate psychological symptoms in a coherent and convincing manner. In the latter instance, the patient typically denies or minimizes cognitive and perceptual abilities. Therefore, the detection strategies must accommodate the style of feigning. At present, no studies have been conducted with the SIRS and feigned cognitive impairment.

One circumscribed application of the SIRS does exist in the assessment of simulated cognitive impairment. Some individuals also feign concomitant psychological symptoms as associated features or sequelae of their putative cognitive impairment. In these instances, the SIRS can be used to assess the plausibility of these psychological symptoms. However, even if evidence of feigning is clearly demonstrated for associated symptoms, it provides only indirect evidence regarding the authenticity of the purported cognitive impairment. In other words, the SIRS cannot be used to comment directly on feigned cognitive impairment.

The second limitation of the SIRS is the lack of validity data on its usefulness with adolescent populations. Limited research on the MMPI (see Herkov, Archer, & Gordon, 1991) has indicated that adolescents may respond to validity-scale items differently from their adult counterparts. For example, Butcher and Williams (1992, p. 212) found that adolescent males and females generally manifested moderate elevations on scale *F* (i.e., *M* scores of approximately 70) when scored on MMPI-2 adult norms. Research is needed with the SIRS and MMPI-2 to investigate their usefulness with adolescents.

In summary, the clinical data clearly support the use of the SIRS in the evaluation of malingering and related response styles. Comprehensive assessments of feigning integrate structured interview data from the SIRS with MMPI/MMPI-2, traditional interviews (Cornell & Hawk, 1989), and other relevant data from patients' backgrounds. As a focused interview, the SIRS provides extensive data on the extent and style of feigning. Beyond its intended scope, the SIRS offers relatively little information of diagnostic relevance.[12]

---

[12]To maximize the differentiation between feigners and bona fide patients, SIRS items were generated that minimized symptom endorsement by patients responding honestly. As a result, the SIRS is unlikely to facilitate differential diagnosis.

13

Other Structured Interviews for Specific Disorders

Structured interviews have been developed to address many specific disorders (Wiens, 1990). Many such efforts were targeted at particular research questions and lack the necessary validation to be considered in this relatively brief chapter. Instead of attempting an encyclopedic coverage, I will focus on recent measures that are likely to have (a) broad appeal to psychologists, and (b) some evidence of psychometric rigor.

The following structured interviews will be considered: the Structured Clinical Interview for *DSM-IV*–Dissociative Disorders (SCID-D; Steinberg, 1993), the Comprehensive Drinker Profile (CDP; Marlatt & Miller, 1984), the Anxiety Disorders Interview Schedule (ADIS; DiNardo, O'Brien, Barlow, Waddell, & Blanchard, 1982), the Psychosocial Pain Inventory (PSPI; Heaton, Lehman, & Getto, 1980), and the Eating Disorder Examination (EDE; Cooper & Fairburn, 1987). The organization of each structured interview will follow the standard outline: (a) description, (b) reliability and validity, and (c) clinical applications.

Structured Clinical Interview for *DSM-IV*– Dissociative Disorders (SCID-D)

Description

The Structured Clinical Interview for *DSM-IV*–Dissociative Disorders (SCID-D) was first developed by Steinberg in 1985 and was involved in field studies from 1989 to 1992. With the advent of the *DSM-IV*, the SCID-D was subsequently modified to reflect changes in inclusion criteria for dissociative disorders (Steinberg, 1993). The SCID-D is a semistructured interview which may be administered alone or in conjunction with the full SCID (Spitzer et al., 1990b).

The SCID-D is organized into eight sections: Psychiatric History, Amnesia, Depersonalization, Derealization, Identity Confusion, Identity Alteration, Associated Features of Identity Disturbance, and Follow-Up Sections. Questions are organized into standard questions, branching questions, and optional probes. Optional probes are identified either by (a) asterisks (inquiries that provide additional clinical data not necessary for diagnosis) or by (b) placement in parentheses (inquiries intended to provide clarification of ambiguous responses).

Multiple rating systems are employed by the SCID-D on 277 items. Symptoms are classified into three categories: 1 for "absent," 3 for "present," and

4 for "inconsistent information." Obviously, no provision is made for subclinical ratings. Characteristics of symptoms are rated on 5- or 6-point scales with respect to frequency or onset. A summary sheet is provided to facilitate diagnosis.

Reliability and Validity

Steinberg, Rounsaville, and Cicchetti (1990) performed an interrater reliability study with 48 outpatients, of whom approximately one-half had dissociative disorders. They found that the SCID-D yielded excellent reliability for the two disorders that were adequately represented: multiple personality disorder (κ = .90) and dissociative disorder NOS (κ =.82). Agreement of symptom scales was generally good (weighted κs = .59 – .88, median = .78).

Steinberg (1992; summarized in Steinberg, 1993, in press-a) conducted a large-scale test-retest reliability study using 140 psychiatric patients from three research centers who showed a wide range of psychiatric disorders. In addition, the diagnostic stability of 50 patients was assessed by a third SCID-D interview at a 6-month interval. Steinberg reported that the reliability coefficients were good to excellent for the five core dissociative symptoms as well as for dissociative diagnoses. Unfortunately, the precise estimates are not published, which makes independent examination of the reliability coefficients impossible.

Several other investigators (Boon & Draijer, 1991; Goff, Olin, Jenike, Baer, & Buttolph, 1992) have also examined SCID-D reliability. Boon and Draijer (1991) employed a Dutch translation of the SCID-D with 44 patients who had been referred for an evaluation of dissociative symptoms. With approximately 50% of the sample warranting a diagnosis of either multiple personality disorder or dissociative disorder NOS, the two authors achieved nearly perfect agreement on diagnosis (97.7%), but did not report any reliability estimates. Goff et al. (1992) conducted a small study of SCID-D interrater reliability using a sample of 16 patients with obsessive-compulsive disorders (OCD) and dissociative symptoms. For the three disorders with any representation, the kappas were .66, .73, and 1.00. More impressive were the reliability coefficients for the severity of dissociative symptoms, which ranged from .85 to .96, with a median of .92. Finally, Bremmer, Steinberg, Southwick, Johnson, and Charney (1993) achieved nearly perfect agreement on total SCID-D scores (ICC = .95) for 55 Vietnam veteran patients.

Steinberg et al. (1990), in the first validity study, examined differences in symptom scores for patients with and without dissociative disorders and found significant differences both for symptoms and for total scores. This study did not address the discriminant validity of the SCID-D in differentiating among specific dissociative disorders.

Boon and Draijer (1991) found highly significant differences, in the expected direction, for specific symptoms on the SCID-D. Given the fact that the SCID-D was employed in making the diagnoses, these differences are not surprising. As modest evidence of convergent validity, Goff et al. (1992) examined the dissociative symptoms of OCD patients who scored high on the Dissociative Experiences Scale (DES; Bernstein & Putnam, 1986) and found that approximately one-half had symptoms of depersonalization, amnesia, and identity confusion.[1]

---

[1]Without comparisons to low scorers on the DES, the interpretation of this finding is very limited.

Steinberg (in press-b) and Steinberg, Cicchetti, Buchanan, Hall, and Rounsaville (1993) summarized data on the discriminant validity of the SCID-D with specific dissociative disorders. Comparisons of SCID-D core symptoms with clinical diagnosis indicated predicted symptom patterns. In addition, patients with dissociative disorders evidenced greater severity on these symptoms (*M*s = 3.0 – 3.7) than patients with other disorders (1.7 – 2.2) or normal controls (0 – 1.4). While obviously significant, statistical comparisons with sensitivity and specificity rates were not presented.

Clinical Applications

The SCID-D would appear to be the semistructured interview of choice in the investigation of dissociative disorders. Steinberg and her colleagues have devoted considerable effort to developing a highly standardized tool to assess dissociative disorders. As noted by Steinberg (in press-a), the alternative measures may be useful in examining dimensions of dissociative experiences but are limited in their diagnostic applications. The SCID-D is a relatively new diagnostic interview that certainly deserves further reliability and validity studies. The present status of the literature is very encouraging with respect to interrater reliability and discriminant validity.

The SCID-D was developed to be compatible with the *DSM-IV* and appears to be completely congruent with *DSM-IV* criteria for dissociative disorders. In addition, the SCID-D includes all the criteria for the provisional diagnosis of dissociative trance disorder.

My endorsement of the SCID-D for clinical practice is largely pragmatic. Although I would like to see further research by other investigators, as well as a full reporting of all reliability and validity data, I find the SCID-D to be presently the best measure available for dissociative disorders. I would, therefore, recommend its use in cases where dissociative disorders are suspected. Clinicians may wish to use self-report measures, such as the DES and the Questionnaire of Experiences of Dissociation (QED; Riley, 1988), for screening measures. As noted by Gilbertson, et al. (1992), these self-report measures are very vulnerable to feigning.

An important feature of the SCID-D is the attention paid to integrating clinical data and writing a comprehensive report. Steinberg et al. (1993) and Steinberg, Cicchetti, et al. (1993) show an enviable thoroughness in describing how the SCID-D is employed and in ensuring that clinical formulations are coherent and well-reasoned.

The limitations of the SCID-D to clinical practice are readily apparent. As previously noted, more data are needed in detailing its reliability and validity. In addition, the reported studies do not describe the psychometric characteristics of associated symptoms and features. In other words, we know very little about the SCID-D items that address the onset and frequency and whether they reliably assess these important dimensions of dissociative disorders.

Steinberg, Bancroft, and Buchanan (1993) discussed the forensic applications of the SCID-D in evaluating dissociative disorders and, particularly, multiple personality disorder in criminal cases. They concluded that the SCID-D is particularly well-suited for such evaluations based on (a) good interrater reliability,

(b) standardized format that allows cross-comparisons, and (c) longitudinal perspective which enables an investigation of the course of the dissociative disorder. This final feature might also aid in the assessment of malingering, since patients would need to create a logical history, not just prominent symptoms at the time of the offense. Moreover, the SCID-D would facilitate the comparison of informant and self-reports in retrospective assessments (e.g., insanity and personal injury).

Comprehensive Drinker Profile (CDP)

Description

Marlatt and Miller (1984) developed the Comprehensive Drinker Profile (CDP) as a structured interview to assess alcoholism and potential for alcoholic treatment. In addition, Miller and Marlatt (1987) devised several related measures: an abbreviated version (Brief Drinker Profile), a treatment outcome version (Follow-up Drinker Profile), and a corroborative version (Collateral Interview Form).

The CDP is composed of 88 items, many of which have multiple subcomponents, and is organized into three sections: demographic information (including family, employment, and educational history), drinking history (alcohol consumption, beverage preference, alcohol-related life problems, drinking settings, other substance abuse, and related medical history), and motivational information (reasons and effects of drinking, and motivation for treatment). Most inquiries require nominal ratings (presence or absence). One notable exception is the computation of alcohol consumption, which is calculated in Standard Ethanol Content (SEC) units across days and episodes. From these data, estimates of blood alcohol concentrations (BAC) are derived. Embedded in the alcohol-related problems are two scales: the Michigan Alcoholism Screening Test (MAST; Selzer, 1971) and a 12-item Ph score for physical dependence.

Reliability and Validity

Miller, Crawford, and Taylor (1979) summarized the level of agreement on ethanol consumption between alcoholics and corroborative reports, using an early version of the CDP. Across four studies, they found modest correlations at intake (median r = .44, range = .06 – .64), with substantial increases at the completion of treatment (median r = .53, range = .42 – .80), and good agreement at a 3-month follow-up (median r = .72, range = .68 – .92). Interestingly, informants were as likely to overestimate as underestimate alcohol consumption. Two issues constrain the generalizability of these findings: First, alcoholics were aware that an informant would be used, which may account for an increasing accuracy in self-reporting. Second, three of the four studies involved self-referred alcoholics, who may be more accurate than others in self-reporting.[2]

Miller, Leckman, Delaney, and Tinkcom (1992) employed the CDP in a treatment outcome study of 140 alcoholics. In a subsample of 116 subjects,

---

[2]The one sample that included court-referred alcoholics (37.0%) had substantially lower correlations.

collateral reports of weekly alcohol consumption were as high as .76.[3] Cross-informant estimates of BAC and alcohol-related problems were modest (*r*s = .39 and .38, respectively). As evidence of interrater reliability, 26 CDP interviews were audiotaped and independently rated on 22 quantitative indices, with excellent agreement (*r*s = .86 – 1.00).

Brown and Miller (in press) examined cross-informant agreement for 28 patients admitted to a private psychiatric facility for alcohol dependence. They found very high rates of agreement for SEC (.91 at intake and .96 at follow-up) and good agreement on BAC (.69 and .94). In contrast, Miller, Benefield, and Tonigan (1992) found low level of agreement for problem drinkers' weekly consumption at intake (*r* = .31) and a moderate level at a 12-month follow-up (*r* = .65).

In summary, the single study of interrater reliability indicated a high level of agreement among clinicians. In contrast, studies of cross-informant consistency appear to be mixed in their results. In general, however, self-referred clients who continue in treatment are likely to evidence a good to high level of agreement with their chosen informants. However, alcoholics at intake, particularly those who are not self-referred, are likely to evidence little correspondence with their informants.

An interesting question is whether the knowledge that an informant will be used "keeps alcoholics honest." Preliminary data by Graber and Miller (1988) on 24 self-referred alcoholics were encouraging, since no significant differences were found, for those underestimating alcohol use, between those aware that an informant would be used and those unaware.[4] Given the paucity of data on this critical issue, psychologists may elect to use openly corroborative sources of data.

Test manuals for the CDP (Miller & Marlatt, 1984, 1987) do not directly address validity. From one perspective, the convergence of self-report and informant data could be perceived as convergent validity, particularly with respect to alcohol consumption and peak BAC. However, evidence of how different scores on the CDP result in dissimilar outcomes would provide useful diagnostic validity. In this regard, a substantial body of treatment literature exists (e.g., Bien, Miller, & Boroughs, 1993; Harris & Miller, 1990; Miller, 1978; Miller & Dougher, 1989; Miller, Gribskov, & Mortell, 1981; Miller, Sovereign, & Krege, 1988; Miller & Taylor, 1980; Miller, Taylor, & West, 1980), of which several studies suggest that persons with higher SEC and BAC scores at intake, in spite of treatment improvement, often continue to yield poorer results than those with less alcohol consumption. Miller, Hedrick, and Taylor (1983) found predicted changes in the alcohol-related life problems component of the CDP that appeared to be associated with concomitant decreases in alcohol use.

---

[3]In approximately two-thirds of the cases, more than one collateral report was available. In these instances, the researchers used only the largest estimates of alcohol consumption, thereby skewing the results.

[4]A chi-squared analysis of under- versus overestimation does not really address the issue of accuracy of self-reporting. A more pertinent issue is the degree of correspondence between the two reports, which could be tested through correlational procedures.

Research has also demonstrated that alcoholics' beliefs about drinking (e.g., Miller, Benefield, & Tonigan, 1992) and treatment goals (Graber & Miller, 1988) as measured by the CDP produced expected differences in treatment outcome. Moreover, these differences in outcome appear to be related to scores on the Alcoholism Use Inventory (AUI; Horn, Wanberg, & Foster, 1990). Miller, Leckman, et al. (1992) predicted long-term outcome through the integration of four earlier studies. In a discriminant analysis, they found that data from the CDP (i.e., Jellinek stage, self-acceptance of alcoholism, alcohol dependence, familial alcoholism, and intake goal) predicted long-term outcome. Interestingly, MAST scores at intake did not predict outcome.

Concurrent validity studies, with direct comparisons of the CDP and such diagnostic measures as the DIS and the SCID, would be most helpful. In addition, research on the CDP and self-report measures would provide important evidence of convergent validity. Such studies should include the AUI and the Substance Abuse Subtle Screening Inventory (SASSI; Miller, 1985). Studies with the SASSI would be particularly helpful, since research has suggested its efficacy with alcoholics denying their abuse.

Clinical Applications

The CDP appears to be particularly effective as an adjunct to treatment with self-referred alcoholics. A substantial literature describes its efficacy, especially as treatment continues, in accurately assessing alcohol use (SEC and BAL) and related life problems. Moreover, the CDP appears, at least in general terms, to document overall improvement and decreased likelihood of relapse.

The advent of *DSM-IV* is unlikely to have any adverse effect on the use of the CDP, which is more descriptive than diagnostic. In addition, the criteria for alcohol abuse and dependence have not changed substantially in the *DSM-IV*. The CDP provides adequate data for their diagnosis.

The focus of the CDP in documenting alcohol use by time of day, day of the week, and type of alcohol is likely to assist problem drinkers in not glossing over the amount of alcohol consumed. Without such structure, alcoholics are likely to overlook or disregard important elements of their drinking patterns. Of course, alcoholics who choose to grossly minimize their consumption are unlikely to be affected by this or any other structured interview. As a protection against minimization, psychologists may elect to routinely conduct corroborative interviews. As previously mentioned, data from the SASSI is encouraging with respect to its detection of underreporting. I recommend both corroborative CDPs and SASSIs with patients who are not self-referred.

The structure of the CDP allows the patient to develop his/her own goals with respect to drinking and to acknowledge its effects on personal and social functioning. In this respect, the simple administration of the CDP may set the stage for treatment interventions. I would see this as a chief advantage of the CDP over substance abuse components of Axis I interviews (e.g., the SCID). As a focused interview, the CDP obviously does not address complex issues of comorbidity in alcoholics. Therefore, psychologists may wish to screen patients for other mental disorders and employ the CDP in cases where alcohol abuse or dependence is the primary diagnosis.

Anxiety Disorders Interview Schedule (ADIS)

Description

The Anxiety Disorders Interview Schedule (ADIS) was developed by DiNardo and his colleagues (DiNardo et al., 1982) after the emergence of *DSM-III* to meet the following objectives: to provide differential diagnosis of anxiety disorders, to rule out other disorders (e.g., psychotic, substance abuse, and mood disorders), and to supply additional clinical data regarding anxiety (see DiNardo, O'Brien, Barlow, Waddell, & Blanchard, 1983). The ADIS was derived in part from other diagnostic interviews, notably the SADS and the PSE. In addition, items from the Hamilton Anxiety Scale (Hamilton, 1959) and the HDRS were also interspersed throughout the ADIS.

The ADIS is a semistructured interview which is organized by diagnosis (i.e., generalized anxiety disorder, PTSD, panic disorder, agoraphobia, simple and social phobias, and obsessive-compulsive disorder), with sections for ruling out depressive and manic episodes, substance abuse, and psychosis. Unlike most structured interviews, the ADIS does not use a consistent rating scale for all items; instead, the ratings of responses vary widely across the ADIS. Many symptoms are rated on a nominal (yes or no) scale. Symptoms integrated from the Hamilton scales are evaluated on 5-point scales (0 = none, 1 = mild, 2 = moderate, 3 = severe, 4 = very severe/grossly disabling). Questions related to phobias are scored on a similar 5-point scale that integrates the severity of the fear with the level of avoidance. Still other inquiries require descriptive responses which are not rated according to any quantitative criteria.

The responses to the ADIS are reviewed by an experienced clinician, who assigns diagnoses on the basis of *DSM-III* criteria. In addition, the Hamilton scales are scored according to standard criteria. Overall level of impairment is rated on an 8-point scale.

Reliability and Validity

DiNardo et al. (1983) conducted the original reliability study of the ADIS using 60 referrals to the Phobia and Anxiety Disorders Clinic. The design was a test-retest reliability with a variable interval (generally < 3 weeks) and the use of pairs of interviewers. For five anxiety disorders, the kappa coefficients ranged from .47 to .85 (median = .69). Clinicians also evidenced moderate reliability in diagnosing non-anxiety disorders (major depression, κ = .57; other disorders, κ = .69).

The ADIS was revised in 1985 (ADIS-R; DiNardo, O'Brien, Barlow, Waddell, & Blanchard, 1985), although it maintained the same basic structure. DiNardo and Barlow (1989; cited in Sanderson, DiNardo, Rapee, & Barlow, 1990), in an unpublished study, administered the ADIS-R to 125 consecutive patients in a test-retest design. They established generally high reliability for five anxiety disorders, with a range from .50 to .92 and a median of .86. Paradis, Friedman, Lazar, Grubea, and Kesselman (1992) examined interscorer reliability (i.e., ADIS-R protocols were evaluated by a second clinician) for 93 primarily African-American patients. Not surprisingly, the rate of agreement was high (median κ = .82).[5]

---

[5]As interscorer reliability, these findings merely reflect the ability of clinicians to take already recorded ADIS-R data and render a diagnosis on the basis of *DSM-III-R*.

In general, the two studies of test-retest reliability indicate a moderate to high level of agreement over variable intervals. These studies did not include patients with PTSD. Also, the samples appeared to be relatively homogeneous, with a high proportion of anxiety disorders (prevalence for combined studies of 83%), especially agoraphobia with panic attacks (n = 64, or 43% of all anxiety disorders). Additional research from other centers with more heterogeneous diagnostic groups would be helpful in confirming ADIS-R reliability.

One shortcoming of the DiNardo et al. (1983) study was the absence of patients with PTSD. To remedy this weakness, Blanchard, Gerardi, Kolb, and Barlow (1986) administered the ADIS to 43 male Vietnam combat veterans who were compared on clinical diagnosis by a psychiatrist experienced in evaluating PTSD. Although not a study of reliability, since different methods (ADIS vs. clinical interview) were employed, the agreement between the ADIS and the psychiatric diagnosis was very high (93.0%, κ = .86). Given the limited diagnostic task (PTSD vs. non-PTSD), this level of agreement is likely to be inflated. In addition, the use of a sole interviewer for the ADIS and a single psychiatrist for the criterion diagnosis severely constrains the generalizability of its results.

The initial validation of the ADIS (DiNardo et al., 1983) compared clinicians' ratings of severity to scores on the Hamilton Anxiety (r = .56) and Depression (r = .77) scales. These correlations are confounded, since the clinician was not blind to the Hamilton when completing the ADIS. This problem could have been reduced, but not eliminated by using the ADIS ratings of one interviewer compared with the Hamilton scores of the second interviewer.

Several studies (Barlow, DiNardo, B. B. Vermilyea, J. A. Vermilyea, & Blanchard, 1986; Sanderson et al., 1990) have employed the ADIS and ADIS-R in the examination of diagnostic overlap. For example, Barlow et al. (1986), in a study of 126 referrals to an anxiety disorder clinic, found that the majority also qualified for additional disorders, including phobias and depression. For example, of the 41 patients with agoraphobia, 18 qualified for other anxiety disorders and 16 for mood disorders. As evidence of construct validity, scores on the Hamilton anxiety scale were compared to specific diagnoses. As might be expected, more circumscribed disorders (simple and social phobias) had lower scores than their more pervasive counterparts (generalized anxiety, obsessive-compulsive disorder, and agoraphobia). Other self-report measures were also administered, including the State-Trait Anxiety Inventory (STAI; Spielberger, Gorsuch, & Lushene, 1970), the Middlesex (Crown & Crisp, 1966), the Fear Questionnaire (Marks & Mathews, 1978), the Cognitive and Somatic Anxiety Questionnaire (CASQ; Spielberger et al., 1970), and the Beck Depression Inventory (BDI). Summarizing across comparisons of 16 scale scores and seven diagnoses, several observations can be made: (a) the Fear Questionnaire offered specific empirical support for agoraphobia and partial support for social phobia; (b) differences on the Middlesex, STAI, and CASQ were relatively modest and often comparable to scores of depressed patients; and (c) with the exception of obsessive-compulsive disorder, anxiety patients received lower scores on the BDI than did depressed patients.

Sanderson et al. (1990) evaluated 130 anxiety-disordered patients with the ADIS-R to test for diagnostic overlap. They found that approximately 70% of patients qualified for an additional anxiety disorder and 33% for a mood disorder. Other Axis I and II disorders were not sufficiently evaluated to know how much additional overlap occurs. Combining the results of Barlow et al. (1986) and Sanderson et al. (1990), the diagnostic validity of anxiety disorders as measured by the ADIS is called into question, since inclusion and exclusion criteria do not appear to clearly differentiate specific disorders. Alternatively, since both studies were conducted at a specialized clinic, their samples may reflect more demanding and complicated cases and have limited generalizability to other out-patient samples.

In summary, like many structured interviews, the ADIS appears to assume that the *DSM-III* and *DSM-III-R* are gold standards of diagnosis. Unlike most other interviews, however, the ADIS has not been adequately compared to other diagnostic interviews or clinical diagnosis. Problems with diagnostic overlap are common with anxiety disorders and, at best, current studies provide only indirect evidence of diagnostic validity. Finally, the comparisons by Barlow et al. (1986) offer only modest evidence of convergent validity.

Clinical Applications

Because of limited ADIS validity data, psychologists may wish to consider more general diagnostic interviews with anxiety disorder sections, such as the SADS-LA and the SCID. However, the ADIS and ADIS-R provide a thorough review of anxiety symptoms in greater detail than that found on more general interviews. In addition, the ADIS method of assessing specific information regarding phobias and related symptoms is likely to facilitate clinical interventions. In addition, this same attention to detail may provide psychologists with specific information on the efficacy of treatment. The ADIS and ADIS-R would appear best suited for specialized treatment units where the emphasis is treatment of specific anxiety symptoms and associated problems rather than differential diagnosis. Although significant changes have been implemented in the *DSM-IV* anxiety disorders, the use of the ADIS and ADIS-R for descriptive and treatment purposes remains largely unaffected.

Psychosocial Pain Inventory (PSPI)

Description

Heaton et al. (1980) constructed the Psychosocial Pain Inventory (PSPI) as a semistructured interview to assess psychological and social factors in patients with chronic pain. As articulated by Getto and Heaton (1985), factors complicating treatment may include primary and secondary reinforcement (social, financial) for assuming the patient role, which interact with dimensions of personality, substance abuse, and iatrogenic influences.

The PSPI is composed of 25 items, many of which consist of multiple components. Most items are scored on a 4-point scale from 0 to 3, with higher scores reflecting increased severity. These scores are totaled and compared to the results of two validity studies that are summarized below. In general, scores that exceed 30 indicate a strong psychosocial component to chronic pain and suggest that customary medical interventions (medications, physical therapy, and surgery) are unlikely to be effective.

The PSPI addresses five general dimensions of pain and pain-related behavior. First, the PSPI assesses environmental stresses through the incorporation of the Social Adjustment Rating Scale (Holmes & Rahe, 1967), which is scored for three time periods: 6 months prior to the injury, 6 months prior to the most significant worsening of pain, and the last 6 months.[6] Second, home activities and the family's awareness and response to the patient's pain are evaluated. Third, treatments for pain, as well as the patient's initiated interventions, are considered. Fourth, the patient's prior work history and current disability status are assessed. Fifth, background information about previous medical and psychological problems, treatment, and substance abuse are investigated.

The PSPI is intended to be used in conjunction with other measures in a comprehensive assessment of pain and its correlates. For instance, Getto and Heaton (1985) advocate the use of the MMPI to assess psychopathology as it relates to pain. In this regard, MMPI elevations are taken into consideration in scoring several responses on the PSPI. In addition, the McGill Pain Questionnaire (Melzack, 1975) provides useful descriptive data on the range and severity of pain experiences.

Getto, Heaton, and Lehman (1983) conducted two studies of the PSPI and its ability to predict treatment outcome. In the first study, 35 patients (primarily with chronic lower back pain) were involved in standardized medical interventions. Nearly all the sample had elevated PSPI scores and failed to respond to treatment at a 9-month follow-up. Three who did respond to treatment were approximately two standard deviations below the sample's mean. In the second study, the PSPI was utilized for 32 patients who were evaluated for pain-related surgery. With a cutting score of 30, the PSPI accurately predicted 72.3% of treatment successes and 78.6% of treatment failures.

Reliability and Validity

Getto and Heaton (1985, p. 12) provide data on a small interrater reliability sample ($N = 24$). They reported high overall agreement on PSPI scores ($r = .98$) but no data on individual items. Unfortunately, we do not have a description of the sample or the procedures employed. Although no data are presented on internal consistency, Getto and Heaton (1985) related that the average item-to-scale correlation was .30.

Little research has been conducted on the PSPI and convergent measures of pain and psychopathology. As part of the standardization, Getto and Heaton (1985) administered the PSPI to 169 consecutive chronic pain patients evaluated at the University of Colorado Pain Clinic. As a component of the evaluation, patients were also given the McGill Pain Questionnaire and the MMPI. The relationship between described pain on the McGill (i.e., intensity and number of descriptors) and total PSPI score was very modest ($r = .26$). Likewise, the PSPI evidenced a few statistically significant but low correlations ($rs \leq .30$) with MMPI scales of F, K, and 1. Although higher correlations among the three measures

---

[6]The focus of these ratings is on how stress may affect pain. Therefore, life events that are caused by pain are supposed to be excluded. Given the multidimensionality of many stress events, this demarcation may sometimes be difficult to achieve.

would be desirable, the authors assert that these instruments measure different facets of pain and psychological impairment.

Clinical Applications

Wiens (1990, p. 335) described the PSPI as a "standardized and reliable method of evaluating a number of psychosocial factors considered important in maintaining and exacerbating chronic pain problems." Certainly, the PSPI offers a greater level of standardization than is typically found in pain evaluations. Data from a relatively small sample suggest that the total scores of the PSPI are reliable. No data are available on the individual ratings or the stability of ratings (test-retest reliability).

Probably the most disappointing dimension of PSPI validity is the absence of any further validation studies, either by its authors or by other investigators, during the last decade. Computer searches failed to reveal any cross-validation of the PSPI.

When should the PSPI be used in clinical practice? Pragmatically speaking, psychologists may wish to employ the PSPI as part of a battery in the assessment of chronic pain, particularly when medical interventions are being considered. Despite the lack of cross-validation, its cutting score may offer a tentative indicator with respect to the potential effectiveness of treatment. Unfortunately, the absence of any systematic research on high scorers and their response to psychological and behavioral treatment methods limits the usefulness of the PSPI. Nevertheless, in the absence of any rival measures, psychologists may find this standardized format useful.

High scorers on the PSPI may be exaggerating their problems, although this issue has not been formally investigated. Data from the standardization sample suggest that high PSPI scorers tend to have higher scores on F and lower scores on K than do low PSPI scorers. Therefore, psychologists may wish to look for corroborative data in addition to MMPI validity indices in cases of elevated PSPI scores. One reason, of course, for poor treatment response could be the use of interventions with bogus or exaggerated pain complaints.

Successive modifications (see APA, 1991) have occurred in the conceptualization and criteria for psychologically influenced pain: the *DSM-III* referred to this syndrome as "psychogenic pain disorder," which was subsequently broadened in *DSM-III-R* with changes in etiologic criteria. The diagnosis was most recently changed to "pain disorder," with psychological factors designated as having an important role in the onset, severity, exacerbation, or maintenance of the pain. Since the PSPI is not recommended for formal diagnoses, these changes should have only a peripheral effect on its circumscribed clinical application.

Eating Disorder Examination (EDE) and Related Measures

Description

Cooper and Fairburn (1987) developed the Eating Disorder Examination (EDE) as a semistructured interview for the assessment of psychopathology associated with eating disorders. Among the 62 ratings are items that address behavioral (e.g., diet, self-induced vomiting, and exercise) and attitudinal (preoccupation with food, fear of fatness, guilt about eating) dimensions of eating. With few exceptions, individual items are measured on a 7-point scale of increasing severity.

The EDE was refined through nine editions to improve the clarity of questions and the ability of individual items to differentiate among four criterion groups: (a) patients with anorexia nervosa, (b) patients with bulimia nervosa, (c) age-matched controls with current concerns about weight and shape, and (d) age-matched controls without such concerns. Because of problems of accurate long-term recall, the EDE is intended to assess only current (i.e., last 4 weeks) characteristics of eating disorders.

Reliability and Validity

Cooper and Fairburn (1987) reported very high interrater reliability for a small sample of three raters and 12 subjects. Although precise figures were not presented, the median *r* was clearly greater than .90, and perfect agreement was attained on 41.9% of the items. These high reliability estimates were corroborated by other investigators (see Wilson & Smith, 1989).

Validation of the EDE includes research on its relationship to criterion groups and related measures. For example, Garfinkel (1992) found that among 104 eating disordered-patients, most, as measured by the EDE, were overweight and overly concerned with physical shape. Similarly, Z. Cooper, P. J. Cooper, and Fairburn (1989) found highly significant differences between 100 eating-disordered patients and 42 controls on EDE subscales related to weight and shape concerns. Marcus, Smith, Santelli, and Kaye (1992) found highly significant differences between eating-disordered and control groups on the EDE subscales, although only one modest difference was observed between subgroups of eating disorders (i.e., obese binge eaters vs. bulimia nervosa patients).

Rosen, Vara, Wendt, and Leitenberg (1990) conducted an external validity study using 106 undergraduate females. From this and a previous study, 20 women were identified as suffering from bulimia nervosa and 29 women were selected as eating-restrained controls. As evidence of criterion-related validity, EDE results were related to eating records and caloric intake, although the correlations were often modest (< .40). EDE scales associated with weight and shape concerns were highly correlated with the Body Shape Questionnaire (P. J. Cooper, Taylor, Z. Cooper, & Fairburn, 1987).

Fitchner et al. (1991) compared the EDE to the Structured Interview for Anorexia and Bulimia Nervosa (SIAB) for a sample of 50 German residents referred to an eating disorders clinic. They found only modest correlations (see discussion of the SIAB).

Investigators have reported mixed results on the usefulness of the EDE in predicting treatment outcome. For example, Wilson and Eldredge (1991) divided eating-disordered patients into poor and good outcome categories as a result of 20 sessions of cognitive-behavioral treatment. They found that EDE scores were not related to outcome.[7] Employing pre- and postmeasures, Smith, Marcus, and Kaye (1992) found the EDE useful in recording changes that occurred as a result of cognitive-behavioral treatment.

Wilson, Nonas, and Rosenblum (1993) described a self-report version of the EDE, the Eating Disorder Examination–Questionnaire or EDE-Q. Results were compared for 31 binge eaters and 139 nonbinge eaters, with significant differences observed in the predicted directions. Unfortunately, no studies are reported which directly compare the EDE-Q with the EDE. Therefore, its comparability remains to be established.

Other Structured Interviews for Eating Disorders

A variety of structured and diagnostic interviews have been developed in the last decade for the assessment of eating disorders. These measures include supplements to general diagnostic interviews, such as the SADS (Schedule of Eating Disorders, Affective Disorders and Schizophrenia-L or EAT-SADS-L; Keller, Nielsen, Herzog, & Stasior, undated) and focused interviews such as the Clinical Eating Disorders Rating Instrument (CEDRI; Palmer, Christie, Cordle, Davis, & Kedrick, 1987) and the SIAB (Fitchner et al., 1991).

The CEDRI (Palmer et al., 1987) is a semistructured interview composed of 31 ratings, of which 22 items cover symptomatology associated with eating disorders. The CEDRI was tested in two small reliability studies, one with 10 and one with 11 female subjects. Employing four raters, the authors established Kendall's coefficients of concordance that ranged from .40 to 1.00. For the 22 items that specifically address eating-disorders symptomatology, the median coefficient was .88, indicating excellent agreement.

The SIAB (Fitchner et al., 1991) was constructed to assess a broader range of individual and family psychopathology than is found on most eating disorder measures. Psychopathology is evaluated with reference to both *DSM-III-R* and ICD-10 diagnoses. The SIAB is organized into two components: the SIAB-P for psychopathology (62 items) and the SIAB-FAM for family interaction and pathology (25 items). Items are scored on a 5-point scale and interpreted in relationship to diagnosis and factor scores. SIAB reliability was established by using six videotapes and six undergraduate interviewers to assess interrater reliability. Kendall's coefficient of concordance was employed across all items, with high levels of agreement obtained for past (.96) and present (.94) symptoms. Family pathology was also highly reliable (i.e., past symptoms = .84 and present symptoms = .89).

Examination of SIAB validity included a separate factor analysis of the SIAB-P with a sample of 347 eating-disordered patients from four clinics. Results indicated a six-factor solution was optimal, with items loading on the following dimensions and with negligible overlap: body image (12% of the variance), social integration (12%), depression (11%), anxiety/compulsion (7%), bulimic behavior (6%), and laxative abuse (5%). As evidence of convergent validity, the SIAB-P was

---

[7] Interestingly, improvement appeared to be related to overall level of psychopathology as measured by SCL-90; these scores were reduced in the successful patients. Therefore, the results may suggest a potential confound in testing the usefulness of the EDE.

correlated with the EDE, although the degree of association was generally modest (< .40).

Morgan and Russell (1975) developed the Morgan-Russell Assessment Schedule for evaluating treatment outcome in eating-disordered patients. In this brief measure, 14 ratings are performed on 5-point scales in covering symptoms associated with anorexia nervosa. According to Morgan and Hayward (1988), the interview may be helpful to busy clinicians in assessing overall recovery/ impairment in a simple but standardized manner. Strein, Ham, and Engeland (1992) provided initial data on the usefulness of the Morgan–Russell interview in assessing treatment drop-outs over a 4-year period. Its psychometric properties have not been formally evaluated.

Clinical Applications of the EDE and Related Interviews

The EDE, among focused interviews of eating disorders, stands out as a reliable diagnostic measure that parallels *DSM-III-R* criteria and may easily be adapted to *DSM-IV*. Although the EDE is described as the gold standard of eating disorders (e.g., Wilson et al., 1993), psychologists may wish to base their decisions regarding a gold standard on specific diagnosis, rather than on the complete category of eating disorders.

Validity data consistently demonstrate highly significant differences between eating-disordered and noneating-disordered subjects. Less-pronounced differences are found between specific diagnoses; this may reflect either (a) limitations in the differential diagnosis of *DSM* eating disorders, or (b) constraints in EDE diagnostic validity.

DSM-IV has introduced several minor changes in the wording of bulimia nervosa. These changes in *DSM-IV* are unlikely to affect the diagnostic validity of the structured interviews developed specifically for eating disorders. The provisional diagnostic category of binge-eating disorder was set forth in the *DSM-IV* appendix for further investigation.

The EDE also provides substantial literature on its use with treatment programs, especially cognitive-behavioral interventions. The EDE would appear to be clinically appropriate for the assessment of eating disorders. Naturally, patients should also be screened for comorbidity, since other disorders (see Wilson & Eldredge, 1991) may negatively affect treatment. Overall, the EDE would appear to be a top candidate as a focused interview for eating disorders.

Psychologists may also wish to consider the newly developed SIAB (Fitchner et al., 1991) for the assessment of eating disorders, as well as for individual and family pathology. Despite a high level of interrater reliability and data on a large sample of eating-disordered patients, however, the SIAB has not been cross-validated by other investigators. As a German instrument, the validation of its English translation also needs to be undertaken. Still, the SIAB is worthy of consideration, particularly in treatment settings that focus on family issues and psychopathology.

Synopsis of Other Structured Interviews

Substance Use Disorders Diagnostic Schedule

Harrison and Hoffman (1985) developed the Substance Use Disorders Diagnostic Schedule (SUDDS) to assess the 23 substance abuse and dependence disorders covered by *DSM-III-R*. The SUDDS is a 99-item structured interview for assessing all major symptoms related to either current or lifetime substance abuse including onset, duration, and effects on functioning. Kruedelbach, McCormick, Schulz, and Grueneich (1993) employed the SUDDS with 34 borderline and 89 nonborderline patients evaluated at a VA substance abuse treatment center. They found that patterns of polysubstance abuse ($\geq$ 3 drugs) were more common among borderline than nonborderline patients. More systematic research is needed to demonstrate the clinical utility of this interview and its ability to establish substance abuse disorders. Diagnosis is greatly complicated by pervasive problems with response styles, typically involving denial and minimization.

Structured and Scaled Interview to Assess Maladjustment (SSIAMI)

Gurland, Yorkston, Stone, Frank, and Fleiss (1982) developed the Structured and Scaled Interview to Assess Maladjustment (SSIAMI) as an overall measure of impaired functioning. Unlike other focused interviews, the SSIAMI assesses not specific disorders, but rather the effects of mental disorders on general adjustment. Life adjustment is measured on five general dimensions: work, social, family, marriage, and sex. The interview component of the SSIAMI consists of 45 items that evaluate three facets for each of the five dimensions: behavior, friction, and distress. Each item is rated on an 11-point scale, with anchoring definitions provided at 5 points.

Gurland et al. (1982) performed an initial reliability study with three raters and 15 patients; they reported good reliability on SSIAMI's factor scores (median ICC = .86, range = .78 – .97). Factor analysis rotated to a varimax solution yielded six factors: social isolation, work inadequacy, friction with the family, dependence on the family, sexual dissatisfaction, and friction outside the family. Factor scores on 89 psychiatric patients were correlated with informant scores (median r = .48). Although the SSIAMI has shown promise as a measure of overall adjustment, it has not been widely used in clinical practice.

Structured Interview of Sleep Disorders (SIS-D)

Schramm et al.(1993) developed the Structured Interview of Sleep Disorders (SIS-D) for the standardized assessment of sleep-wake disorders in accordance with *DSM-III-R* criteria. The SIS-D was modeled after the SCID and is composed of (a) a semistructured component for assessing physical health, substance abuse, medications, and mental health; and (b) a structured component for assessing sleep disorders. With an initial validation study of 68 patients from sleep laboratories and an inpatient psychiatric unit, two interviewers were able to achieve good test-retest reliability[8] at 1- to 3-day intervals (κs = .49 – .91, median = .79). Initial data on 30 patients suggest that the diagnosis was confirmed by sleep laboratory findings in 90.0% of the cases. The SIS-D shows considerable promise as a potential measure for the evaluation of sleep disorders.

---

[8]These reliability estimates apply only to patients who are prescreened for a current sleep disturbance.

Part IV

Summary Chapters

14

Clinical Applications

Fundamental changes in the health care system are resulting in increased competition and greater requirements for accountability. The identity of psychologists as uniquely qualified to provide diagnostic and clinical assessment is clearly brought into question as a host of other mental health service providers vie for consultations.[1] I believe that psychologists, steeped in psychometric traditions, have adopted a relatively insular approach to evaluations, based on familiar tests and scales (e.g., see Meyer, 1993). While not casting aside traditional assessment methods, I am convinced that psychologists must "fight for the edge" in their knowledge of innovative assessment methods and overall sophistication in psychometric and diagnostic evaluations.

Use of structured interviews is not a renouncement of traditional tests but an acknowledgement that other evaluative tools are also important to psychological assessments. As observed in the introductory chapter, the "either/or fallacy" unnecessarily polarizes both psychologists and their styles of evaluation. The following discusses how structured interviews can play a crucial role in psychological assessments.

Goals of Assessment

The goals of an assessment depend on the type and quality of desired information that are needed to address the referral. Is the referral issue a matter of differential diagnosis? Alternatively, if the diagnosis has been firmly established, is the referral issue a comprehensive description and/or systematic rating of critical symptoms or syndromes? Differing goals of the evaluation have important implications to the use of structured interviews.

One simple and convenient model of assessment goals is presented in Table 14.1. Often, the primary goal of treatment is the reduction of symptom severity. Because of their chronic course, mental health professionals typically do not expect that certain Axis I and most Axis II disorders will completely remit. Rather, the goal of assessment is systematic examination of targeted symptoms. As noted in Table 14.1, assessments at the symptom level primarily address the consistency of clinical ratings through interrater and test-retest reliability. For

---

[1]As a compelling example, I recently received from Western Psychological Services a catalog of "clinical tools" for social workers that includes multiscale inventories and projective tests.

Table 14.1
Targeted Assessments: Symptoms, Syndromes/Scales, and Disorders

Type of assessment	Typical validation
Symptoms	Interrater and test-retest reliability
Syndromes/scales	Interrater and test-retest reliability, internal consistency, and convergent validity
Disorders	Interrater and test-retest reliability; internal consistency; convergent, concurrent, diagnostic, and predictive validity

evaluations in which accurate appraisal of symptoms is a primary concern, selective use of structured interviews would appear to be essential to the assessment.

Psychologists are often interested in the use of syndromes and scales in their assessment of psychiatric populations. This approach typically has the advantage of offering dimensional ratings that are related to either a constellation of symptoms (syndrome) or a relevant construct (scale). Validation of syndromes and scales frequently involves not only reliability, but also internal consistency and convergent validity. Syndromes and scales are generally "method-specific" (i.e., different measures are likely to define similar constructs in related but unique ways). Therefore, validation often emphasizes convergent validity rather than concurrent validity. In addition, some scales also have predictive validity. For example, elevations on certain MMPI scales have treatment implications (Butcher & Williams, 1992). Moreover, some structured interviews have scales (e.g., SADS summary scales) which have proved useful in evaluating treatment effectiveness.

Evaluations which emphasize dimensional ratings of psychopathology with respect to syndromes and scales may not require structured interviewing. Depending on the referral question, a number of structured interviews, as noted in previous chapters, offer dimensional ratings that have direct relevance to the evaluation, treatment, and overall management of patient care. I would, therefore, recommend that psychologists consider the potential usefulness of structured interviewing in such cases where dimensions of psychopathology constitute the primary clinical issue.

Many psychological evaluations focus on complex issues of differential diagnosis. For this purpose, structured interviews address nearly all aspects of validation, including convergent, concurrent, diagnostic, and predictive validity. Carefully selected structured interviews are likely to be the centerpiece of these evaluations. In other words, the best structured interview within a specific group (e.g., Axis I and Axis II interviews) almost invariably has the optimal reliability and validity of *any* measure for that particular diagnostic group. Structured interviews for differential diagnosis can be further augmented by multiscale inventories, unstructured interviews, informant interviews and, occasionally, projective methods.

Selection of Structured Interviews

Psychologists have dozens of structured interviews from among which to choose. The determination of the optimal structured interview is highly dependent on the referral question. For Axis I disorders, the three primary measures are the DIS, SADS, and SCID. Additional Axis I interviews include the CASH (promising but presently not well-validated), the PSE (ICD-based interview which is very different in structure and format) and other lesser-used measures. I have summarized in Table 14.2 the general and psychometric characteristics for the DIS, SADS, SCID, and CASH. As a general caution, the data in this and subsequent tables are highly distilled; psychologists should review the actual chapters on specific structured interviews, prior to making their selections.

Major Axis I Interviews

DIS. When should psychologists employ the DIS? As summarized in Table 14.2, the DIS has three distinct advantages over other Axis I interviews. First and foremost, the DIS is the only interview which has been adequately validated for Hispanic populations. For assessments of monolingual Mexican-Americans in particular, the DIS is the obvious interview of choice. Second, the DIS is the only Axis I measure that was designed to be used by nonprofessionals. Psychologists who utilize B.A.-level interviewers for diagnostic assessment are likely to choose the DIS, given its track record with nonprofessionals. Third, the DIS surpasses all other measures in epidemiological studies and cross-cultural applications. For English-speaking persons from other cultures, the DIS is a likely candidate for Axis I assessment.

Table 14.2
Comparison of Axis I Structured Interviews: Characteristics and Psychometric Properties

Variable	DIS	SADS	SCID	CASH
General characteristics				
Semistructured	no	yes	yes	yes
Professional interviewer	no	yes	yes	yes
Use of an informant	opt	opt	opt	opt
Congruent with *DSM* criteria	yes[a]	no[b]	yes	yes[c]
Present diagnosis	yes	yes	yes	yes
Lifetime diagnosis	yes	yes	yes	yes
Severity of symptoms	yes[d]	yes[e]	yes[f]	yes[g]
Etiology of symptoms	yes	no	no	no
Questions grouped by diagnosis	yes	yes[h]	yes	no[i]
Reliability[j]				
Individual symptoms	?	+	?	+
Scales	NA	+	NA	NA
Diagnosis	=	+	=	?
Lifetime diagnosis	=	=	=	?

Table 14.2   (continued)
Comparison of Axis I Structured Interviews: Characteristics and Psychometric Properties

Variable	DIS	SADS	SCID	CASH
Validity[j]				
Clinical diagnosis	=	=	?	?
Convergent validity	–	+	=	?
Longitudinal dimensions				
Risk factors	=	=	=	?
Course of the disorder	+	+	+[k]	?
Response to treatment	?	+	+[k]	?
Applications				
Inpatients	yes	yes	yes	yes
Outpatients	yes	yes	yes	yes
Epidemiological	yes	yes	no	no
Hispanic version	yes[l]	no	no	no

Note. DIS = Diagnostic Interview Schedule; SADS = Schedule of Affective Disorders and Schizophrenia; SCID = Structured Clinical Interview of *DSM-III-R* Disorders; CASH = Comprehensive Assessment of Symptoms and History; opt = optional; NA = not applicable. [a]The DIS also allows for Feighner and RDC diagnostic criteria. [b]The SADS was developed on the basis of RDC diagnostic criteria. Given the correspondence between RDC and *DSM*, clinicians are often able to make *DSM* diagnosis directly from the SADS. [c]The CASH is broader than *DSM-III-R* and includes RDC and other criteria. [d]Three-point scale consists of 1 for "not present," 2 for "subclinical," and 3, 4, or 5 for "clinically relevant" (different scores reflect apparent etiology and not severity). [e]Six-point scale for most symptoms, (not at all, slight or subclinical, mild, moderate, severe, or extreme). Psychotic and past symptoms are rated on a 3-point scale (for not at all, suspected or likely, and definite). [f]Three-point scale (for absent, subthreshold, and threshold or present). [g]Six-point scale for most symptoms (not at all, questionable, mild, moderate, marked, and severe). [h]Part I of the SADS is organized by syndromes and Part II by diagnosis. [i]Organized by syndromes. [j]Comparative data are coded in the following manner: ? for insufficient studies to make a comparison; – for poor, or weaker than other measures; = for average, or comparable to other measures; + for superior, or stronger than other measures. [k]These studies are limited, however, to panic and mood disorders. [l]The DIS has well-validated versions based on Mexican, Mexican-American, and Puerto Rican translations.

The DIS offers a broad coverage of mental disorders and criteria that are directly translatable into *DSM-III-R* and, with anticipated revisions, *DSM-IV* criteria. The DIS distinguishes itself from other interviews by its inclusion of a cognitive screen, specifically the MMSE. Moreover, the DIS optimistically attempts to establish the etiology (i.e., emerging from an entirely functional origin, arising from a medical condition, or resulting from substance abuse) of specific symptoms. Finally, unlike the SADS and the CASH, the DIS limits most of its questions to those related to the DSM inclusion criteria.

SADS. When is the SADS the optimal Axis I interview? The SADS is the interview of choice when psychologists are interested in the comprehensive assessment of mood disorders. In such cases, the SADS offers comprehensive data on symptom severity that is unparalleled by other interview measures. The SADS is also excellent in establishing reliably prior episodes of mental disorders. In addition, the SADS provides a wealth of information on the included disorders that extends far beyond the minimum information needed for diagnosis. Lastly, considerable research has been conducted on SADS diagnosis and longitudinal dimensions of diagnostic validity (future course of the disorder and expected treatment response).

The SADS has several limitations in comparison to other Axis I interviews. While affording greater depth to certain disorders, the SADS covers many fewer diagnoses than other general structured interviews. Additionally, the SADS is based on RDC rather than *DSM* criteria. While close correspondence occurs on many disorders, psychologists are required to ask additional inquiries when making a *DSM-IV* diagnosis.

SCID. When should the SCID be employed as an Axis I interview? The SCID has two major advantages over competing measures. First, it was developed in conjunction with the SCID-II, thus affording an opportunity to evaluate the greatest breadth of mental disorders. Second, considerable research has been conducted with the SCID and panic disorders. Clearly, the SCID is the interview of choice in assessing longitudinal dimensions (course and treatment response) of panic disorders.

A substantial limitation of the SCID is in its reliability data, which are constrained by the paucity of studies and modest results. In addition, studies have generally not investigated SCID concurrent validity, either with clinical diagnosis or with other structured interviews. These constraints may lead psychologists to select other interviews, such as the SADS, when preliminary assessments suggest that the working diagnosis is covered by another Axis I interview.

CASH. When should the CASH be considered as an Axis I interview? The answer is relatively simple. The chief advantage of the CASH, based on its current validation, is the systematic description of symptoms and signs. Therefore, the CASH has very good reliability for individual items and has greater breadth in symptom coverage than the SADS. Moreover, the CASH offers meaningful gradations of psychotic symptoms in greater detail than found in other interviews. Presently, the CASH is not recommended in cases which require either *DSM-IV* diagnoses or dimensional ratings.

In summary, psychologists and other mental health professionals may wish to develop expertise in several Axis I interviews, given their respective strengths and limitations. For mainstream evaluations, the SADS and the SCID complement each other with depth and breadth. For bilingual and cross-cultural settings, the DIS is unequalled. Training in several Axis I disorders will provide psychologists with considerable expertise in the overall assessment of major mental disorders.

Child and Adolescent Structured Interviews

Four major diagnostic interviews (K-SADS, CAS, DISC, and DICA) have been validated for children and adolescents and are summarized in Table 14.3. All four interviews were developed for comparable ages, combine child interviews with parent-informant interviews, and yield current diagnoses. New revisions that are *DSM-IV* compatible are anticipated and may facilitate diagnosis. Each diagnostic interview has its own strengths and limitations; these are presented below.

Table 14.3

Comparison of Child and Adolescent Structured Interviews: Characteristics and Psychometric Properties

Variable	K-SADS	CAS	DISC	DICA
General characteristics				
Ages	6–18	7–17	8–17	6–17
Semistructured	yes	no	no	no[a]
Professional interviewer	yes	yes	no	yes
Parallel forms (parent/child)	yes	yes	yes	yes
Parallel form with adult	yes	no	yes	no
Congruent with *DSM* criteria	yes[b]	yes	yes	yes
Present diagnosis	yes	yes	yes	yes
Lifetime diagnosis	no	no	no	yes
Severity of symptoms	yes	no	no	no
Questions grouped by diagnosis	yes	no	no	no
Reliability[c]				
Individual symptoms	+	?	+	–
Scales	+	+	=	?
Diagnosis	+	+	+	=
Total score	?	=	=	?
Parent-child agreement	+	?	?	=
Validity[c]				
Clinical diagnosis	=[d]	?[e]	?[e]	–
Convergent–CBCL/TRF	=	+	=	?
Convergent–other	yes	yes	yes	yes
Longitudinal dimensions				
Risk factors	?	?	+	+
Course of the disorder	=	?	=	?
Response to treatment	?	?	?	?
Applications				
Inpatients	yes	no[f]	yes	yes
Outpatients	yes	yes	yes	yes
Epidemiological	no[g]	no	yes	yes
Hispanic	no	no	yes	no

Note. For more detailed comparisons, see Gutterman et al. (1987) and Hodges (1993). K-SADS = Schedule of Affective Disorders and Schizophrenia for School-Age Children; CAS = Child Assessment Schedule; DISC = Diagnostic Interview Schedule for Children; DICA = Diagnostic Interview for Children and Adolescents.

[a]Although the DICA is described as "structured," clinicians are allowed to make some exceptions. [b]Actually depends on form; the K-SADS-III-R is congruent with *DSM-III-R*. [c]Comparative data are coded in the following manner: ? insufficient studies to make a comparison; – for poor, or weaker than other measures; = for average, or comparable to other measures; + for superior, or stronger than other measures. [d]Limited range of diagnoses was represented. [e]Research addressed level of impairment and not diagnostic concordance. [f]Most studies have been on outpatients and excluded psychotic children. [g]The K-SADS-E was developed for epidemiological studies but was only infrequently used.

K-SADS. The K-SADS parallels the SADS for mood and psychotic disorders but augments the coverage by the inclusion of childhood and developmental disorders. The K-SADS, like the SADS, distinguishes itself with respect to reliability and symptom severity. For reliability, the K-SADS has evidenced superior reliability for symptoms, scales, and diagnosis. For symptom severity, nonpsychotic symptoms are rated on 5- and 6-point scales of increasing severity. Validational studies suggest adequate concurrent and convergent validity.

The K-SADS has paid relatively little attention to longitudinal dimensions of diagnosis, especially risk factors and response to treatment. Likewise, the range of diagnosis covered by the K-SADS is somewhat more circumscribed than that covered by other child interviews. In spite of these limitations, the K-SADS is likely to be a strong candidate as a reliable and valid Axis I child interview.

CAS. The CAS is a topically organized and easily administered diagnostic interview for children. Its primary strengths lie in its reliability and convergent validity with teacher and parent ratings (i.e., TRF and CBCL). Validation has focused predominantly on dimensional ratings rather than on diagnosis itself. Therefore, psychologists may choose not to employ the CAS in circumstances where diagnosis is a primary concern. Rather, the CAS is well suited for determining treatment interventions and assessing dimensions of psychopathology. A chief limitation is the relative absence of validity studies with inpatient children.

DISC. The DISC, like the DIS, was developed as a structured interview for community/epidemiological studies. Towards this end, the DISC is the only child interview to be administered by nonprofessionals. It may, therefore, be useful in clinical settings where paraprofessionals contribute to the assessment process. The DISC has adequate to good reliability and substantial evidence of convergent validity. Psychologists will likely want to employ the DISC with both Spanish-speaking children and English-speaking children from different cultures. In addition, the DISC may be the interview of choice in the early assessment of risk factors for mental disorders. Given its correspondence to the DIS, the DISC may also be useful in assessing family pathology. In summary, the DISC is a carefully validated child interview which is well-suited for a variety of clinical settings, particularly those with multicultural clientele.

DICA. The DICA is the only child interview to pay close attention to the lifetime prevalence of mental disorders. For psychologists attempting to understand the etiology of disorders and/or formulate early intervention programs, this feature is certainly attractive. The chief limitations of the DICA are the data on reliability and validity, which sometimes fall short of the competing structured interviews. For example, comparisons of the DICA with other diagnostic standards raise concerns regarding concurrent validity. The DICA is probably not the interview of choice for making a complex differential diagnosis. Like the CAS, the DICA may be effective as a gauge to treatment effectiveness.

In summary, child interviews face daunting diagnostic challenges, given the divergence of perspectives among children, parents, and interested professionals (e.g., teachers, child-care workers, and health-care professionals). While child interviews often do not manifest the psychometric rigor of adult Axis I interviews, they do provide a standardized and generally reliable method of assessing diagnosis and dimensions of psychopathology. I would strongly recommend the use of a structured interview as an important component of child assessments.

Major Axis II Interviews

The two foremost Axis II interviews (SIDP and PDE) are not well-known by most psychologists and other mental health professionals. Both interviews are supported by a wealth of studies on their reliability and validity. In addition, two other structured interviews, the SCID-II and PDI-IV, show considerable promise. The relatively small number of changes in *DSM-IV* inclusion criteria is a decided asset with respect to the validity of these measures and their usefulness with *DSM-IV* diagnoses. Table 14.4 summarizes the major Axis II interviews.

SIDP. The hallmark of the SIDP is its organization and format, which elicits a broad range of clinical information, often with general questions which have little face validity (i.e., they are not obviously related to specific psychopathology). The SIDP has good reliability and excellent convergent validity. An important feature of its diagnostic validity is the low degree of overlap among personality disorders, a feature that distinguishes the SIDP from all other Axis II measures. Because of the breadth of research, the SIDP is the obvious interview of choice when considering Axis I and II interactions as they affect treatment outcome. Overall, the SIDP is an excellent Axis II interview that should be employed in a wide range of settings.

Table 14.4

Comparison of Axis II Structured Interviews: Characteristics and Psychometric Properties

Variable	SIDP	PDE	CID-II	PDI
General characteristics				
Semistructured	yes	yes	yes	yes
Professional interviewer	yes	yes	yes	no[a]
Use of an informant	yes	opt	no	no
Congruent with *DSM* criteria	yes	yes	yes	yes
Present diagnosis	yes	yes	yes	yes
Past diagnosis	no	yes	no	no
Dimensional scores	no	yes	no	no
Severity of symptoms	yes[b]	yes[c]	yes[d]	yes[e]
Questions grouped by diagnosis	no	no	yes	no[f]
Reliability[g]				
Individual symptoms	=	+	?	?
Scales	NA	+	NA	NA
Diagnosis	+	+	–	=[h]
Validity[g]				
Clinical diagnosis	?	=	?	?
Convergent validity	+	+	?[i]	=
Diagnostic overlap	+	=	=	?
Longitudinal dimensions				
Risk factors	=	=	?	?
Course of the disorder	=	=	?	?
Response to treatment	+	=	?	?

Table 14.4   (continued)
Comparison of Axis II Structured Interviews: Characteristics and Psychometric Properties

Variable	SIDP	PDE	CID-II	PDI
Applications				
Inpatients	yes	yes	?	?
Outpatients	yes	yes	yes	yes
Epidemiological	no	no	no	yes
Multicultural	no	yes[j]	no	no

Note. SIDP = Structured Interview for *DSM-III* Personality Disorders; PDE = Personality Disorder Examination; SCID-II = Structured Clinical Interview for *DSM-III-R*–Axis II Disorders; PDI = Personality Disorder Interview; opt = optional but recommended. [a]Although designed for nonprofessionals, all PDI reliability data appear to have been collected with psychology staff. [b]Three-point scale (1-3) with "2" for meeting criterion and "3" for being severe. [c]Three-point scale: (0-2) with "1" for exaggerated and "2" for meeting criterion. [d]Three-point scale (1-3) with "2" subthreshold and "3" meeting criterion. [e]Earlier versions (PIQ) employed a 9-point scale of increasing severity. The latest version (PDI-IV) uses a 3-point (0-2) scale with "2" for meeting criterion and "3" for severe. [f]A version organized by diagnosis is now available, although validity studies were carried out on the topical version. [g]Comparative data are coded in the following manner: ? for insufficient studies to make a comparison; – for poor, or weaker than other measures; = for average, or comparable to other measures; + for superior, or stronger than other measures. [h]A single study appeared to produce high reliability estimates. [i]Despite weak findings on convergent validity, a large factor-analytic study offered good evidence of construct validity. [j]The international version (IPDE) has been tested in 11 countries; unfortunately a Hispanic version is not currently available.

PDE. The PDE is distinguished from other structured interviews in three important ways. First, the PDE emphasizes dimensional ratings in addition to diagnoses; these ratings are often useful in assessing changes in clinical status. Second, the PDE systematically addresses past Axis II disorders, instead of facilely assuming "once a personality disorder, always a personality disorder." Third, the PDE stands out as an Axis II interview by continued attention to multicultural and cross-cultural issues. The PDE would likely be given preference over the SIDP under circumstances in which an informant is unavailable and when cross-cultural issues must be considered. Like the SIDP, the PDE is an outstanding Axis II interview and applicable to a broad range of clinical settings.

SCID-II. The chief advantage of the SCID-II is its ease of administration in conjunction with the SCID-II-Q. For the psychologist who needs to screen quickly for personality disorders, the SCID-II-Q followed by the SCID-II would appear to be a reasonable method. Other features of the SCID-II include its organization by disorders and its easy combination with the SCID for a relatively comprehensive coverage of mental disorders. However, the usefulness of the SCID-II is severely constrained by less-than-adequate reliability, which does not systematically address the majority of personality disorders. In addition, validity studies for the SCID-II are not on par with either the SIDP or the PDE. Therefore, psychologists may wish to employ the SCID-II as an intermediate screen for personality disorders, but not as well-validated diagnostic measure.

PDI. The PDI offers considerable promise with outpatient and community samples as a useful Axis II interview. The PDI has already been revised to make its inclusion criteria compatible with *DSM-IV*. Although described as intended for use with nonprofessionals, the available reliability data were gathered entirely by psychology staff. Therefore, I cannot presently recommend its use with paraprofessionals. Although there is modest evidence of convergent validity, the PDI has not been sufficiently validated for general clinical use. Given sustained efforts at fully testing its validity, its status as a nonclinical measure may well change.

In summary, psychologists have two excellent measures in the SIDP and PDE. I strongly recommend that clinicians develop an expertise with at least one of these Axis II interviews. As noted in earlier chapters, use of the PDQ-R as a screening measure for selective use of the SIDP and PDE would appear to be particularly effective.

Specialized Structured Interviews

A diverse group of focused interviews have been developed to address intensively single disorders, response styles, or psychological impairment. These measures, because of their specialized nature, often have important yet circumscribed clinical applications. I will summarize a representative sampling of focused disorders (see Table 14.5) and subsequently review the SIRS as a structured interview for response styles.

Table 14.5

An Overview of Structured Interviews for Specific Disorders: Characteristics and Psychometric Properties

Variable	DIB	PCL-R	SCID-D	ADIS
General characteristics				
Semistructured	yes	yes	yes	yes
Professional interviewer	yes	yes	yes	yes
Use of corroborative data	yes	yes	no	yes
Congruent with *DSM* criteria	no	no	yes	yes
Present diagnosis	yes	yes	yes	yes
Past diagnosis	no	no	yes	no
Dimensional scores	yes	yes	no	no
Severity of symptoms	no[a]	yes[b]	yes[c]	yes[d]
Questions grouped by scales or clusters	yes	no	yes	yes
Reliability[e]				
Individual symptoms	=	+	?	?
Scales	=	NA	NA	NA
Diagnosis	=	+	+[f]	=
Validity[e]				
Clinical diagnosis	+	=	?	?
Convergent validity	=	=	–	?
Longitudinal dimensions				
Risk factors	?	+[g]	?	?
Course of the disorder	?	+[g]	?	?
Response to treatment	=	=	?	?

Table 14.5   (continued)
An Overview of Structured Interviews for Specific Disorders:
Characteristics and Psychometric Properties

Variable	DIB	PCL-R	SCID-D	ADIS
Applications				
Inpatients	yes	yes	yes	no
Outpatients	yes	yes	yes	yes
Epidemiological	no	no	no	no
Multicultural	no	–[h]	?	no

Note. DIB = Diagnostic Interview for Borderlines; PCL-R = Psychopathy Checklist-Revised; SCID-D = Structured Clinical Interview for *DSM-IV* Dissociative Disorders; ADIS = Anxiety Disorders Interview Schedule.
[a]Items are rated on a 3-point scale with respect to their certainty (no, probable, and definite). [b]Items are rated on a 3-point scale which combines severity and certainty (no, maybe/in some respects, and yes). [c]Symptoms are categorized as "present" or "absent"; however, frequency, onset, and duration of these symptoms are rated generally on a 5-point scale of severity. [d]Many items are rated on a 5-point scale (none, mild, moderate, severe, very severe/grossly disabling). [e]Comparative data are coded in the following manner: ? for insufficient studies to make a comparison; – for poor, or weaker than other measures; = for average, or comparable to other measures; + for superior, or stronger than other measures. [f]Abstracted information for original studies appears to be excellent, although actual reliability data have not been published. [g]Risk factors and the course of the disorder are related to violence and adjustment. [h]Little data are available on minorities with reference to external validation; moreover, Kosson, Smith, and Newman (1990) found a very different distribution between African-American and White inmates.

DIB. The importance of the DIB to clinical practice lies less in its diagnostic validity and more in its theoretical formulations. In other words, general Axis II interviews provide sufficient reliability and validity for the diagnosis of borderline personality disorders. What the DIB contributes is an operationalization of Gunderson's widely accepted conceptual model of borderlines. Psychologists providing specialized treatment consistent with Gunderson's formulations are likely to find the DIB extremely valuable. Moreover, the DIB extends beyond diagnosis and offers a relatively reliable measure of critical borderline dimensions. From this perspective, the DIB may be a valuable resource in systematically assessing these dimensions.

PCL. The PCL is not intended as diagnostic measure of APD. Like the DIB, the PCL is more driven by theoretical formulations than diagnostic validity. The clinical applications of the PCL are presently limited to white males with a history of either incarceration or maximum-security hospitalization. The PCL's hallmark is its predictive validity. With the previously described population, the PCL is the measure of choice for risk assessment; it has incremental validity over antisocial history in determining which offenders are likely to recidivate and act aggressively. Moreover, the PCL is an effective measure for estimating institutional problems and inmates' willingness to participate in treatment.

SCID-D. Dissociative disorders have not been extensively investigated by Axis I interviews. To address this need, the SCID-D is intended to augment the SCID by systematically evaluating dissociative disorders. The SCID-D appears to have good reliability for diagnosis but only modest evidence of convergent validity. The SCID-D assumes the validity of *DSM-IV* diagnosis. Despite this untested assumption, the SCID-D is the best measure of dissociative disorders, with further work on its validation underway.

ADIS. The ADIS, as one of the first focused interviews, provides extensive information about anxiety disorders and their associated features. The ADIS offers few diagnostic advantages over general Axis I interviews, such as the SADS-LA or the SCID. Its usefulness, like that of the DIB, centers on its treatment implications. The ADIS offers a very extensive outline of symptoms and situations for clinical intervention. In this regard, the ADIS may be useful in centers devoted to the treatment of anxiety disorders, both in delineating symptoms or impairment and in measuring outcome.

SIRS. The SIRS is a focused interview which was developed for the express purpose of assessing response styles rather than mental disorders. The SIRS has excellent reliability and discriminant validity. This measure is recommended for any evaluation where there is substantial concern regarding the feigning or over-reporting of psychopathology.

Use of MSEs

Summaries of comprehensive and cognitive MSEs were presented in Tables 2.1 and 2.2. Both types of MSE should be considered only for screening purposes. Comprehensive MSEs typically provide a brief overview of Axis I symptoms, while cognitive MSEs examine a limited range of cognitive dysfunction that is most frequently associated with dementias. With respect to cognitive MSEs, both the DIS and the CASH include the MMSE within their interview format.

Integrated Evaluations and Reports

General Overview

The overall goal of most evaluations is a well-integrated and coherent report that addresses the referral question and other critical issues. How is this integration achieved? What happens to discordant information? Are all clinical findings treated as if they were equally valid? Is the logic from clinical data to overall conclusions explicit to the informed reader?

The content and organization of any evaluation is largely dependent on the referral source. Reports differ in sophistication if they are written for (a) psychologists, (b) other mental health professionals, (c) professionals outside of mental health, and (d) nonprofessionals. As a backdrop to all evaluations, psychologists should assume that the patient has or could have access to the report. As a guideline to evaluations, endpoints of continua are presented below.

Accuracy Versus Simplicity. At the extremes, overly detailed reports may excruciatingly delineate each and every clinical finding, while overly distilled reports leave large gaps in clinical data. Psychologists must make judgments regarding major and minor findings and treat the clinical data accordingly. For consultations to other psychologists, I prefer to emphasize accuracy so that major findings can be verified. For example, I often provide 2-point MMPI-2 codes in addition to the interpretation. For nonprofessionals, the meaning of the findings, simply stated, is more important than very precise but abstruse language.

Synthesis Versus Syncretism. I am deeply worried when I review a psychological evaluation in which all the pieces appear to fit together. While integration is the goal of evaluations, psychological data are often discordant and lack concinnity. To force disparate information to fit is syncretism, not synthesis. I prefer psychological assessments that openly acknowledge nonconvergent and discrepant findings. I believe that such forthrightness does not detract from the report but adds to its credibility.

Certainty Versus Fallibility. Several related issues emerge from this continuum. Many psychological reports are written with a degree of certitude that is totally unjustified by the data. On the other hand, wallowing in self-doubt, while much rarer among psychologists, provides more confusion than clarity. As I have previously written (Rogers, 1986), one alternative is to provide qualifying descriptors (e.g., "these symptoms are likely to be..." or "this profile is consistent with..."). While I advocate the use of qualifiers, I am very concerned whether the consumers of psychological assessments make any actual discriminations regarding the certainty of conclusions. Perhaps a better solution is to make explicit statements about the certitude of a conclusion (e.g., "While the test results *suggest...*, this finding should be viewed as *preliminary*"). Moreover, if an interpretation is not well-grounded in clinical research, possibly the most prudent course would be to omit it entirely. If rigorous standards were applied (for an example with the MMPI, see Gynther, Altman, & Sletten, 1973), many fewer interpretations would be made.

Structured Interviews in Psychological Assessments

Reporting the results of structured interviews is easily integrated into psychological evaluations. Below, I offer general guidelines for the incorporation of structured interviews.

Description of Structured Interviews. Many psychologists and other mental health professionals lack familiarity with diagnostic and structured interviews. I believe that we need to educate our referral sources regarding the standardized measures that we employ. This description may be accomplished in one or two sentences. For example, a personal injury consultation might include the following statements about the SADS: "I also administered the Schedule of Affective Disorders and Schizophrenia (SADS), an extensive semistructured diagnostic interview. The SADS was an appropriate measure in this case because of its excellent reliability in assessing both current and past episodes and its usefulness at estimating the severity of symptoms at different time periods." Clinical data from structured interviews should probably be separated from that of traditional, unstructured interviews so that the referring professional can clearly distinguish which findings are and which are not standardized.

Diagnosis and Clinical Findings. Clinical data from diagnostic interviews can often be organized with three levels of abstraction:

1. Diagnosis: a clear statement of the mental disorder, with accompanying information on its onset, duration, and course.

2. Diagnostic criteria: an account of *DSM-IV* inclusion criteria met by the patient and the severity of each symptom, as noted in the structured interview.

3. Examples/description: a selective reporting of "raw data" for key symptoms, such as quotes from the patient (e.g., actual words used in a suicide threat) or a distillation of the patient's account (e.g., the specifics of a paranoid delusion, including the "perpetrators" and the "plot").

Adherence to this format ensures that the logic or basis of diagnosis is clearly presented. Multiple perspectives are often presented in complex cases. Psychologists are much more likely to be convincing and credible in such cases when the conclusions and the basis of those conclusions are carefully delineated. With consultations targeted for nonprofessionals, psychologists have the responsibility of defining psychological terms in nontechnical language, so as to facilitate rather than impede understanding.

Predictive Statements. Referring professionals often desire clinical predictions on treatment effectiveness and risk assessment. Unfortunately, neither structured interviewing nor psychological testing frequently yield high-quality predictive information. Typically, the best predictions are rendered from extreme data (e.g., predicting suicide on the basis of dozens of nearly lethal and very recent attempts). In such extreme cases, is the prediction even necessary?[2] In response, I think predictions may be useful although not essential, even in such extreme cases. In other cases, psychologists must be very circumspect in making any predictions. Towards this end, predictive statements should *always* be accompanied by both probability estimates and cautions. Psychologists must make clear the known accuracy of a prediction. If the specific probability is unknown, then the ensuing predictions are more likely to be prejudicial than helpful. In addition to probability estimates, a caution is almost always required, since even the best predictive data probably do not completely correspond to the patient in question and his/her circumstances. Substantive differences either in clinical setting or in diagnosis/symptomatology of the patient are likely to affect the accuracy of prediction.

Regarding probability estimates and cautions, I do make the distinction between positive and negative predictions. Negative predictions involve statements that are likely to curtail opportunities, coerce treatment, and deprive freedoms. In contrast, positive predictions usually concern enabling the patient through the selection of treatments or requested accommodations to a disability. When the "cost" of a positive prediction is relatively low (e.g., recommendation of cognitive-behavioral treatment for an anxiety disorder), I am less concerned about probability estimates and cautions than when the cost is both large and experienced as negative by the patient (e.g., civil commitment). From this context, treatment recommendations for a motivated patient, while based on implicit predictions, are largely determined by comparative effectiveness and availability.

---

[2]For example, a very high scorer on the PCL-R typically has extensive criminal history and considerable documentation of institutional problems within prisons and forensic hospitals. Could not the relevant authorities make these determinations without PCL-R data?

15

Research: Current Models and Future Directions

The previous chapters on structured and diagnostic interviews include a large number of implicit research questions that merit further investigation. Moreover, summary Tables 14.2 through 14.5 provide an overview of the current validation of structured interviews and their future research needs. For this reason, this chapter will make no attempt to recapitulate the considerable array of specific research questions. Rather, the chapter focuses on a broad conceptualization of structured interviews and their role, both current and potential, in clinical research.

The first component of this chapter addresses the assessment of psychopathology and is subdivided into symptoms, scales, and diagnoses. The second component addresses motivational concerns in psychological assessment. The third component offers examples of how structured interviewing may be used in testing theories. The fourth component summarizes other applications of structured interviewing to clinical settings.

Assessment of Psychopathology

A major thrust of clinical research is the accurate appraisal of psychopathology. I am very concerned that the selection of measures in such research is often dictated by brevity and familiarity. As an example of the former, many studies have employed the BDI as a measure of depression when other more comprehensive measures are readily available. As an example of the latter, the Millon Clinical Multiaxial Inventory–II (MCMI-II; Millon, 1982) is sometimes used in research as a substitute for Axis II diagnosis, although its lack of correspondence with *DSM* disorders has been convincingly established. Brevity and familiarity are not adequate criteria for the selection of measures. A small but appreciable improvement could be made throughout clinical research if each published study was required to justify explicitly through systematic comparisons its selection of interviews, tests, or scales.

If brevity and familiarity are not the appropriate watchwords of clinical research, on what basis should measures be selected? The overall validation of any measure is an obvious consideration. Equally important are decisions regarding the type of measurement for psychopathology and its specific validation. For example, the SADS focuses on symptom severity while the DIS attends to the etiology of symptoms. For any study addressing specific symptoms, clear preferences between the SADS and the DIS should be easily established based simply on the type of clinical data required. Measures also differ in the breadth of symptomatology. For instance, in descriptive studies of psychotic patients, clinical researchers may opt for the CASH, given its comprehensive review of relevant symptoms.

The assessment of psychopathology can be simply, but effectively organized along a continuum of abstraction that is composed of symptoms, scales, and disorders. Depending on the purpose of the study, researchers must decide which among these three categories is their primary focus. In turn, this decision will inform the subsequent selection of psychological measures, based on their comparative strengths.

Focus on Specific Symptoms

The primary focus of most longitudinal studies is changes in symptoms, not disorders. As noted in Chapter 1, longitudinal research on schizophrenia might examine alterations in symptoms during prodromal, active, and residual phases. An interesting question is whether symptoms at each phase reflect discrete changes in psychopathology or simply represent observable changes in severity. Are overvalued ideas and delusions essentially the same symptom expressed at different levels?[1] A second question is whether negative symptoms constitute true inclusion criteria or whether they actually indicate the resulting impairment that often arises from the positive symptoms.

The answer to these questions would rely on the systematic assessment of schizophrenic symptoms across short intervals, thus allowing for the investigation of symptom severity as well as the emergence of new symptoms. In other words, the primary focus is symptomatology and its concomitant severity. Structured interviews, such as the SADS and the CASH, might well be considered. In addition, similar questions could be posed for mood disorders (e.g., differentiating dysthymia and major depression based on symptomatic differences).

Treatment studies typically address differences in symptoms. For example, psychopharmacological interventions are aimed at the reduction of targeted symptoms, not the cure or even the remission of mental disorders. For instance, the primary focus of anxiolytic medication is the reduction and control of specific anxiety symptoms. Toward this end, structured interviews that emphasize diagnostic reliability, but not symptom reliability, may not be appropriate measures. In this case, use of focused interviews, such as the ADIS, might be considered.

The importance of symptoms, in their own right, merits further study. Although delusions can be diagnosed in diverse groups of organic, schizophrenic, delusional, schizoaffective, and mood disorders, what about understanding the symptoms themselves? The content of delusions, their complexity,

---

[1]One source of confusion in understanding prodromal psychotic symptoms is that they are rarely diagnosed in the presence of active psychotic symptoms. In other words, overvalued ideas, superstitiousness, and recurrent illusions are typically not recorded in the presence of delusions, paranoid ideation, and hallucinations. Therefore, clinicians are at a serious disadvantage in attempting to assess whether active psychotic symptoms represent new developments or are an accentuation of prodromal symptoms.

and their effects on behavior are all worthy of study. For example, what are the precursors to the emergence of a pseudocommunity? How does cultural relativism affect delusions (see Murphy, 1986) even among ethnic groups within the United States?[2] Do combinations of delusions (e.g., grandiose and paranoid) signal a difference in overall functioning or prognosis?

The severity of symptoms warrants further investigation. Structured interviews have often used a curious admixture of criteria in establishing the severity of symptoms. With mood symptoms, for example, severity is typically evaluated in terms of frequency and subjective distress. For personality disorders, a common criterion is negative effects on others. For psychotic and anxiety disorders, severity is commonly assessed with respect to behavioral consequences (e.g., the patient obeyed the command hallucinations; see Rogers, Gillis, Turner, & Smith, 1990). The assessment of individual symptoms along multiple dimensions would represent a particularly interesting avenue of research. Table 15.1 presents multiple perspectives of symptom severity that could be incorporated into structured interviews and self-report measures.

Table 15.1
Assessment of Symptom Severity from Multiple Perspectives

Indicators of severity	Representative inquiries
Frequency/duration	How often does it occur? How long does it last?
Subjective distress	Does it bother (upset) you? How much?
Behavioral consequences	What do you usually do when it occurs? What is the worst thing you have done?
Effects on others	What do others do when it occurs?
Relative importance	How important is it for you to get help for this problem? Is this (problem or symptom) worse than others?

Focus on Scales

A hallmark of clinical psychology is the intense and sustained research on traditional psychological tests and their relationship to psychopathology. At the same time, psychologists have largely adopted the *DSM* standards for diagnosis. How are these divergent models of mental disorders reconciled? Which predominate in psychological evaluations?

Prior to the *DSM-III*, psychologists provided the optimal standardization to the assessment of psychopathology through systematic comparisons of psychometric data. Rorschach and MMPI data were clearly superior to idiosyncratic interviews and arduous history taking. Even when test data were compared to diagnosis, the lack of strong relationships was often blamed, perhaps rightfully, on the frailties of the *DSM-II*. However, with the emergence of the *DSM-III* and

---

[2]Cultural influences can affect both patients (i.e., the content and style of presentation of delusional material) and mental health professionals (i.e., assessment and interventions regarding similar delusions in patients from different subcultures).

the development of structured interviews, psychologists have often remained insular in their validational methods and eschewed comparisons with well validated interview methods.

How many studies have compared MMPI and MMPI-2 2-point codes to SADS or SCID diagnoses? How many studies have sought convergent validity by comparing patterns of psychopathology between MMPI and structured interviews (e.g., Scale 2 with the relevant summary scales of the SADS)? Or compared the schizophrenic index of the Rorschach with diagnostic data on which the reliability is known? The common answer to all three questions is "less than a handful." A rich opportunity exists for studies to make a substantial impact on psychological evaluations by adopting the most rigorous standards for test validation.

Gynther et al. (1983) set the standard for MMPI validation when they employed systematic data from the MMS (see Chapter 2) in the validation of MMPI codetypes. They only accepted a clinical descriptor if its description could be cross-validated on very large psychiatric populations (>10,000). A similarly rigorous standard employing more sophisticated structured interviews than the MSS could be set for multiscale inventories. Simply put, psychologists need to validate traditional tests against the highest standards for the assessment of symptoms, syndromes, and disorders. These highest standards are almost invariably found in structured interviewing.

Substantial progress has been made on the validation of self-report measures with structured interviews. Interestingly, the *Journal of Personality Disorders* has set a standard for the assessment of Axis II disorders with many studies that employ the SIDP, PDE, and SCID-II. These studies, along with clinical diagnosis, have typically found the MCMI-II lacking any diagnostic equivalence, but have demonstrated the usefulness of the PDQ-R as an effective screening measure. Studies have also underscored the dangers of "descriptor fallacy" (Rogers & Ornduff, in press) which occurs when similar clinical terms are erroneously equated, despite their divergent operational definitions and nonconvergent research.

Researchers on the MMPI/MMPI-2, in particular, should be aware of pervasive problems with "pseudoparallelism." MMPI-2 interpretations typically list diagnoses which are commonly found with 2-point codes. However, a frequent code-type cannot be interpreted diagnostically. For example, a 6-8 code is often associated with schizophrenia. However, many schizophrenics do not have a 6-8 profile and many individuals with 6-8 profiles are not schizophrenic. Although psychologists often carefully couch their reports of such profiles (e.g., a representative statement in a psychological report might be, "the patient's profile is 'consistent with' a schizophrenic disorder"), most referral sources are not likely to make such subtle distinctions. From a research perspective, studies are urgently needed which define the sensitivity and specificity rates for 2-point codes, based on reliable diagnoses. Similar studies are needed with the PAI to determine the actual meaning of its diagnostic scales.

Projective methods frequently fall short in their validation of specific interpretations, which are often theory-based rather than empirically-derived. When studies are conducted, they often address only the degrees of association between two methods. A much more sophisticated model would be the multitrait-multimethod matrix proposed by Campbell and Fiske (1959). For example, components of the Rorschach hypervigilance index (Exner, 1991) could be compared to suspiciousness and paranoid symptoms as measured by structured interviews and other tests (i.e., convergent validity) in combination with the inclusion of other Rorschach and clinical data that are predicted to be unrelated to the hypervigilance index (i.e., discriminant validity). Rorschach interpretation supported by the multitrait-multimethod matrix would be easily defensible on both theoretical and empirical grounds.

This discussion of psychological tests and their validation may seem unduly critical, perhaps even heretical. On the contrary, I see myself as a strong supporter of traditional psychometric methods. By insisting on the highest standards, psychological testing will continue to prosper. By insisting that we confront such perennial problems as overinterpretation, descriptor fallacy, and pseudoparallelism, our goal is the presentation of clinical data that is useful and not misleading.

Focus on Disorders

This section will consider two major facets of diagnostic research, namely, the use of Syndeham's criteria and the comparison of dimensional, categorical, and synthesized models. In addition, I will offer various observations regarding underexplored elements of diagnostic research.

Syndeham's Criteria. What would happen if we truly invoked Syndeham's criteria for disorders? If we allowed only those disorders with clear inclusion and exclusion criteria to be diagnosed? If we insisted that disorders have identifiable outcome criteria that set them apart from other disorders?

The first step in this process, as described in Chapter 1, would be the refinement of inclusion and expansion of exclusion criteria to maximize the differentiation among disorders. Inclusion criteria, which are common to many disorders (e.g., social withdrawal), are obviously not effective. By the same token, nonspecific exclusion criteria provide little assistance in the demarcation of specific disorders. The second and more challenging step would be the demonstration of outcome criteria. For example, are subtypes of schizophrenia justifiable in systematic examinations of their precursors, course, or response to treatment? Moreover, do familial and laboratory correlates exist to support the specific etiology of these subtypes?

As a *Gedanken* or thought experiment, consider what might happen if Syndeham was strictly followed. Many Axis I disorders would become simplified. It is doubtful that psychotic disorders would manifest differential outcomes to such a degree as to warrant more than a few diagnoses. Moreover, most Axis II disorders would cease to exist, given their predicted chronicity and overlap with other disorders. Alternatively, personality disorders might flourish with increased attention to differential outcomes and discriminative responses to treatment. At present, nonspecific treatment generally yields nonspecific results.

Large-scale studies of the SADS and the DIS, already conducted, could assist in the refinement of mental disorders. In other words, the data currently exist to implement Syndeham with some Axis I disorders. This research would likely lead to hierarchical diagnoses, since differential outcome criteria would be next to impossible to establish with multiple disorders. Moreover, the whole focus of diagnostic research could be sharpened simply by insisting that we follow Syndeham's dicta. Genetic and familial studies would provide valuable ancillary data to further refine diagnoses.

Categorical and Dimensional Models. The debate over categorical and dimensional diagnosis is far from resolved. The advantages of the categorical model are well-known for its clinician acceptance and straightforward communication of information (see Gunderson, Links, & Reich, 1991). In contrast, dimensional ratings offer diversity, provide a continuum from normal to abnormal, and provide for diagnostic overlap. In addition, dimensional models offer superior information allowing for more sophisticated analysis than the nominal data of categorical diagnosis (Widiger, 1991).

Widiger (1992), as a proponent of the dimensional approach, is strongly critical of the current categorical paradigm. He argues that the boundaries for establishing mental disorders are largely arbitrary. For example, the *DSM-III-R* Personality Disorder Advisory Committee had no empirical data to guide the establishment of cutting scores for 9 of the 11 personality disorders, but were guided by pragmatism and consensus. He made the cogent observation that often one or two extreme symptoms causing social impairment and distress may likely qualify for a personality disorder.

Widiger (1991) has proposed a synthesis of the categorical and dimensional model through an ordinal organization of symptoms that would be divided into six groups: absent, traits, subthreshold, threshold, moderate, and prototypic. Gunderson et al. (1991) also suggested a synthesized model with dimensional ratings for certain psychotic processes and personality traits and a categorical model for certain other disorders. I propose a third alternative that combines a minimum number of inclusion criteria with severity ratings. In order for a disorder to be a disorder it should consist of a minimum number (4-6) of correlated symptoms; otherwise, only a few isolated symptoms are being represented as a disorder. Second, the symptoms present should not be considered as equal. For conduct symptoms, running away from home overnight should not be equated with arson or sexual assault. Moreover, some consideration needs to be given to the frequency and severity of the behavior. Burning a tool shed cannot be equated with torching a densely-populated apartment building. We could establish a minimum score for mental disorders that would require a minimum number of inclusion criteria and a minimum severity score (inclusion criteria multiplied by severity ratings). A more elaborate model might incorporate prototypic ratings so that frequent arson and frequent lying are differentially scored.

Why this brief discussion of categorical, dimensional, and synthesized diagnostic models? If we could agree on the fundamental criteria, for example Syndeham, I believe the choice of the optimum organization and type of measurement would become obvious. The important lesson from structured interviews is that reliable dimensions for specific inclusion criteria can be established. We have also learned from prototypical analysis that core characteristics of particular mental disorders can be reliably established. These methodologies could be combined to study the most effective model for establishing distinctive outcome criteria. What is now needed is systematic research of different models to establish specific outcome criteria that are understandable in terms of current theory and defensible with respect to treatment outcome. Metamethodological research could have a very real impact on diagnosis if systematic comparisons of different diagnostic models proved the superiority of one paradigm over others.

Other Considerations. A largely ignored facet of the diagnosis is symptom content. Does it matter whether paranoid ideation involves family/friends, governmental agencies, or extraterrestrial beings? Does it matter whether paranoid thoughts involve different forms of killing or simply the discrediting a person's standing in the community? For example, research on hallucinations (Larkin, 1979; Rogers, Gillis, Turner, & Smith, 1990) has suggested that the content of the hallucinations may be closely related to adjustment. Likewise, mood disorders and personality disorders could be categorized by symptom content. Certainly, the excellent work accomplished on the treatment of specific types of anxiety symptoms would recommend further examination of this approach. In other words, symptom content, such as that found with delusional disorders, may have merit in establishing diagnostic validity for other disorders.

Research in Chapter 7 (e.g., see Reich & Troughton, 1988b) demonstrated the potential effect that Axis I diagnoses may have on the assessment of Axis II disorders. What remains unexplored is the reverse: the effect of Axis II disorders on the assessment of major mental disorders. For example, does the presence of a narcissistic personality disorder limit the disclosure of major depression? How does a preexisting avoidant personality disorder affect the diagnosis of generalized anxiety disorder? Certainly, more research is needed to fully understand Axis I–Axis II interactions, as well as the effects of substance abuse disorders on both. With respect to the latter, are functional disorders underdiagnosed because of attributions made by patients (or psychologists) about the presence of substance abuse?

Diagnostic research, in general, is appallingly simplistic in its cross-cultural considerations. This research typically assumes that all African-Americans and Hispanics are similar and will respond similarly to the same psychometric measure. Many studies of minorities naively assume that comparable norms justify the generalization of external validity data from one cultural group to another. Other studies compare test data across groups to establish cultural differences without having objective external criteria. Given the differential stigmas attached to psychological treatment, we should not conclude that self-referrals to counseling centers represent similar levels of distress across cultural groups. For example, certain ethnic groups may have higher elevations on MMPI profiles, not because of cultural differences on the test itself but because of differences in their referral patterns. Many studies need to be conducted on intragroup differences (e.g., first vs. second generation Asian-Americans) as well as on establishing external validity among minorities.

A final consideration might be "diagnosis by treatment." If we accepted that the overriding objective of assessment is the effective treatment of mentally disordered persons, then the logical conclusion would be to link diagnosis to treatment. What would be the implications of this radical departure from our current nosology? First and foremost, "untreatable" disorders would no longer be unnecessarily stigmatized. As noted by Rogers and Lynett (1991), the diagnosis of APD typically signals to the criminal justice system an untreatable person who is, therefore, likely to receive very punitive criminal sanctions. Of course, the obvious limitation of this approach is that treatment methods might never be developed. An apparent solution would be the development of provisional disorders that would be "sunsetted" if effective treatment was not forthcoming after a specified period of time. Research on a treatment-typology might offer an incisive approach to diagnosis and militate against diagnostic overrefinement.

Motivational Issues in Psychological Assessment

Nearly all psychological measures are based on three rebuttable assumptions: (a) that each patient is psychologically engaged in the assessment process, (b) that each patient shares the same goals as the examining psychologist, and (c) that each patient will cooperate with the psychologist's methods of achieving these goals. Research directly on these assumptions might offer valuable insights on their viability in psychological assessments. For example, we could attempt to assess patients' motivations, understanding of the psychologists' motivations, and agreement with the methods for achieving their own as well as the psychologists' objectives.

The first assumption, psychological engagement in the assessment process, has been systematically evaluated with several multiscale inventories (e.g., MMPI and PAI). With these measures, the patient's responses are evaluated as to whether items are being read and responded to consistently. The response style inherent in this approach is "irrelevant responding" (see Rogers, 1988). Irrelevant responding has not been systematically explored with structured interviewing or with most types of psychological testing. Research which combines interview and self-report measures (e.g., the SCID-II and SCID-II-Q) might be particularly effective in assessing consistency of self-report, which would be the underlying strategy in the detection of irrelevant responding.

The patient's motivation, as the second assumption, may correspond to that of the examining psychologist in an accurate appraisal of psychopathology and diagnosis. Alternatively, the patient may be motivated to exaggerate/fabricate symptoms in light of an external goal (i.e., malingering and factitious disorders), to minimize/deny symptoms (defensiveness), or to acknowledge only symptoms which are less stigmatizing (social desirability). Two additional and largely unexplored response styles in clinical assessment include (a) "role assumption" (Kroger & Turnbull, 1975), in which the patient assumes the role of a different person as a method of foiling the evaluation, and (b) "impression management" (Tetlock & Mansard, 1985), in which individuals attempt to create desired social images and identities. In addition, patients may develop hybrid response styles in which they combine more than one of the previous styles. The classic example of a hybrid response style is the pedophile who is often self-disclosing about most aspects of his/her life, but highly defensive about his/her interest in and sexual arousal toward children.

Research on response styles has proceeded rather unevenly. Concerted attention has been paid to malingering in the last decade, with a proliferation of studies. In contrast, a relatively small literature has been established on defensiveness and social desirability. Very little clinical research has been conducted on role assumption and impression management. Certainly, more systematic research is needed on all forms of response style, particularly as they relate to structured interviewing and projective techniques.

The third assumption is that patients agree with psychologists in the selection of assessment methods. Patients' willingness or unwillingness to engage in certain forms of assessment has yet to be systematically studied. Although "resistance" has been described in patients who give only minimal responses to projective techniques, perhaps the more basic issue is the agreement, explicit or implicit, between examiner and examinee. The effects of negotiated versus non-negotiated assessments has yet to be empirically investigated. In other words, how does coercion, whether acknowledged or not, affect participation and results?

Test conditions have long been known to affect motivation and performance, particularly on aptitude tests (Cronbach, 1970). How do situational characteristics affect patients' performance on clinical measures? For example, we could compare symptoms and diagnoses for children tested in juvenile detention facilities with the same children as tested in the community. By the same token, we could also compare diagnoses made from videotapes by mental health professionals who were blind to the location of the testing. In this way, we could test for "real" differences in motivation and self-reporting while simultaneously estimating the situational effects on the examining psychologists. My point is that much more sophisticated research is possible on the relationship of situational characteristics to reported psychopathology. Likewise, internal states (e.g., fatigue or tiredness) could be experimentally manipulated and rigorously tested.

Unfamiliarity with testing procedures may represent a related confound to psychological assessment. In several ongoing studies involving the assessment of Mexicans and Mexican-Americans, my colleagues and I have found that lack of acquaintance with multiple-choice and Likert-type ratings was often an impediment to their cooperation and compliance. Lack of enculturation in American-style schooling may have profound effects on performance, especially when the format of the assessment differs substantially from past educational experiences.

Theory Testing

Like many of my academic colleagues, I have frequent occasions to review dissertations and am struck by how many are simply isolated empirical exercises that proliferate in the absence of theory. Although perhaps draconian, I would like to see an additional standard imposed by assessment journals: at a minimum, the results should be tied to theory. Atheoretical assessment studies are not accidental. Indeed, the *DSM-III* promulgated this stance as an attempt to reconcile differences between dynamic and biological schools (see Faust & Miner, 1986). Theory extends beyond etiology to diagnostic models (e.g., categorical vs. dimensional), diagnostic validity (e.g., Syndeham's criteria), response styles and motivation, and, of course, treatment methods.

A resurgence of interest in the assessment of personality, per se, with greater sophistication, especially in methodology, has been observed in the last two decades (Jackson & Paunonen, 1980). The relationship of personality to Axis I and II disorders has recently generated considerable theoretical interest. For example, the NEO Personality Inventory has been related to diagnosis and treatment (Costa & McCrae, 1992), particularly with regard to personality disorders (Schroeder, Wormworth, & Livesley, 1992). The theoretical possibilities of integrating personality and disorders are exciting. Moreover, much assessment research with dimensional ratings provides a basis for theoretical exploration of normality versus abnormality.

Longitudinal research is the *sine qua non* of theory testing and building. While the systematic comparisons of measures may further our understanding of important theory-based relationships, only through repeated measures can these relationships be fully understood. Even the best-crafted cross-sectional study offers but a single time perspective, although this may be augmented by the use of structured interviews that gather data regarding previous episodes. For example, Meehl's (1990) theory of schizotaxia as the etiological basis of schizophrenia should optimally be tested through longitudinal research. Best efforts at theory testing require stable samples with longitudinal assessments. A laudable goal for nearly all researchers is the identification of a clinical sample which is likely to remain relatively accessible to research across time.

Some theoretically based research may not require exhaustive efforts; it simply waits to be conducted. For example, could social-labeling theory be empirically tested? In many mental health clinics with case-management organization, diagnosis is deemphasized. Research with diagnostic interviews could establish "true" diagnoses and compare these to "working diagnoses" of the clinicians' and patients' self descriptions. By comparing the relative utility of each in predicting current functioning, we could test in a naturalistic design, the potential effects, both salutary and harmful, of social-labeling theory.

Theory-based interventions represent a vibrant component of treatment outcome research. In addition to its obvious merits, the vitality of cognitive-behavioral treatment lies in systematic research, which tests its relative efficacy with specific patient populations. Many other theoretical schools have languished, partly because of this inattention to theory-based research. Psychologists, searching to make important contributions, would do well to consider other theory-based interventions and systematic investigations into their treatment potential for clinical samples.

Other Applications

The use and application of structured interviews extends far beyond the reaches of general clinical practice. Standardized interview data have formed the basis of many attempts to evaluate individual competencies. As an example, forensic psychologists have developed several structured interviews for systematically assessing the legal construct of competency to stand trial. Dozens of studies have examined the validity of such measures as the Competency to Stand Trial Assessment Instrument (CAI; Laboratory of Community Psychiatry, 1973), the Interdisciplinary Fitness Interview (IFI; Golding, Roesch, & Schreiber, 1984), and the Georgia Court Competency Test (GCCT; Wildman et al., 1978). Comprehensive reviews of these competency measures are readily available (Bagby, Nicholson, Rogers, & Nussbaum, 1992; Nicholson & Kugler, 1991). Certainly, these efforts could be enlarged to address a host of equally complex forensic competencies (Grisso, 1986).

Research on structured interviews could easily be expanded beyond clinical issues to include educational and vocational applications. Standardization of interview and other data may improve predictive validity regarding important decisions, such as graduate student success, even when less than elegant models are employed (Dawes, 1979). By the same token, standardized interviews could be tested for the measurement of interpersonal functioning and its underlying dimensions; this might lead to a more comprehensive understanding of different types of relationships. Even such vague constructs as "adjustment" or "superior functioning" could be operationalized and assessed.

Psychologists have emphasized scale development, sometimes to the exclusion of other potentially valuable methods. I am advocating an expansion of assessment and not the jettisoning of inventories, scales, and ratings. By invoking a multimethod approach to assessment, I am recommending that we review important assessment domains which are typically measured by paper and pencil measures and consider the possibilities of structured interviews to complement these existing methods.

Concluding Comments

The separateness of clinical practice and applied research is often experienced in both our training and professional lives. This division of professional psychology has profound implications for the unnecessary and often detrimental compartmentalization of practice and research. In its own small way, I hope that the structured interview methods embraced by this book may forge a common ground, selectively employed by practitioners and vigorously tested by researchers.

References

References

Abrams, R. C., Alexopoulos, G. S., & Young, R. C. (1987). Geriatric depression and DSM-III-R personality disorder criteria. *Journal of the American Geriatrics Society, 35*, 383-386.

Achenbach, T. M. (1985). Clinical data systems: Rating scales and interviews. In R. Michels, J. O. Cavenar, A. M. Cooper, S. B. Guze, L. L. Judd, G. L. Klerman, & A. J. Solnit (Eds.), *Psychiatry* (Vol. 2, Chap. 23). Philadephia: J. B. Lippincott.

Achenbach, T. M., & Edelbrock, C. S. (1979). The child behavior profile: II. Boys aged 12-16 and girls aged 6-11 and 12-16. *Journal of Consulting and Clinical Psychology, 47*, 223-233.

Achenbach, T. M., & Edelbrock, C. S. (1983). *Manual for the Child Behavior Checklist and Revised Child Behavior Profile*. Burlington, VT: University of Vermont, Department of Psychiatry.

Achenbach, T. M., & Edelbrock, C. S. (1986). *Manual for the Teacher's Report Form and Teacher Version of the Child Behavior Profile*. Burlington, VT: University of Vermont, Department of Psychiatry.

Achenbach, T. M., & Edelbrock, C. S. (1987). *Manual for the Youth Self-Report and profile*. Burlington, VT: University Associates in Psychiatry.

Achenbach, T. M., McConaughy, S. H., & Howell, C. T. (1987). Child/adolescent behavioral and emotional problems: Implications of cross-informant correlations for situational specificity. *Psychological Bulletin, 101*, 213-232.

Albert, M., Smith, L. A., Scherr, P. A., Taylor, J. O., Evans, D. A., & Funkenstein, H. H. (1991). Use of brief cognitive tests to identify individuals in the community with clinically diagnosed Alzheimer's disease. *International Journal of Neuroscience, 57*, 167-178.

Allen-Meares, P. (1991). A study of depressive characteristics in behaviorally disordered children and adolescents. *Children and Youth Services Review, 13*, 271-286.

Alnaes, R., & Torgersen, S. (1988). The relationship between DSM-III symptom disorders (Axis I) and personality disorders (Axis II) in an outpatient population. *Acta Psychiatrica Scandinavica, 78*, 485-492.

Alnaes, R., & Torgersen, S. (1989a). Clinical differentiation between major depression only, major depression with panic disorder, and panic disorder only: Childhood, personality, and personality disorder. *Acta Psychiatrica Scandinavica, 79*, 370-377.

Alnaes, R., & Torgersen, S. (1989b). Personality and personality disorders among patients with major depression in combination with dysthymic and cyclothymic disorders. *Acta Psychiatrica Scandinavica, 79*, 363-369.

Alnaes, R., & Torgersen, S. (1990). DSM-III personality disorders among patients with major depression, anxiety disorders, and mixed conditions. *Journal of Nervous and Mental Disease, 178*, 693-698.

Alnaes, R., & Torgersen, S. (1991). Personality and personality disorders among patients with various affective disorders. *Journal of Personality Disorders, 5*, 107-121.

Alterman, A. I., Cacciola, J. S., & Rutherford, M. J. (1993). Reliability of the Revised Psychopathy Checklist in substance abuse patients. *Psychological Assessment, 5*, 442-448.

Altman, H., Angle, H. B., Brown, M. L., & Sletten, I. W. (1972a). Prediction of hospital stay. *Comprehensive Psychiatry, 13*, 471-480.

Altman, H., Angle, H. B., Brown, M. L., & Sletten, I. W. (1972b). Prediction of unauthorized absence. *American Journal of Psychiatry, 128*, 1460-1463.

Altman, H., Evenson, R. C., & Cho, D. W. (1976). New discriminant functions for computer diagnosis. *Multivariate Behavioral Research, 11*, 367-376.

Altman, H., Evenson, R. C., & Cho, D. W. (1977). *Predicting danger to self and others among psychiatric patients*. Unpublished technical report, Missouri Institute of Psychiatry, Mental Health Systems Research Unit, St. Louis.

Altman, H., Evenson, R. C., Hedlund, J. L., & Cho, D. W. (1978). Missouri actuarial report system (MARS). *Comprehensive Psychiatry, 19*, 185-192.

Altman, H., Evenson, R. C., & Sletten, I. W. (1973). Comparison of psychotropic drug assignment by psychiatrists and by a multivariate computer model. *International Research Communications System, 73*, 32-27-1.

Ambrosini, P. J. (1992). *Schedule for Affective Disorders and Schizophrenia for School Age Children (6-18 years): Kiddie-SADS (K-SADS) (Present state version)*. Philadelphia: Medical College of Pennsylvania.

Ambrosini, P. J., Metz, C., Prabucki, K., & Lee, J. C. (1989). Videotape reliability of the third revised edition of the K-SADS. *Journal of the American Academy of Child and Adolescent Psychiatry, 28*, 723-728.

American Psychiatric Association. (1968). *Diagnostic and statistical manual of mental disorders* (2nd. ed.). Washington, DC: Author.

American Psychiatric Association. (1980). *Diagnostic and statistical manual of mental disorders* (3rd ed.). Washington, DC: Author.

American Psychiatric Association. (1987). *Diagnostic and statistical manual of mental disorders* (3rd ed., rev.). Washington, DC: Author.

American Psychiatric Association. (1991). *DSM-IV options book: Work in progress*. Washington, DC: Author.

American Psychiatric Association. (1994). *Diagnostic and statistical manual of mental disorders* (4th ed.). Washington, DC: Author.

Anastasi, A. (1988). *Psychological testing* (6th ed.). New York: Macmillan.

Anderson, J. C., Williams, S., McGee, R., & Silva, P. A. (1987). DSM-III disorders in preadolescent children. *Archives of General Psychiatry, 42*, 69-76.

Andreasen, N. C. (1977). Reliability of proverbs: Interpretation to assess mental status. *Comprehensive Psychiatry, 18*, 465-473.

Andreasen, N. C. (1984a). *Scale for the Assessment of Negative Symptoms (SANS)*. Iowa City: University of Iowa College of Medicine.

Andreasen, N. C. (1984b). *Scale for the Assessment of Positive Symptoms (SAPS)*. Iowa City: University of Iowa College of Medicine.

Andreasen, N. C. (1987). *Comprehensive Assessment of Symptoms and History*. Iowa City: University of Iowa College of Medicine.

Andreasen, N. C., Flaum, M., & Arndt, S. (1992). The Comprehensive Assessment of Symptoms and History (CASH): An instrument for assessing diagnosis and psychopathology. *Archives of General Psychiatry, 49*, 615-623.

Andreasen, N. C., Grove, W. M., Shapiro, R. W., Keller, M. B., Hirschfield, R. A., & McDonald-Scott, P. (1981). Reliability of lifetime diagnosis. *Archives of General Psychiatry, 35*, 400-405.

Andreasen, N. C., McDonald-Scott, P., Grove, W. M., Keller, M. B., Shapiro, R. W., & Hirschfield, R. M. A. (1982). Assessment of reliability in multicenter collaborative research with a videotape approach. *American Journal of Psychiatry, 139*, 876-882.

Andreasen, N. C., & Olsen, S. (1982). Negative vs. positive schizophrenia. *Archives of General Psychiatry, 39*, 789-794.

Anduaga, J. C., Forteza, C. G., & Lira, L. R. (1991). Concurrent validity of the DIS: Experience with psychiatric patients in Mexico City. *Hispanic Journal of Behavioral Sciences, 13*, 63-77.

Angold, A., Cox, A., Prendergast, M., Rutter, M., & Simonoff, E. (1987). *The Child and Adolescent Psychiatric Assessment (CAPA)*. Unpublished manuscript.

Angus, L. E., & Marziali, E. (1988). A comparison of three measures for the diagnosis of borderline personality disorder. *American Journal of Psychiatry, 145*, 1453-1454.

Anthony, J. C., Folstein, M., Romanoski, A. J., Von Korff, M. R., Nestadt, G. R., Chahal, R., Merchant, A., Brown, H., Shapiro, S., Kramer, M., & Gruenber, E. M. (1985). Comparison of the lay Diagnostic Interview Schedule and a standardized psychiatric diagnosis. *Archives of General Psychiatry, 42*, 667-675.

Anthony, J. C., LeResche, L., Niaz, U., Von Korff, M. R., & Folstein, M. F. (1982). Limits of the Mini-Mental state as a screening test for dementia and delirium among hospital patients. *Psychological Medicine, 12*, 397-408.

Apter, A., Bleich, A., Plutchik, R., Mendelsohn, S., & Tyrano, S. (1988). Suicidal behavior, depression, and conduct disorder in hospitalized adolescents. *Journal of the American Academy of Child and Adolescent Psychiatry, 27*, 696-699.

Apter, A., Orvaschel, H., Laseg, M., Moses, R., & Tyano, S. (1989). Psychometric prop-erties of the K-SADS-P in an Israeli adolescent inpatient population. *Journal of the American Academy of Child and Adolescent Psychiatry, 28,* 61-65.

Arnold, L., & Smeltzer, D. (1974). Behavior checklist factor analysis for children and adolescents. *Archives of General Psychiatry, 30,* 799-804.

Aronen, E. A., Noam, G. G., & Weinstein, S. R. (1993). Structured diagnostic inter-views and clinicians' discharge diagnoses in hospitalized adolescents. *Journal of the American Academy of Child and Adolescent Psychiatry, 32,* 674-681.

Bachneff, S. A., & Engelsmann, F. (1983). Correlates of cerebral event-related slow potentials and psychopathology. *Psychological Medicine, 13,* 763-770.

Baer, L., Jenike, M. A., Black, D. W., Treece, C., Rosenfeld, R. & Griest, J. (1992). Effect of Axis II diagnosis on treatment outcome with clomipramine in 55 patients with obsessive-compulsive disorder. *Archives of General Psychiatry, 49,* 862-866.

Baer, L., Jenike, M. A., Ricciardi, J. N., Holland, A. D., Seymour, R. J., Minichiello, W. E., & Buttolph, M. L. (1990). Standardized assessment of personality disorders in obsessive-compulsive disorder. *Archives of General Psychiatry, 47,* 826-830.

Bagby, R. M., Nicholson, R. A., Rogers, R., & Nussbaum, D. (1992). Domains of com-petency to stand trial. *Law and Human Behavior, 16,* 491-507.

Bailey, B., West, K. Y., Widiger, T. A., & Freiman, K. (1993). The convergent and dis-criminant validity of the Chapman scales. *Journal of Personality Assessment, 61,* 121-135.

Bailine, S., Katzoff, A., & Rau, J. H. (1977). Diagnosis of schizophrenia by computer and clinicians: A pilot study. *Comprehensive Psychiatry, 18,* 141-145.

Baker, F. M. (1990). Screening tests for cognitive impairment. *Hospital and Community Psychiatry, 40,* 339-340.

Baldelli, M. V., Toschi, A., Motta, M., Marra, R., & Muratori, C. (1991). Cognitive assessment of the elderly patients: The choice of suitable assessment tools. *Archives of Gerontology and Geriatrics, 2,* 91-94.

Ballenger, J. C., Burrows, G. D., DuPont, R. L., Jr., Lesser, I. M., Noyes, R., Pecknold, J. C., Rifkin, A., & Swinson, R. P. (1988). Alprazolam in panic disorder and agora-phobias: Results from a multicenter trial. I. Efficacy in short-term treatment. *Archives of General Psychiatry, 45,* 413-422.

Banks, M. H. (1983). Validation of the General Health Questionnaire in a young com-munity sample. *Psychological Medicine, 13,* 349-353.

Barlow, D. H. (1991). Diagnoses, dimensions, and DSM-IV: The science of classifica-tion [Special issue]. *Journal of Abnormal Psychology, 100*(4).

Barlow, D. H., DiNardo, P. A., Vermilyea, B. B., Vermilyea, J. A., & Blanchard, E. B. (1986). Comorbidity and depression among the anxiety disorders: Issues in classi-fication and diagnosis. *Journal of Nervous and Mental Disease, 174,* 63-72.

Baron, M. (1980). *The Schedule for Interviewing Borderlines (SIB).* New York: New York State Psychiatric Institute.

Barrash, J., Kroll, J., Carey, K., & Sines, L. (1983). Discriminating borderline disorder from other personality disorders: Cluster analysis of the Diagnostic Interview for Borderlines. *Archives of General Psychiatry, 40*, 1297-1302.

Barrash, J., Pfohl, B., & Blum, N. (1993). "Unstable" personality disorders: Prognostic implications for major depression. *Journal of Personality Disorders, 7*, 155-167.

Barrett, E. T., & Gleser, G. C. (1987). Development and validation of the Cognitive Status Examination. *Journal of Consulting and Clinical Psychology, 55*, 877-882.

Bartlett, J. A., Schleifer, S. J., Johnson, R. L., & Keller, S. E. (1991). Depression in inner city adolescents attending an adolescent medicine clinic. *Journal of Adolescent Health, 12*, 316-318.

Bateman, A. W. (1989). Borderline personality in Britain: A preliminary study. *Comprehensive Psychiatry, 30*, 385-390.

Beaber, J. R., Marston, A., Michelli, J., & Mills, M. J. (1985). A brief test for measuring malingering in schizophrenic individuals. *American Journal of Psychiatry, 142*, 1478-1481.

Bebbington, P. E., Hurry, J., & Tennant, C. (1988). Adversity and the symptoms of depression. *International Journal of Social Psychiatry, 34*, 163-171.

Bebbington, P. E., Hurry, J., Tennant, C., Sturt, E., & Wing, J. K. (1981). Epidemiology of mental disorders in Camberwell. *Psychological Medicine, 11*, 561-579.

Bebbington, P. E., Sturt, E., & Kumakura, N. (1983). The study of depressive disorders using the PSE-ID-CATEGO system. *Acta Psychiatrica Scandinavica, 72*, 55-64.

Beck, A. T., Ward, C. H., Mendelson, M., Mock, J. E., & Erbaugh, J. (1961). An inventory for measuring depression. *Archives of General Psychiatry, 4*, 561-571.

Beck, A. T., Weissman, A., Lester, D., & Trexler, L. (1974). The measurement of pessimism: The Hopelessness Scale. *Journal of Consulting and Clinical Psychology, 42*, 861-865.

Bell, R., & Hall, R. C. W. (1977). The mental status examination. *American Family Physician, 16*, 145-152.

Bell, R. C., & Jackson, H. J. (1992). The structure of personality disorders in DSM-III. *Acta Psychiatrica Scandinavica, 85*, 279-287.

Bender, L. (1938). *A visual motor gestalt test and its clinical use.* New York: American Orthopsychiatric Association.

Benjamin, R. S., Costello, E. J., & Warren, M. (1990). Anxiety disorders in a pediatric sample. *Journal of Anxiety Disorders, 4*, 293-316.

Benton, A. L. (1967). Problems of test construction in the field of aphasia. *Cortex, 3*, 32-58.

Berg, G., Edwards, D. F., Danzinger, W. L., & Berg, L. (1987). Longitudinal change in three brief assessments of SDAT. *Journal of the American Geriatrics Society, 35*, 205-212.

Berman, W. H., Berman, E. R., Heymsfield, S., Fauci, M., & Ackerman, S. (1992). The incidence and comorbidity of psychiatric disorders in obesity. *Journal of Personality Disorders, 6*, 168-175.

Berner, P., Gabriel, E., Katschnig, H., Kieffer, W., Koehler, K., Lenz, G., & Semhandl, C. (1983). *Diagnostic criteria for schizophrenic and affective psychoses.* Vienna: World Psychiatric Association.

Bernstein, E. M., & Putnam, F. W. (1986). Development, reliability, and validity of a dissociation scale. *Journal of Nervous and Mental Disease, 174,* 727-734.

Berry, D. T. R., Baer, R. A., & Harris, M. J. (1991). Detection of malingering on the MMPI: A meta-analytic review. *Clinical Psychology Review, 11,* 585-598.

Berwick, D. M., Murphy, J. M., Goldman, P. A., Ware, J. E., Jr., Barsky, A. J., & Weinstein, M. C. (1991). Performance of a five-item mental health screening test. *Medical Care, 29,* 169-176.

Biederman, J., Farone, S. V., Doyle, A., Lehman, B. K., Kraus, I., Perrin, J., & Tsuang, M. T. (1993). Convergence of the Child Behavior Checklist with a structured interview-based psychiatric diagnosis of ADHD children with and without comorbidity. *Journal of Child Psychology and Psychiatry, 34,* 1241-1251.

Biederman, J., Keenan, K., & Farone, S. G. (1990). Parent-based diagnosis of attention deficit disorder predicts a diagnosis based on teacher report. *Journal of the American Academy of Child and Adolescent Psychiatry, 29,* 698-701.

Biederman, J., Rosenbaum, J. F., Hirshfeld, D. R., Faraone, S. V., Bolduc, E. A., Gersten, M., Meminger, S. R., Kagan, J., Snidman, N., & Reznick, J. S. (1990). Psychiatric correlates of behavioral inhibition in young children of parents with and without psychiatric disorders. *Archives of General Psychiatry, 47,* 21-26.

Bien, T. H., Miller, W. R., & Boroughs, J. M. (1993). *Motivational interviewing with alcohol outpatients.* Manuscript submitted for publication.

Bird, H. R., Canino, G., Gould, M. S., Ribera, J., Rubio-Stipec, M., Woodbury, M., Huertas-Goldman, S., & Sesman, M. (1987). Use of the Child Behavior Checklist as a screening instrument of epidemiological research in child psychiatry: Results of a pilot study. *Journal of the American Academy of Child and Adolescent Psychiatry, 26,* 207-213.

Bird, H. R., Canino, G., Rubio-Stipec, M. R., Gould, M. S., Ribera, J., Sesman, M., Woodbury, M., Huertas-Goldman, S., Pagan, A., Sanchez-Lacay, A., & Moscoso, M. (1988). Estimates of the prevalence of childhood maladjustment in a community survey in Puerto Rico. *Archives of General Psychiatry, 45,* 1120-1126.

Bird, H. R., Canino, G., Rubio-Stipec, M. R., & Shrout, P. (1987). Use of the Mini-Mental State Examination in a probability sample of a Hispanic population. *Journal of Nervous and Mental Disease, 175,* 731-737.

Bird, H. R., Gould, M. S., & Staghezza, B. (1992). Aggregating data from multiple informants in child psychiatry epidemiological research. *Journal of the American Academy of Child and Adolescent Psychiatry, 31,* 78-85.

Bird, H. R., Gould, M. S., Yager, T., Staghezza, B., & Cannino, G. (1989). Risk factors for maladjustment in Puerto Rican children. *Journal of the American Academy of Child and Adolescent Psychiatry, 28,* 847-850.

Blanchard, E. B., Gerardi, R. J., Kolb, L. C., & Barlow, D. H. (1986). The utility of the Anxiety Disorders Interview Schedule (ADIS) in the diagnosis of post-traumatic stress disorder (PTSD) in Vietnam veterans. *Behavioral Research and Therapy, 24,* 577-580.

Blashfield, R. K. (1992, August). *Are there any prototypical patients with personality disorders?* Paper presented at the American Psychological Association convention, Washington, DC.

Blashfield, R. K., & Livesley, W. J. (1991). Metaphorical analysis of psychiatric classification as a psychological test. *Journal of Abnormal Psychology, 100*, 262-270.

Bleecker, M. L., Bolla-Wilson, K., Kawas, C., & Agnew, J. (1988). Age-specific norms for the Mini-Mental State Exam. *Neurology, 38*, 1565-1568.

Blessed, G., Tomlinson, B. E., & Roth, M. (1968). The association between quantitative measures of dementia and senile change in the cerebral grey matter of elderly subjects. *British Journal of Psychiatry, 114*, 797-811.

Blouin, A. G., Perez, E. L., & Blouin, J. H. (1988). Computerized administration of the Diagnostic Interview Schedule. *Psychiatry Research, 23*, 335-344.

Bonato, D. P., Cyr, J. J., Kalpin, R. A., Prendergast, P., & Sanhueza, P. (1988). The utility of the MCMI as a DSM-III Axis I diagnostic tool. *Journal of Clinical Psychology, 44*, 867-875.

Boon, S., & Draijer, N. (1991). Diagnosing dissociative disorders in the Netherlands: A pilot study with the Structured Clinical Interview for DSM-III-R Dissociative Disorders. *American Journal of Psychiatry, 148*, 458-462.

Borgherini, G., Bernasconi, G., & Magni, G. (1992). Personality disorders in peptic ulcer disease: A preliminary report. *Journal of Personality Disorders, 6*, 241-245.

Borst, S. R., Noam, S. G., & Bartok, J. A. (1991). Adolescent suicidality: A clinical-development approach. *Journal of the American Academy of Child and Adolescent Psychiatry, 30*, 796-803.

Boyd, J. H., Weissman, M. M., Thompson, W. D., & Myers, J. K. (1983). Different definitions of alcoholism, I: Impact of seven definitions on prevalence rates in a community sample. *American Journal of Psychiatry, 140*, 1309-1313.

Boyle, M. H., Byles, J. A., Offord, D. R., Hofmann, H. G., & Catlin, G. P. (1987). Ontario child health study: Methodology. *Archives of General Psychiatry, 44*, 826-831.

Brandt, J., Strauss, M. E., Lucas, J., Jensen, B., Folstein, S. E., & Folstein, M. F. (1984). Clinical correlates of dementia and disability in Huntington's disease. *Journal of Clinical Neuropsychology, 6*, 401-412.

Brawman-Mintzer, O., Lydiard, R. B., Emmanuel, N., Payeur, R., Johnson, M., Roberts, J., Jarrell, M. P., & Ballenger, J. C. (1993). Psychiatric comorbidity in patients with generalized anxiety disorder. *American Journal of Psychiatry, 150*, 1216-1218.

Brayne, C., & Calloway, P. (1989). An epidemiological study of dementia in a rural population of elderly women. *British Journal of Psychiatry, 155*, 214-219.

Brayne, C., & Calloway, P. (1990). The case identification of dementia in the community: a comparison of methods. *International Journal of Geriatric Psychiatry, 5*, 309-316.

Bremmer, J. D., Steinberg, M., Southwick, S. M., Johnson, D. R., & Charney, D. S. (1993). Use of the Structured Clinical Interview for DMS-IV Dissociative Disorders for systematic assessment of dissociative symptoms in post-traumatic stress disorder. *American Journal of Psychiatry, 150*, 1011-1014.

Brent, D. A., Zelenak, J. P., Busstein, O., & Brown, R. V. (1990). Reliability and validity of the Structured Interview for Personality Disorders in adolescents. *Journal of the American Academy of Child and Adolescent Psychiatry, 29*, 349-354.

Breslau, N. (1987). Inquiring about the bizarre: False positives in Diagnostic Interview Schedule for Children (DISC)—Ascertainment of obsessions, compulsions, and psychotic symptoms. *Journal of the American Academy of Child and Adolescent Psychiatry, 26*, 639-644.

Breslau, N., Davis, G. C., Prabucki, K. (1987). Searching for evidence on the validity of generalized anxiety disorder: Psychopathology in children of anxious mothers. *Psychiatry Research, 20*, 285-297.

Bromet, E. J., Bunn, L. O., Connell, M. M., Dew, M. A., & Schulberg, H. C. (1986). Long-term reliability of diagnosing lifetime major depression in a community sample. *Archives of General Psychiatry, 43*, 435-440.

Brooks, R. B., Baltazar, P. L., McDowell, D. E., Munjack, D. J., & Bruns, J. R. (1991). Personality disorders co-occurring with panic disorder with agoraphobia. *Journal of Personality Disorders, 5*, 328-336.

Broughton, R. (1990). The prototype concept in personality assessment. *Canadian Psychology, 31*, 26-37.

Brown, J. M., & Miller, W. R. (in press). Impact of motivational interviewing on participation and outcome in residential alcoholism treatment. *Psychology of Addictive Behaviors*.

Brunshaw, J. M., & Szatmari, P. (1988). The agreement between behavior checklists and structured psychiatric interviews for children. *Canadian Journal of Psychiatry, 33*, 474-481.

Bucholz, K. K., Robins, L. N., Shayka, J. J., Przybeck, T. R., Helzer, J. E., Goldring, E., Klein, M. H., Griest, J. H., Erdman, H. P., & Skare, S. S. (1991). Performance of two forms of a computer psychiatric screening interview: Version I of the DISSI. *Journal of Psychiatric Research, 25*, 117-129.

Burnam, M. A., Hough, R. L., Karno, M., Escobar, J. I., & Telles, C. A. (1987). Acculturation and lifetime prevalence of psychiatric disorders among Mexican-Americans in Los Angeles. *Journal of Health and Social Behavior, 28*, 89-102.

Burnam, M. A., Karno, M., Hough, R. L., Escobar, J. I., & Forsythe, A. B. (1983). The Spanish Diagnostic Interview Schedule: Reliability and comparison with clinical diagnoses. *Archives of General Psychiatry, 40*, 1189-1196.

Bushnell, J. A., Wells, J. E., Hornblow, A. R., Oakley-Browne, M. A., & Joyce, P. (1990). Prevalence of three bulimia syndromes in the general population. *Psychological Medicine, 20*, 671-680.

Buss, A. H. (1966). *Psychopathology*. New York: Wiley.

Butcher, J. N., & Williams, C. L. (1992). *Essentials of MMPI-2 and MMPI-A interpretation*. Minneapolis, MN: University of Minnesota Press.

Buydens-Branchey, L., Branchey, M. H., & Noumair, D. (1989). Age of alcoholism onset: I. Relationship to psychopathology. *Archives of General Psychiatry, 46*, 225-230.

Byrne, P. (1984). Psychiatric morbidity in a gynecology clinic: An epidemiological survey. *British Journal of Psychiatry, 144*, 28-34.

Cacciola, J. S., Rutherford, M. J., & Alterman, A. I. (1990, June). *Use of the Psychopathy Checklist with opiate addicts.* Paper presented to Committee on Problems in Drug Dependence, National Drug Administration, Richmond, VA.

Campbell, D. T., & Fiske, D. W. (1959). Convergent and discriminant validation by the multitrait-multimethod matrix. *Psychological Bulletin, 56,* 81-105.

Canino, G. J., Bird, H. R., Shrout, P. E., Rubio-Stipec, M., Bravo, M., Martinez, R., Sesman, M., Guzman, A., & Guevara, L. M. (1987). The prevalence of specific psychiatric disorders in Puerto Rico. *Archives of General Psychiatry, 44,* 727-735.

Canino, G. J., Bird, H. R., Shrout, P. E., Rubio-Stipec, M., Bravo, M., Martinez, R., Sesman, M., Guzman, A., Guevara, L. M., & Costas, H. (1987). The Spanish Diagnostic Interview Schedule: Reliability and concordance with clinical diagnoses in Puerto Rico. *Archives of General Psychiatry, 44,* 720-726.

Carlson, G. A., Kashani, J. H., Thomas, M. D. F., Vaidya, A., & Daniel, A. E. (1987). Comparison of the DISC and the K-SADS-P interviews in an epidemiological sample of children. *Journal of the American Academy of Child and Adolescent Psychiatry, 26,* 645-648.

Carnes, M., Gunter-Hunt, G., & Rodgers, E. (1987). The effect of an interdisciplinary geriatrics clinic visit on mental status. *Journal of the American Geriatrics Society, 35,* 1035-1036.

Carpenter, W. T., Jr., & Gunderson, J. G. (1977). Five year follow-up comparison of borderline and schizophrenic patients. *Comprehensive Psychiatry, 18,* 567-571.

Carson, R. C. (1991). Dilemmas in the pathway of the DSM-IV. *Journal of Abnormal Psychology, 100,* 302-307.

Casey, P. R., Tyrer, P. J., & Platt, S. (1985). The relationship between social functioning and psychiatric symptomatology in primary care. *Social Psychiatry, 20,* 5-9.

Catalan, J., Gath, D., Bond, A., & Martin, P. (1984). The effects of non-prescribing anxiolytics in general practice: II. Factors associated with outcome. *British Journal of Psychiatry, 144,* 603-610.

Cavanaugh, S. V., & Wettstein, R. M. (1989). Emotional and cognitive dysfunction associated with medical disorders. *Journal of Psychosomatic Research, 33,* 505-514.

Chambers, W. J., Puig-Antich, J., Hirsch, M., Paez, P., Ambrosini, P. J., Tabrizi, M. A., & Davies, M. (1985). The assessment of affective disorders in children and adolescents by semistructured interview: Test-retest reliability of the Schedule for Affective Disorders and Schizophrenia for School-Aged Children, present episode version. *Archives of General Psychiatry, 42,* 696-702.

Chapman, L. J., & Chapman, J. P. (1987). The search for symptoms predictive of schizophrenia. *Schizophrenia Bulletin, 13,* 497-503.

Chapman, L. J., Chapman, J. P., Numbers, J. S., Edell, W. S., Carpenter, B. N., & Beckfield, D. (1984). Impulsive nonconformity as a trait contributing to the prediction of psychotic-like and schizotypal symptoms. *Journal of Nervous and Mental Disease, 172,* 681-691.

Chapman, T. F., Mannuzza, S., Klein, D. F., & Fyer, A. J. (1994). Effects of informant mental disorder of psychiatric family history. *American Journal of Psychiatry, 151,* 574-579.

Christensen, H., Hadzi-Pavlovic, D., & Jacomb, P. (1991). The psychometric differentiation of dementia from normal aging: A meta-analysis. *Psychological Assessment: A Journal of Clinical and Consulting Psychology, 3,* 147-155.

Clark, L. A. (1992). Resolving taxonomic issues in personality disorders: The value of large-scale analyses of symptom data. *Journal of Personality Disorders, 6,* 360-376.

Clark, L. A., & Watson, D. (1991). Tripartite model of anxiety and depression: Psychometric evidence and taxonomic implications. *Journal of Abnormal Psychology, 100,* 316-336.

Clarkin, J. F., Hull, J. W., & Hurt, S. W. (1993). Factor structure of borderline personality disorder criteria. *Journal of Personality Disorders, 7,* 137-143.

Cleckley, H. (1976). *The mask of insanity* (4th ed.). St. Louis, MO: Mosby.

Cloninger, C. R., Martin, R. L., Guze, S. B., & Clayton, P. J. (1985). Diagnosis and prognosis in schizophrenia. *Archives of General Psychiatry, 42,* 15-25.

Cohen, J. (1960). A coefficient of agreement for nominal scales. *Educational and Psychological Measurement, 20,* 37-46.

Cohen, P., Kasen, S., Brook, J. S., & Struening, E. L. (1991). Diagnostic predictors of treatment patterns in a cohort of adolescents. *Journal of the American Academy of Child and Adolescent Psychiatry, 30,* 989-993.

Cohen, P., O'Conner, P., Lewis, S., Veliz, C. N., & Malachowski, B. (1987). Comparison of DISC and K-SADS-P interviews of an epidemiological sample of children. *Journal of the American Academy of Child and Adolescent Psychiatry, 26,* 662-667.

Coie, J. D., Watt, N. F., West, S. G., Hawkins, J. D., Asarnow, J. R., Markman, H. J., Ramey, S. L., Shure, M. B., & Long, B. (1993). The science of prevention: A conceptual framework and some directions for a national research program. *American Psychologist, 48,* 1013-1022.

Colsher, P. L., & Wallace, R. B. (1990). Are hearing and visual dysfunction associated with cognitive impairment? A population-based approach. *Journal of Applied Gerontology, 9,* 91-105.

Connell, D. K. (1991). *The SIRS and the M Test: The differential validity and utility of two instruments designed to detect malingered psychosis in a correctional sample.* Unpublished doctoral dissertation, University of Louisville, KY.

Conners, C. (1969). A teacher rating scale for use in drug studies in children. *American Journal of Psychiatry, 126,* 152-156.

Cooney, N. L., Kadden, R. M., & Litt, M. D. (1990). A comparison of methods for assessing sociopathy in male and female alcoholics. *Journal of Studies on Alcohol, 51,* 42-48.

Cooper, J. E., Copeland, J. R. M., Brown, G. W., Harris, T., & Gourlay, A. J. (1977). Further studies on interviewer training and interrater reliability of the Present State Examination (PSE). *Psychological Medicine, 7,* 517-523.

Cooper, Z., Cooper, P. J., & Fairburn, C. G. (1989). The validity of the Eating Disorder Examination. *British Journal of Psychiatry, 154,* 808-812.

Cooper, J. E., Kendell, R. E., Gurland, B. J., Sharpe, L., Copeland, J. R. M., & Simon, R. (1972). *Psychiatric diagnosis in New York and London*. London: Oxford University Press.

Cooper, P. J., Taylor, M. J., Cooper, Z., & Fairburn, C. G. (1987). The development and validation of the Body Shape Questionnaire. *International Journal of Eating Disorders, 6*, 1-8.

Cooper, Z., & Fairburn, C. G. (1987). The Eating Disorder Examination: A semi-structured interview for the assessment of the specific psychopathology of eating disorders. *International Journal of Eating Disorders, 6.*

Copolov, D. L., Rubin, R. T., Stuart, G. W., Poland, R. E., Mander, A. J., Sashidharan, S. P., Whitehouse, A. M., Blackburn, I. M., Freeman, C. P., & Blackwood, D. H. R. (1989). Specificity of the salivary cortisol dexamethasone suppression test across psychiatric diagnoses. *Biological Psychiatry, 25*, 879-893.

Cornell, D. G., Silk, K. R., Ludolph, P. S., & Lohr, N. E. (1983). Test-retest reliability of the diagnostic interview for borderlines. *Archives of General Psychiatry, 40*, 1307-1310.

Coryell, W. H., Akiskal, H. S., Leon, A. C., Winokur, G., Maser, J. D., Mueller, T. I., & Keller, M. B. (1994). The time course of nonchronic major depressive disorder. *Archives of General Psychiatry, 51*, 405-410.

Coryell, W. H., & Noyes, R. (1988). Placebo response in panic disorder. *American Journal of Psychiatry, 145*, 1138-1140.

Coryell, W. H., & Zimmerman, M. (1989). Personality disorder in the families of depressed, schizophrenic, and never-ill probands. *American Journal of Psychiatry, 146*, 496-502.

Costa, P. T., Jr., & McCrae, R. R. (1985). *NEO Personality Inventory: Professional manual*. Odessa, FL: Psychological Assessment Resources.

Costa, P. T., Jr., & McCrae, R. R. (1992). Normal personality assessment in clinical practice: The NEO Personality Inventory. *Psychological Assessment, 4*, 5-13.

Costello, A. J., Edelbrock, C. S., Dulcan, M. K., Kalas, R., & Klaric, S. H. (1984). *Development and testing of the NIMH Diagnostic Interview Schedule for Children on a clinical population: Final report*. Rockville, MD: Center for Epidemiological Studies, National Institute of Mental Health.

Costello, E. J. (1989). Child psychiatric disorders and their correlates: A primary care pediatric sample. *Journal of the American Academy of Child and Adolescent Psychiatry, 28*, 851-855.

Costello, E. J., Benjamin, R., Angold, A., & Silver, D. (1991). Mood variability in adolescents: A study of depressed, nondepressed and comorbid patients. *Journal of Affective Disorders, 23*, 199-212.

Costello, E. J., Costello, A. J., Edelbrock, C., Burns, B. J., Dulcan, M. K., Brent, D., & Janiszewski, S. (1988). Psychiatric disorders in pediatric primary care: Prevalence and risk factors. *Archives of General Psychiatry, 45*, 1107-1116.

Costello, E. J., Edelbrock, C. S., & Costello, A. J. (1985). Validity of the NIMH Diagnostic Interview Schedule for Children: A comparison between psychiatric and pediatric referrals. *Journal of Abnormal and Child Psychology, 13*, 579-595.

Cote, G., & Hodgins, S. (1989). *Psychopathy Checklist: Validation of a French version*. Unpublished manuscript, Institute Philippe Pinel, Montreal, Canada.

Couch, A., & Keniston, K. (1960). Yeasayers and naysayers: Agreeing response set as a personality variable. *Journal of Abnormal and Social Psychology, 60,* 151-174.

Craft, M. J. (1965). *Ten studies into psychopathic personality*. Bristol, England: John Wright.

Cromwell, R. L. (1988). *Behavior genetics of schizophrenia: New research perspectives*. Paper presented as the inaugural address of the M. Erik Wright Professorship in Clinical Psychology, University of Kansas, Lawrence.

Cronbach, L. J. (1970). *Essentials of psychological testing* (3rd ed.). New York: Harper & Row.

Crook, T., Gilbert, J. G., & Ferris, S. H. (1980). Operationalizing memory impairment in elderly persons: The Guild Memory Test. *Psychological Reports, 47,* 1315-1318.

Crown, S., & Crisp, A. H. (1966). A short diagnostic self-ratings scale for psychoneurotic patients. *British Journal of Psychiatry, 112,* 917-923.

Cunnien, A. J. (1988). Psychiatric and medical syndromes associated with deception. In R. Rogers (Ed.), *Clinical assessment of malingering and deception* (pp. 13-33). New York: Guilford.

Dahl, A. A., & Bordahl, P. E. (1993). Obstetric complications as a risk factor for subsequent development of personality disorders. *Journal of Personality Disorders, 7,* 22-27.

Dalton, J. E., Pederson, S. L., Blom, B. E., & Holmes, N. R. (1987). Diagnostic errors using the Short Portable Mental Status Questionnaire with a mixed clinical population. *Journal of Gerontology, 42,* 512-514.

David, A. S., Jeste, D. V., Folstein, M. F., & Folstein, S. E. (1987). Voluntary movement dysfunction in Huntington's disease and tardive dyskinesia. *Acta Neurologica Scandinavica, 75,* 130-139.

Davidson, J. R. T., & Foa, E. B. (1991). Diagnostic issues in posttraumatic stress disorder: Considerations for DSM-IV. *Journal of Abnormal Psychology, 100,* 346-355.

Davies, W., & Feldman, P. (1981). The diagnosis of psychopathy by forensic specialists. *British Journal of Psychiatry, 138,* 329-331.

Dawes, R. M. (1979). Robust beauty of improper linear model in decision making. *American Psychologist, 34,* 571-582.

Dean, C., Surtees, P. G., & Sahsidharan, S. P. (1983). Comparison of research diagnostic systems in an Edinburgh community sample. *British Journal of Psychiatry, 142,* 247-256.

Denicoff, K. D., Joffe, R. T., Lakshmanan, M. C., Robbins, J., & Rubinow, D. R. (1990). Neuropsychiatric manifestations of altered thyroid state. *American Journal of Psychiatry, 147,* 94-99.

DePaulo, J. R., & Folstein, M. F. (1978). Psychiatric disturbances in neurological patients: Detection, recognition, and hospital course. *Annals of Neurology, 4,* 225-228.

Derksen, J. (1990). An exploratory study of borderline personality disorder in women with eating disorders and psychoactive substance abuse patients. *Journal of Personality Disorders, 4,* 372-380.

Derogatis, L. R. (1977). *The SCL-90, R version manual: Scoring administration and procedures for the SCL-90.* Baltimore: Johns Hopkins University Press.

Derogatis, L. R., & Spencer, P. M. (1982). *The Brief Symptom Inventory (BSI): Administration, scoring and procedures manual.* Baltimore: Johns Hopkins University Press.

Deykin, E. Y., Buka, S. L., & Zeena, T. H. (1992). Depressive illness among chemically dependent adolescents. *American Journal of Psychiatry, 149,* 1341-1347.

Dick, J. P. R., Guiloff, R. J., Stewart, A., Blackstock, J., Bielawska, C., Paul, E. A., & Marsden, C. D. (1984). Mini-Mental State Examination in neurological patients. *Journal of Neurology, Neurosurgery, and Psychology, 47,* 496-499.

DiNardo, P. A., O'Brien, G. T., Barlow, D. H., Waddell, M. T., & Blanchard, E. B. (1982). *Anxiety Disorders Interview Schedule (ADIS).* Albany, NY: Center for Stress and Anxiety Disorders, State University of New York at Albany.

DiNardo, P. A., O'Brien, G. T., Barlow, D. H., Waddell, M. T., & Blanchard, E. B. (1985). *Anxiety Disorders Interview Schedule–Revised (ADIS-R).* Albany, NY: Center for Stress and Anxiety Disorders, State University of New York at Albany.

DiNardo, P. A., O'Brien, G. T., Barlow, D. H., Waddell, M. T., & Blanchard, E. B. (1983). Reliability of DSM-III anxiety disorders using a new structured interview. *Archives of General Psychiatry, 40,* 1070-1074.

Donnelly, J., Rosenberg, M., & Fleeson, W. P. (1970). The evolution of the mental status: Past and future. *American Journal of Psychiatry, 126,* 121-126.

Dubro, A. F., Wetzler, S., & Kahn, M. W. (1988). A comparison of three self-report questionnaires for the diagnosis of DSM-III personality disorders. *Journal of Personality Disorders, 2,* 256-266.

Duncan, D. K. (1987). A comparison of two structured diagnostic interviews (Doctoral dissertation, York University, 1987). *Dissertation Abstracts International, 48,* 3109B.

Earls, R., Reich, W., Jung, K. G., & Cloninger, C. R. (1988). Psychopathology in children of alcoholic and antisocial parents. *Alcoholism: Clinical and Experimental Research, 12,* 481-487.

Earls, F., Smith, E., Reich, W., & Jung, K. G. (1988). Investigating psychopathological consequences of a disaster in children: A pilot study incorporating a structured diagnostic interview. *Journal of the American Academy of Child and Adolescent Psychiatry, 27,* 90-95.

Eaton, W. W., Kramer, M., Anthony, J. C., Dryman, A., Shapiro, S., & Locke, B. Z. (1989). The incidence of specific DIS/DSM-III mental disorders: Data from the NIMH epidemiologic catchment area program. *Acta Psychiatrica Scandinavica, 79,* 163-178.

Eckblad, M., & Chapman, L. J. (1986). Development and validation of a scale for hypomanic personality. *Journal of Abnormal Psychology, 95,* 214-222.

Edelbrock, C., & Costello, A. J. (1988). Convergence between statistically derived behavior problem syndromes and child psychiatric diagnoses. *Journal of Abnormal Child Psychology, 16,* 219-231.

Edelbrock, C., & Costello, A. J. (1990). Structured interviews for children and adolescents. In G. Goldstein & M. Hersen (Eds.), *Handbook of psychological assessment* (2nd ed.) (pp. 308-323). New York: Pergamon Press.

Edelbrock, C., Costello, A. J., Dulcan, M. K., Kalas, R., & Conover, N. C. (1985). Age differences in the reliability of the psychiatric interview of the child. *Child Development, 56,* 265-275.

Edell, W. S., Joy, S. P., & Yehuda, R. (1990). Discordance between self-report and observer-rated psychopathology in borderline patients. *Journal of Personality Disorders, 4,* 381-390.

Edwards, D. F., Baum, C. M., & Deuel, R. K. (1991). Constructional apraxia in Alzheimer's disease: Contributions to functional loss. *Physical and Occupational Therapy in Geriatrics, 9,* 53-68.

Endicott, J., Cohen, J., Nee, J., Fleiss, J., & Sarantakos, S. (1981). Hamilton Depression Rating Scale: Extracted from regular and change versions of the Schedule for Affective Disorders and Schizophrenia. *Archives of General Psychiatry, 38,* 98-103.

Endicott, J., Nie, J., Cohen, J., Fleiss, J. L., & Simon, R. (1986). Diagnosis of schizophrenia: Prediction of short-term outcome. *Archives of General Psychiatry, 43,* 13-19.

Endicott, J., & Spitzer, R. L. (1972). Current and Past Psychopathology Scales (CAPPS): Rationale, reliability, and validity. *Archives of General Psychiatry, 27,* 678-687.

Endicott, J., & Spitzer, R. L. (1978). A diagnostic interview: The Schedule of Affective Disorders and Schizophrenia. *Archives of General Psychiatry, 35,* 837-844.

Endicott, J., & Spitzer, R. L. (1979). Use of the Research Diagnostic Criteria and the Schedule of Affective Disorders and Schizophrenia to study affective disorders. *American Journal of Psychiatry, 136,* 52-56.

Endicott, J., Spitzer, R. L., & Fleiss, J. L. (1975). The Mental Status Evaluation Record (MSER): Reliability and validity. *Comprehensive Psychiatry, 16,* 285-301.

Endicott, J., Spitzer, R. L., Fleiss, J. L., & Cohen, J. (1976). The Global Assessment Scale: A procedure for measuring overall severity of psychiatric disturbance. *Archives of General Psychiatry, 33,* 766-771.

Engel, I. M. (1979). The mental status examination in psychiatry: Origin, use, and content. *Journal of Psychiatric Education, 3,* 99-108.

Erdman, H. P., Klein, M. H., Greist, J. H., Bass, S. M., Bires, J. K., & Machtinger, P. E. (1987). A comparison of the Diagnostic Interview Schedule and clinical diagnosis. *American Journal of Psychiatry, 144,* 1477-1480.

Erdman, H. P., Klein, M. H., Greist, J. H., Skare, S. S., Husted, J. J., Robins, L. N., Helzer, J. E., Goldring, E., Hamburger, M., & Miller, J. P. (1992). A comparison of two computer-administered versions of the NIMH Diagnostic Interview Schedule. *Journal of Psychiatric Research, 26,* 85-95.

Erkinjuntti, T., Sulkava, R., Wikstrom, J., & Autio, L. (1987). Short Portable Mental Status Questionnaire as a screening test for dementia and delirium among the elderly. *Journal of the American Geriatrics Society, 35,* 412-416.

Escobar, J. I., Burnham, A., Karno, M., Forsythe, A., Landsverk, J., & Golding, J. M. (1986). Use of the Mini-Mental State Examination (MMSE) in a community population of mixed ethnicity: Cultural and linguistic artifacts. *Journal of Nervous and Mental Disease, 174,* 607-614.

Evenson, R. C. (1976). *Community Adjustment Profile Scales (CAPS); Manual* (rev.). Unpublished manuscript, Missouri Institute of Psychiatry, Mental Health Systems Research Unit, St. Louis, MO.

Evenson, R. C., Altman, H., Cho, D. W., & Sletten, I. W. (1974a). The relationship of diagnosis and target symptoms to psychotropic drug assignment. *Comprehensive Psychiatry, 15,* 173-178.

Evenson, R. C., Altman, H., Cho, D. W., & Sletten, I. W. (1974b). Simple algorithms for predicting psychotropic drugs assigned to psychiatric inpatients. *Diseases of the Nervous System, 35,* 80-83.

Evenson, R. C., Altman, H., Sletten, I. W., & Cho, D. W. (1973a). Accuracy of actuarial and clinical predictions for length of stay and unauthorized absence. *Diseases of the Nervous System, 36,* 250-252.

Evenson, R. C., Altman, H., Sletten, I. W., & Cho, D. W. (1973b). Clinical judgment versus multivariate formulae in assignment of psychotropic drugs. *Journal of Clinical Psychology, 29,* 332-337.

Exner, J. E., Jr. (1991). *The Rorschach: A comprehensive system, Volume 2: Interpretation* (2nd ed.). New York: Wiley.

Famularo, R., Kinscherff, R., & Fenton, T. (1992). Psychiatric diagnoses of maltreated children: Preliminary findings. *Journal of the American Academy of Child and Adolescent Psychiatry, 31,* 863-867.

Farber, J. F., Schmitt, F. A., & Logue, P. E. (1988). Predicting intellectual level from the Mini-Mental State Examination. *Journal of the American Geriatrics Society, 36,* 509-510.

Farmer, A. E., Katz, R., McGuffin, P., & Bebbington, P. A. (1987). A comparison of the Present State Examination and the Composite International Diagnostic Interview. *Archives of General Psychiatry, 44,* 1064-1068.

Farrer, L. A., Florio, L. P., Bruce, M. L., Leaf, P. J., & Weissman, M. A. (1989). Reliability of self-reported age at onset of major depression. *Journal of Psychiatric Research, 23,* 35-47.

Faust, D., & Mine, R. A. (1986). The empiricist and his new clothes: DSM-III in perspective. *American Journal of Psychiatry, 143,* 962-967.

Faustman, W. O., Moses, J. A., & Csernansky, J. G. (1990). Limitations of the Mini-Mental State Examination in predicting neuropsychological functioning in a psychiatric sample. *Acta Psychiatrica Scandinavica, 81,* 126-131.

Feighner, J. P., Robins, E., Guze, S. B., Woodruff, R. A., Jr., Winokur, G., & Munoz, R. (1972). Diagnostic criteria for use in psychiatric research. *Archives of General Psychiatry, 26,* 57-63.

Fields, S. D., Fulop, G., Sachs, C. J., Strain, J., & Fillit, H. (1992). Usefulness of the neurobehavioral cognitive status examination in the hospitalized elderly. *International Psychogeriatrics, 4,* 93-102.

Fillenbaum, G. G. (1980). Comparison of two brief tests of organic impairment, the MSQ and the Short Portable MSQ. *Journal of the American Geriatrics Society, 28,* 381-384.

Fisher, P. W., Shaffer, D., Piacentini, J. C., Lapkin, J., Kafantaris, V., Leonard, H., & Herzog, D. B. (1993). Sensitivity of the Diagnostic Interview Schedule for Children, 2nd edition (DISC-2.1) for specific diagnoses of children and adolescents. *Journal of the American Academy of Child and Adolescent Psychiatry, 32,* 666-673.

Fisk, A. A., & Pannill, F. C., III. (1987). Assessment and care of the community-dwelling Alzheimer's disease patient. *Journal of the American Geriatrics Society, 35,* 307-311.

Fisk, J. D., Braha, R. E. D., Walker, A., & Gray, J. (1991). The Halifax Mental Status Scale: Development of a new test of mental status for use with elderly clients. *Psychological Assessment: A Journal of Clinical and Consulting Psychology, 3,* 162-167.

Fitchner, M. M., Elton, M., Engel, K., Meyer, A. E., Mall, H., & Poustka, F. (1991). Structured Interview for Anorexia and Bulimia Nervosa (SIAB): Development of a new instrument for the assessment of eating disorders. *International Journal of Eating Disorders, 10,* 571-592.

Fleiss, J. L., & Cohen, J. (1973). The equivalence of weighted kappa and the intraclass correlation coefficient as measures of reliability. *Educational and Psychological Measurement, 33,* 613-619.

Fleming, M. F., & Barry, K. L. (1991). The effectiveness of alcoholism screening in an ambulatory setting. *Journal of Studies on Alcohol, 52,* 33-36.

Folks, D. G., & Rabin, P. L. (1985). Residents' structured versus nonstructured assessment of cognitive function. *Journal of Psychiatric Education, 9,* 60-65.

Folstein, M. F. (1983). The Mini-Mental Status Examination. In T. Crook, S. Ferris, & R. Bartus (Eds.), *Assessment in geriatric psychopharmacology* (pp. 137-143). New Canaan, CT: Mark Powley.

Folstein, M. F., Anthony, J. C., Parhad, I., Duffy, B., & Gruenberg, E. M. (1985). The meaning of cognitive impairment in the elderly. *Journal of the American Geriatrics Society, 33,* 228-235.

Folstein, M. F., Folstein, S. E., & McHugh, P. R. (1975). Mini-mental state: A practical method of grading cognitive state of patients for the clinician. *Journal of Psychiatric Research, 12,* 189-198.

Folstein, M. F., Romanoski, A. J., Nestadt, G., Chahal, R., Merchant, A., Shapiro, S., Kramer, M., Anthony, J., Gruenberg, E. M., & McHugh, P. R. (1985). Brief report on the clinical reappraisal of the Diagnostic Interview Schedule carried out at the Johns Hopkins site of the epidemiological catchment area program of the NIMH. *Psychological Medicine, 15,* 809-814.

Folstein, S. E., Jensen, B., Leigh, R. J., & Folstein, M. F. (1983). The measurement of abnormal movement: Methods developed for Huntington's disease. *Neurobehavioral Toxicology and Teratology, 5,* 605-609.

Ford, C. V., King, B. R., & Hollender, M. H. (1988). Lies and liars: Psychiatric aspects of prevarication. *American Journal of Psychiatry, 145,* 554-562.

Ford, J., Hillard, J. R., Giesler, L. J., Lassen, K. L., & Thomas, H. (1989). Substance abuse/mental illness: Diagnostic issues. *American Journal of Drug and Alcohol Abuse, 15,* 297-305.

Foreman, M. D. (1987). Reliability and validity of mental status questionnaires in elderly hospitalized patients. *Nursing Research, 36,* 216-220.

Forth, A. E., Hart, S. D., & Hare, R. D. (1990). Assessment of psychopathy in male young offenders. *Psychological Assessment: A Journal of Consulting and Clinical Psychology, 2,* 342-344.

Foster, J. R., Sclan, S., Welkowitz, J., Boksay, I., & Seeland, I. (1988). Psychiatric assessment in medical long-term care facilities: Reliability of commonly used rating scales. *International Journal of Geriatric Psychiatry, 3,* 229-233.

Frances, A. J. (1982). Categorical and dimensional systems of personality disorders: A comparison. *Comprehensive Psychiatry, 23,* 516-527.

Frances, A. J. (1985). Introduction to personality disorders. In R. Michels, J. O. Cavenar, A. M. Cooper, S. B. Guze, L. L. Judd, G. L. Klerman, & A. J. Solnit (Eds.), *Psychiatry* (Vol. 1, Chap. 14). Philadelphia: J. B. Lippincott.

Frances, A., Clarkin, J. F., Gilmore, M., Hurt, S. W., & Brown, R. (1984). Reliability of criteria for borderline personality disorder: A comparison of DSM-III and the Diagnostic Interview for Borderline Patients. *American Journal of Psychiatry, 141,* 1080-1084.

Freeman, H., Cheadle, A. J., & Korer, J. R. (1979). Use of hospital services by chronic schizophrenics in the community. *British Journal of Psychiatry, 134,* 417-421.

Freeman, T. W., Clothier, J. L., Pazzaglia, P., Sesem, M. D., & Swann, A. C. (1992). A double-blind comparison of valproate and lithium in the treatment of acute mania. *American Journal of Psychiatry, 149,* 108-111.

Fyer, A. J., Endicott, J., Manuzza, S., Klein, D. F. (1985). *Schedule of Affective Disorders and Schizophrenia—Lifetime version* (modified for the study of anxiety disorders). New York: Anxiety Disorder Clinic, New York State Psychiatric Institute.

Fyer, A. J., Mannuzza, S., Martin, L. Y., Gallops, M. S., Endicott, J., Schleyer, B., Gorman, J. M., Liebowitz, M. R., & Klein, D. F. (1989). Reliability of anxiety assessment. II: Symptom agreement. *Archives of General Psychiatry, 46,* 1102-1110.

Gacono, C. B., & Hutton, H. E. (in press). Suggestions for the clinical and forensic use of the Hare Psychopathy Checklist–Revised (PCL-R). *International Journal of Psychiatry.*

Gacono, C. B., & Meloy, J. R. (1991). A Rorschach investigation of attachment and anxiety in antisocial personality disorder. *Journal of Nervous and Mental Disease, 179,* 546-552.

Gadow, K. D., & Sprafkin, J. (1987). *Stony Brook Child Psychiatric Checklist–3R.* Stony Brook, NY: State University of New York at Stony Brook, Department of Psychiatry.

Gaffney, F. A., Fenton, B. J., Lane, L. D., & Lake, R. (1988). Hemodynamic, ventilatory, and biochemical responses of panic patients and normal controls with sodium lactate infusion and spontaneous panic attacks. *Archives of General Psychiatry, 45,* 53-60.

Galasko, D., Klauber, M. R., Hofstetter, H., Salmon, D. P., Lasker, B., & Thal, L. J. (1990). The Mini-Mental State Examination in the early diagnosis of Alzheimer's disease. *Archives of Neurology, 47,* 49-52.

Gallagher, D. E., & Thompson, L. W. (1983). Effectiveness of psychotherapy for both endogenous and nonendogenous depression in older adult outpatients. *Journal of Gerontology, 38,* 707-712.

Gallager, R. E., Flye, B. L., Hurt, S. W., Stone, M. H., & Hull, J. W. (1992). Retrospective assessment of traumatic experiences (RATE). *Journal of Personality Disorders, 6,* 99-107.

Ganellen, R. J., Matuzas, W., Uhlenhuth, E. H., Glass, R., & Easton, C. R. (1986). Panic disorder, agoraphobia, and anxiety-relevant cognitive style. *Journal of Affective Disorders, 11,* 219-225.

Garfinkel, P. E. (1992). Evidence in support of attitudes to shape and weight as a diagnostic criterion of bulimia nervosa. *International Journal of Eating Disorders, 11,* 321-325.

Gartner, A. R., Marcus, R. N., Halmi, K., & Loranger, A. W. (1989). DSM-III-R personality disorders in patients with eating disorders. *American Journal of Psychiatry, 146,* 1585-1591.

Garyfallos, G., Karastergiou, A., Adamopoulou, A., Moutzoukis, C., Alagiozidou, E., Mala, D., & Garyfallos, A. (1991). Greek version of the general health questionnaire: Accuracy of translation and validity. *Acta Psychiatrica Scandinavica, 84,* 371-378.

Gasperini, M., Provenza, M., Ronchi, P., Scherillo, P., Bellodi, L., & Smeraldi, E. (1989). Cognitive processes and personality disorders in affective patients. *Journal of Personality Disorders, 3,* 63-71.

Gauron, E. F., & Dickinson, J. K. (1966). Diagnostic decision-making in psychiatry: Information usage. *Archives of General Psychiatry, 14,* 225-232.

Gavin, D. R., Ross, H. E., & Skinner, H. A. (1989). Diagnostic validity of the Drug Abuse Screening Test in the assessment of DSM-III drug disorders. *British Journal of Addictions, 84,* 301-307.

Getto, C. J., & Heaton, R. K. (1985). *Psychosocial Pain Inventory manual*. Odessa, FL: Psychological Assessment Resources.

Getto, C. J., Heaton, R. K., & Lehman, A. W. (1983). PSPI: A standardized approach to the evaluation of psychosocial factors in chronic pain. In J. J. Bonica (Ed.), *Advances in pain research and therapy* (Vol. 5, pp. 885-889). New York: Ravens Press.

Gilbertson, A., Torem, M., Cohen, R., Newman, I., Radojicic, C,. & Patel, S. (1992). Susceptibility of common self-report measures of dissociation to malingering. *Dissociation, 5,* 216-220.

Gillis, J. J., Gilger, J. W., Pennington, B. F., & DeFries, J. C. (1992). Attention deficit disorder in reading-disabled twins: Evidence for a genetic etiology. *Journal of Abnormal Child Psychology, 20,* 303-315.

Gillis, L. S., Elk, R., Ben-Arie, O., & Teggin, A. (1982). The Present State Examination: Experiences with Xhosa-speaking psychiatric patients. *British Journal of Psychiatry, 141,* 143-147.

Goekoop, J. G., Knoppert-Van der Klein, E. A. M., Hoeksema, T., Klinkhamer, R. A., Van Gaalen, H. A. E., & Van der Velde, E. A. (1991). The interrater reliability of a Dutch version of the Comprehensive Psychopathological Rating Scale. *Acta Psychiatrica Scandinavica, 83,* 202-205.

Goff, D. C., Olin, J. A., Jenike, M. A., Baer, L., & Buttolph, M. L. (1992). Dissociative symptoms in patients with obsessive-compulsive disorder. *Journal of Nervous and Mental Disease, 180,* 332-337.

Goldberg, D. (1978). *Manual for the General Health Questionnaire*. Windsor, Great Britain: NFER Publishing.

Goldberg, P. A., & Miller, S. J. (1966). Structured personality tests and dissimulation. *Journal of Projective Techniques and Personality Assessment, 30,* 452-455.

Golden, C. J., Sawicki, R. R., & Franzen, M. S. (1984). Test construction. In A. S. Bellack & M. Hersen (Eds.), *Research methods in clinical psychology* (pp. 233-265). New York: Pergamon Press.

Golding, S. L., Roesch, R., & Schreiber, J. (1984). Assessment and conceptualization of competency to stand trial: Preliminary data on the Interdisciplinary Fitness Interview. *Law and Human Behavior, 8,* 321-334.

Goldsmith, S. J., Anger-Friedfeld, K., Beren, S., Rudolph, D., Boeck, M., & Aronne, L. (1992). Psychiatric illness in patients presenting for obesity treatment. *International Journal of Eating Disorders, 12,* 63-71.

Goodman, W. K., Price, L. H., Rasmussen, S. A., Mazure, C., Delgado, P., Henigner, G. R., & Charney, D. S. (1989). The Yale-Brown Obsessive Compulsive Scale (YBOCS), I: Development, use, and reliability. *Archives of General Psychiatry, 46,* 1006-1011.

Gorham, D. R. (1956). Use of the Proverbs Test for differentiating schizophrenics from normals. *Journal of Consulting Psychology, 20,* 435-440.

Gothard, S. (1993). *Detection of malingering in mental competency evaluations*. Unpublished doctoral dissertation, California School of Professional Psychology, San Diego.

Graber, R. A., & Miller, W. R. (1988). Abstinence or controlled drinking goals for problem drinkers: A randomized clinical trial. *Psychology of Addictive Behaviors, 2,* 20-33.

Grad, L. R., Pelcovitz, D., Olson, M., Matthews, M., & Grad, G. J. (1987). Obsessive-compulsive symptomatology in children with Tourette's syndrome. *Journal of the American Academy of Child and Adolescent Psychiatry, 26,* 69-73.

Gray, K. C., & Hutchinson, H. C. (1964). The psychopathic personality: A survey of Canadian psychiatrists' opinions. *Canadian Psychiatric Association Journal, 9,* 452-461.

Grayson, P., & Carlson, G. A. (1991). The utility of a DSM-III-R based checklist in screening child psychiatric patients. *Journal of the American Academy of Child and Adolescent Psychiatry, 30,* 669-673.

Green, C. J. (1987). The Structured Interview for DSM-III Personality Disorders (SIDP): A review. *Journal of Personality Disorders, 1,* 288-290.

Green, C. J. (1989). The Personality Disorder Examination. *Journal of Personality Disorders, 3,* 352-354.

Greenbaum, P. E., Prange, M. E., Friedman, R. M., & Silver, S. E. (1991). Substance abuse prevalence and comorbidity with other psychiatric disorders among adolescents with severe emotional disturbances. *Journal of the American Academy of Child and Adolescent Psychiatry, 30,* 575-583.

Greene, R. L. (1988). Assessment of malingering and defensiveness by objective personality measures. In R. Rogers (Ed.), *Clinical assessment of malingering and deception* (pp. 123-158). New York: Guilford.

Greene, R. L., & Price, T. R. P. (1986). Procedural validity of an abbreviated version of the SADS/RDC diagnostic process. *Psychiatry Research, 18,* 379-391.

Greenwald, J., & Satow, Y. (1978). A short social desirability scale. *Psychological Reports, 27,* 131-135.

Gregory, R. J. (1987). *Adult intellectual assessment.* Boston: Allyn & Bacon.

Griest, J. H., Klein, M. H., Erdman, H. P., Bires, J., Bass, S., Machtinger, P., & Kresge, D. (1987). Psychiatric diagnosis via direct patient-computer interview. *Hospital and Community Psychiatry, 38,* 1305-1311.

Griest, J. H., Mathisen, K. S., Klein, M. H., Benjamin, L. S., Erdman, H. P., & Evans, F. J. (1984). Psychiatric diagnosis: What role for the computer. *Hospital and Community Psychiatry, 35,* 1089-1093.

Griffin, M. L., Weiss, R. D., Mirin, S. M., Wilson, H., & Bouchard-Voelk, B. (1987). The use of the Diagnostic Interview Schedule in drug-dependent patients. *American Journal of Drug and Alcohol Abuse, 13,* 281-291.

Grinker, R. R., Werble, B., & Drye, R. (1968). *The borderline syndrome: A behavioral study of ego functions.* New York: Basic Books.

Grisso, T. (1986). *Evaluating competencies: Forensic assessments and instruments.* New York: Plenum.

Grove, W. M., Andreasen, N. C., McDonald-Scott, P., & Keller, M. B. & Shapiro, R. W. (1981). Reliability studies of psychiatric diagnoses. *Archives of General Psychiatry, 38,* 408-413.

Grove, W. M., & Tellegen, A. (1991). Problems in the classification of personality disorders. *Journal of Personality Disorders, 5,* 31-41.

Gunderson, J. G. (1982). *Diagnostic interview with borderline patients* (2nd ed.). New York: Roerig-Pfizer.

Gunderson, J. G., Carpenter, W. T., Jr., & Strauss, J. S. (1975). Borderline and schizophrenic patients: A comparative study. *American Journal of Psychiatry, 132,* 1257-1264.

Gunderson, J. G., & Kolb, J. E. (1976, May). *Diagnosing borderlines: A semi-structured interview.* Paper presented at the American Psychiatric Association convention, Miami Beach.

Gunderson, J. G., & Kolb, J. E. (1978). Discriminating features of borderline patients. *American Journal of Psychiatry, 135,* 792-796.

Gunderson, J. G., Kolb, J. E., & Austin, V. (1981). The diagnostic interview for borderline patients. *American Journal of Psychiatry, 138,* 896-903.

Gunderson, J. G., Links, P. S., & Reich, J. H. (1991). Competing models of personality disorders. *Journal of Personality Disorders, 5,* 60-68.

Gunderson, J. G., & Singer, J. T. (1975). Defining borderline patients. *American Journal of Psychiatry, 132,* 1-10.

Gunderson, J. G., & Zanarini, M. C. (1992). *Revised Diagnostic Interview for Borderlines (DIB-R).* Boston: Harvard Medical School.

Gurland, B. J., Cote, L. J., Cross, P. S., & Toner, J. A. (1987). The assessment of cognitive function in the elderly. *Clinics in Geriatric Medicine, 3,* 53-63.

Gurland, B. J., Yorkston, N. J., Goldberg, K., Fleiss, J. L., Sloane, R. B., & Cristol, A. H. (1982). The Structured and Scaled Interview to Assess Maladjustment (SSIAM): II. Factor analysis, reliability, and validity. *Archives of General Psychiatry, 27,* 264-267.

Gurland, B. J., Yorkston, N. J., Stone, A. R., Frank, J. D., & Fleiss, J. L. (1982). The Structured and Scaled Interview to Assess Maladjustment (SSIAM): I. Description, rationale and development. *Archives of General Psychiatry, 27,* 259-264.

Gutterman, E. M., O'Brian, J. D., & Young, J. G. (1987). Structured diagnostic interviews for children and adolescents: Current status and future directions. *Journal of the American Academy of Child and Adolescent Psychiatry, 26,* 621-630.

Gynther, M. D., Altman, H., & Sletten, I. W. (1973). Replicated correlates of MMPI two-point code types: The Missouri actuarial system (monograph). *Journal of Clinical Psychology, 29,* 363-289.

Haddad, L. B., & Coffman, T. L. (1987). A brief neuropsychological screening exam for psychiatric-geriatric patients. *Clinical Gerontologist, 6,* 3-10.

Haley, G. M. T., Fine, S., & Marriage, K. (1988). Psychotic features in adolescents with major depression. *Journal of the American Academy of Child and Adolescent Psychiatry, 27,* 489-493.

Hammen, C. (1988). Self-cognitions, stressful events, and the prediction of depression in children of depressed mothers. *Journal of Abnormal Child Psychology, 16,* 347-360.

Hammen, C., Gordon, D., Burge, D., Adrian, C., Jaenicke, C., & Hiroto, D. (1987). Maternal affective disorders, illness, and stress: Risk for children's psychopathology. *American Journal of Psychiatry, 144,* 736-741.

Hamilton, M. (1959). The assessment of anxiety states by rating. *British Journal of Medical Psychology, 32,* 50-55.

Hamilton, M. (1960). A rating scale for depression. *Journal of Neurology, Neurosurgery, and Psychiatry, 23,* 56-62.

Hamparian, D. (1987). How well can we predict for juveniles? Juvenile delinquency and adult crime. In F. N. Dutile & C. H. Foust (Eds.), *The prediction of criminal violence* (pp. 169-184). Springfield, IL: C.C. Thomas.

Hare, R. D. (1980). A research scale for the assessment of psychopathy in criminal populations. *Personality and Individual Differences, 1,* 111-119.

Hare, R. D. (1985a). Comparison of procedures for the assessment of psychopathy. *Journal of Consulting and Clinical Psychology, 53,* 7-16.

Hare, R. D. (1985b). *The Psychopathy Checklist.* Unpublished manuscript, University of British Columbia, Vancouver, Canada.

Hare, R. D. (1991). *Manual for the Revised Psychopathy Checklist.* Toronto: Multi-Health Systems.

Hare, R. D., & Cox, D. N. (1978). Clinical and empirical conceptions of psychopathy, and the selection of subjects for research. In R. D. Hare & S. Schalling (Eds.), *Psychopathic behavior: Approaches to research.* Chichester, England: Wiley.

Hare, R. D., Cox, D. N., & Hart, S. D. (1989). *Preliminary manual for the Psychopathy Checklist: Clinical Version (PCL:CV).* Unpublished manuscript, University of British Columbia, Vancouver, Canada.

Hare, R. D., Cox, D. N., & Hart, S. D. (in press). *Manual for the Screening Version of Psychopathy Checklist—Revised (PCL-SV).* Toronto, Canada: Multi-Health Systems.

Hare, R. D., Harpur, T. J., Hakstian, A. R., Forth, A. E., Hart, S. D., & Newman, J. P. (1990). The revised Psychopathy Checklist: Reliability and factor structure. *Psychological Assessment: A Journal of Consulting and Clinical Psychology, 2,* 338-341.

Hare, R. D., & Hart, S. D. (1993). Psychopathy, mental disorder and crime. In S. Hodgins (Ed.), *Mental disorder and crime* (pp. 104-115). Newbury Park, CA: Sage.

Hare, R. D., & Hart, S. D. (in press). A comment on the DSM-IV antisocial personality disorder field trial. In W. J. Livesley (Ed.), *DSM-IV personality disorders.* New York: Guilford Press.

Hare, R. D., Hart, S. D., & Harpur, T. J. (1991). Psychopathy and the DSM-IV criteria for antisocial personality disorder. *Journal of Abnormal Psychology, 100,* 391-398.

Hare, R. D., & McPherson, L. M. (1984). Violent and aggressive behavior by criminal psychopaths. *International Journal of Law and Psychiatry, 7,* 35-50.

Hare, R. D., McPherson, L. M., & Forth, A. E. (1988). Male psychopaths and their criminal careers. *Journal of Clinical and Consulting Psychology, 56,* 710-714.

Harkness, A. R. (1992, August). *Multiply diagnosable patient: Hierarchical personality models and clinical judgment*. Paper presented at the American Psychological Association convention, Washington, DC.

Harpur, T. J., Hakstian, R., & Hare, R. D. (1988). Factor structure of the Psychopathy Checklist. *Journal of Consulting and Clinical Psychology, 56,* 741-748.

Harpur, T. J., Hare, R. D., & Hakstian, A. R. (1989). Two-factor conceptualization of psychopathy: Construct validity and assessment implications. *Psychological Assessment: A Journal of Consulting and Clinical Psychology, 1,* 6-17.

Harris, G. T., Rice, M. E., & Cormier, C. A. (1991). Length of detention in matched groups of insanity acquittees and convicted offenders. *Law and Human Behavior, 15,* 625-637.

Harris, K. B., & Miller, W. R. (1990). Behavioral self-control training for problem drinkers: Components of efficacy. *Psychology of Addictive Behavior, 4,* 82-90.

Harrison, P. A., & Hoffman, N. G. (1985). *The Substance Use Disorders Diagnostic Schedule*. St Paul, MN: Ramsey Clinic.

Hart, S. D., Forth, A. E., & Hare, R. D. (1991). The MCMI-II and psychopathy. *Journal of Personality Disorders, 5,* 318-327.

Hart, S. D., & Hare, R. D. (1989). Discriminant validity of the Psychopathy Checklist in a forensic psychiatric population. *Psychological Assessment: A Journal of Consulting and Clinical Psychology, 1,* 211-218.

Hart, S. D., & Hare, R. D. (1994). Psychopathy and the Big 5: Correlations between observer's ratings of normal and pathological personality. *Journal of Personality Disorders, 8,* 32-40.

Hart, S. D., Hare, R. D., & Cox, D. N. (1991, August). *Recent advances in the assessment of psychopathy*. Paper presented at the American Psychological Association convention, San Francisco.

Hart, S. D., Hare, R. D., & Forth, A. E. (in press). Psychopathy as a risk marker for violence: Development and validation of a screening version of the revised psychopathy checklist. In J. Monahan & H. J. Steadman (Eds.), *Violence and mental disorder: Developments in risk assessment*. Chicago: University of Chicago Press.

Hart, S. D., Hare, R. D., & Harpur, T. J. (1992). The Psychopathy Checklist—Revised (PCL-R): An overview for researchers and clinicians. In J. C. Rosen & P. McReynold (Eds.), *Advances in psychological assessment* (Vol. 8, pp. 103-130). New York: Plenum.

Hart, S. D., Kropp, P. R., & Hare, R. D. (1988). Performance of male psychopaths following conditional release from prison. *Journal of Consulting and Clinical Psychology, 56,* 227-232.

Hasin, D. S., & Grant, B. F. (1987a). Assessment of specific drug disorders in a sample of substance abuse patients: A comparison of the DIS and the SADS-L procedures. *Drugs and Alcohol Dependence, 19,* 165-176.

Hasin, D. S., & Grant, B. F. (1987b). Diagnosing depressive disorders in patients with alcohol and drug problems: A comparison of the SADS-L and the DIS. *Journal of Psychiatric Research, 21,* 301-311.

Hasin, D. S., & Grant, B. F. (1987c). Psychiatric diagnosis of patients with substance abuse problems: A comparison of two procedures, the DIS and the SADS-L. *Journal of Psychiatric Research, 21,* 7-22.

Hayward, C., Killen, J. D., Hammer, L. D., Litt, I. F., Wilson, D. M., Simmonds, B., & Taylor, C. B. (1992). Pubertal stage and panic attack history in sixth- and seventh-grade girls. *American Journal of Psychiatry, 149,* 1239-1243.

Hayward, C., & King, R. (1990). Somatization and personality disorder traits in non-clinical volunteers. *Journal of Personality Disorders, 4,* 402-406.

Heaton, R. Q., Lehman, R. A. W., & Getto, C. J. (1980). *Psychosocial Pain Inventory.* Odessa, FL: Psychological Assessment Resources.

Hedlund, J. L., Evenson, R. C., Sletten, I. W., & Cho, D. W. (1980). The computer and clinical prediction. In J. B. Sidowski, J. Johnson, & T. A. Williams (Eds.), *Technology in mental health care delivery systems* (pp. 201-235). Norwood, NJ: Ablex.

Hedlund, J. L., Sletten, I. W., Altman, H., & Evenson, R. C. (1973). Prediction of patients who are dangerous to others. *Journal of Clinical Psychology, 29,* 443-447.

Heilbrun, K., Gustaffson, D., Hart, S. D., & Hare, R. D. (1992). *Psychopathy and the prediction of violence in forensic patients.* Unpublished manuscript.

Helzer, J. E. (1981). The use of a structured interview for routine psychiatric evaluations. *Journal of Nervous and Mental Disease, 169,* 45-49.

Helzer, J. E., Brockington, I. F., & Kendell, R. E. (1981). Predictive validity of the DSM-III and Feighner definitions of schizophrenia. *Archives of General Psychiatry, 38,* 791-797.

Helzer, J. E., Clayton, P. J., Pambakian, R., Reich, T., Woodruff, R. A., & Reveley, M. A. (1977). Reliability of psychiatric diagnosis. *Archives of General Psychiatry, 34,* 136-141.

Helzer, J. E., & Robins, L. N. (1988). The Diagnostic Interview Schedule: Its development, evolution, and use. *Social Psychiatry and Psychiatric Epidemiology, 23,* 6-16.

Helzer, J. E., Robins, L. N., Croughan, J. L., & Welner, A. (1981). Renard Diagnostic Interview: Its reliability and procedural validity with physicians and lay interviewers. *Archives of General Psychiatry, 38,* 393-398.

Helzer, J. E., Robins, L. N., McEnvoy, L. T., Spitznagel, E. L., Stoltzman, R. K., Farmer, A., & Brockington, I. F. (1985). A comparison of clinical and Diagnostic Interview Schedule diagnoses. *Archives of General Psychiatry, 42,* 657-666.

Helzer, J. E., Spitznagel, E. L., & McEnvoy, L. (1987). The predictive validity of lay Diagnostic Interview Schedule diagnoses in the general population: A comparison with physician examiners. *Archives of General Psychiatry, 44,* 1069-1077.

Hemphill, J. F., Hart, S. D., & Hare, R. D. (1990, May). *Self-reported frequency and age of first substance use in criminal psychopaths.* Paper presented at the annual meeting of the Canadian Psychological Association, Ottawa.

Henderson, S., Duncan-Jones, P., Byrne, D. G., Scott, R., & Adcock, S. (1979). Psychiatric disorder in Canberra: A standardized study of prevalence. *Acta Psychiatrica Scandinavica, 60,* 355-374.

Hendrie, H. C., Hall, K. S., Brittain, H. M., Austrom, M. G., Farlow, M., Parker, J., & Kane, M. (1988). The CAMDEX: A standardized instrument for the diagnosis of mental disorder in the elderly—A replication with a U.S. sample. *Journal of the American Geriatrics Society, 36,* 402-408.

Herjanic, B., & Campbell, W. (1977). Differentiating psychiatrically disturbed children of the basis of a structured interview. *Journal of Abnormal Child Psychology, 5,* 127-134.

Herjanic, B., Herjanic, M., Brown, F., & Wheatt, T. (1975). Are children reliable reporters? *Journal of Abnormal and Child Psychology, 3,* 41-48.

Herjanic, B., & Reich, W. (1982). Development of a structured psychiatric interview for children: Agreement between child and parent on individual symptoms. *Journal of Abnormal Child Psychology, 10,* 307-324.

Herjanic, B., & Reich, W. (1983a). *Diagnostic Interview for Children and Adolescents (DICA-C): Child version.* St. Louis, MO: Washington University School of Medicine.

Herjanic, B., & Reich, W. (1983b). *Diagnostic Interview for Children and Adolescents (DICA-P): Parent version.* St. Louis, MO: Washington University School of Medicine.

Herkov, M. J., Archer, R. P., & Gordon, R. A. (1991). MMPI response sets among adolescents: An evaluation of the limitations of the subtle-obvious subscales. *Psychological Assessment: A Journal of Clinical and Consulting Psychology, 3,* 424-426.

Herrmann, D. J. (1982). Know thy memory: The use of questionnaires to assess and study memory. *Psychological Bulletin, 92,* 434-452.

Hersch, E. L., Kral, V. A., & Palmer, R. B. (1978). Clinical value of the London psychogeriatric rating scale. *Journal of the American Geriatrics Society, 26,* 348-354.

Hershey, L. A., Jaffe, D. F., Greenough, P. G., & Yang, S. L. (1987). Validation of cognitive and functional assessment instruments in vascular dementia. *International Journal of Psychiatry in Medicine, 17,* 183-192.

Herst, L. D., Voss, C. B., & Waldman, J. (1990). Cortical function assessment in the elderly. *Journal of Neuropsychiatry and Clinical Neurosciences, 2,* 385-390.

Herz, M. I., Spitzer, R. L., Gibbon, M., Greenspan, K., & Reibel, S. (1974). Individual versus group aftercare treatment. *American Journal of Psychiatry, 131,* 808-812.

Herzog, D. B., Keller, M. B., Sacks, N. R., Yeh, C. J., & Lavori, P. W. (1992). Psychiatric comorbidity in treatment-seeking anorexics and bulimics. *Journal of the American Academy of Child and Adolescent Psychiatry, 31,* 810-818.

Hesselbrock, V., Stabenau, J., Hesselbrock, M., Mirkin, P., & Meyer, R. (1982). A comparison of two interview schedules: The Schedule of Affective Disorders and Schizophrenia—Lifetime and the National Institute of Mental Health Diagnostic Interview Schedule. *Archives of General Psychiatry, 39,* 674-677.

Heumann, K. A., & Morey, L. C. (1990). Reliability of categorical and dimensional judgments of personality disorder. *American Journal of Psychiatry, 147,* 498-500.

Hill, R. D., Gallagher, D., Thompson, L. W., & Ishida, T. (1988). Hopelessness as a measure of suicidal intent in the depressed elderly. *Psychology and Aging, 3,* 230-232.

Hirschfeld, R. M. A., Klerman, G. L., Clayton, P. J., Keller, M. B., McDonald-Scott, P., & Larkin, B. H. (1988). Assessing personality: Effects of the depressive state on trait measurement. *American Journal of Psychiatry, 140,* 695-699.

Hodges, K. (1990). Depression and anxiety in children: A comparison of self-report questionnaires to clinical interview. *Psychological Assessment: A Journal of Clinical and Consulting Psychology, 2,* 376-381.

Hodges, K. (1993). Structured interviews for assessing children. *Journal of Child Psychology and Psychiatry, 34,* 49-68.

Hodges, K., Cools, J., & McKnew, D. (1989). Test-retest reliability of a clinical research interview for children: The Child Assessment Schedule (CAS). *Psychological Assessment: A Journal of Consulting and Clinical Psychology, 1,* 317-322.

Hodges, K., & Craighead, W. E. (1990). Relationship of children's depression inventory factors to diagnosed depression. *Psychological Assessment: A Journal of Clinical and Consulting Psychology, 2,* 489-492.

Hodges, K., Gordon, Y., & Lennon, M. P. (1990). Parent-child agreement on symptoms assessed via a clinical research interview for children: The Child Assessment Schedule (CAS). *Journal of Child Psychology and Psychiatry, 31,* 427-436.

Hodges, K., Kline, J., Fitch, P., McKnew, D., & Cytryn, L. (1981). The Child Assessment Schedule: A diagnostic interview for research and clinical use. *Catalog of Selected Documents in Psychology, 17,* 56.

Hodges, K., Kline, J., Stern, L., Cytryn, L., & McKnew, D. (1982). The development of a Child Assessment Interview for research and clinical use. *Journal of Abnormal and Child Psychology, 10,* 173-189.

Hodges, K., McKnew, D., Burbach, D. J., & Roebuck, L. (1987). Diagnostic concordance between the Child Assessment Schedule (CAS) and the Schedule for Affective Disorders and Schizophrenia for School-Age Children (K-SADS) in an outpatient sample using lay interviewers. *Journal of American Academy of Child and Adolescent Psychiatry, 26,* 654-661.

Hodges, K., McKnew, D., Cytryn, L., Stern, L., & Kline, J. (1982). The Child Assessment Schedule (CAS) diagnostic interview: A report on reliability and validity. *Journal of the American Academy of Child Psychiatry, 21,* 468-473.

Hodges, K., & Plow, J. (1990). Intellectual ability and achievement in psychiatrically hospitalized children with conduct, anxiety, and affective disorders. *Journal of Clinical and Consulting Psychology, 58,* 589-595.

Hodges, K., & Saunders, W. (1989). Internal consistency of a diagnostic interview for children: The Child Assessment Schedule. *Journal of Abnormal Child Psychology, 17,* 691-701.

Hodiamont, P., Peer, N., & Sybern, N. (1987). Epidemiological aspects of psychiatric disorder in the Dutch health area. *Psychological Medicine, 17,* 495-505.

Hogg, B., Jackson, H. J., Rudd, R. P., & Edwards, J. (1990). Diagnosing personality disorders in recent-onset schizophrenia. *Journal of Nervous and Mental Disease*, *178*, 194-199.

Hokanson, J. E., Rubert, M. P., Welker, R. A., Hollander, G. R., & Hedeen, C. (1989). Interpersonal concomitants and antecedents of depression among college students. *Journal of Abnormal Psychology*, *98*, 209-217.

Holcomb, W. R., & Ahr, P. R. (1988). Arrest rates among young adult psychiatric patients treated in inpatient and outpatient settings. *Hospital and Community Psychiatry*, *39*, 52-57.

Holmes, T. H., & Rahe, R. H. (1967). The Social Readjustment Rating Scale. *Journal of Psychosomatic Research*, *11*, 213-218.

Holzman, P. S., Kringlen, E., & Mathysse, S. (1988). A single dominant gene can account for eye-tracking dysfunction and schizophrenia in offspring of discordant twins. *Archives of General Psychiatry*, *45*, 641-650.

Horn, J. L., Wanberg, K. W., & Foster, F. M. (1990). *Guide to the Alcohol Use Inventory*. Minneapolis: National Computer Systems.

Hout, M. A., & Griez, E. (1984). Validity and utility of the Present State Examination in assessing neurosis: Empirical findings and critical considerations. *Journal of Psychiatric Research*, *18*, 161-172.

Hunt, C., & Andrews, A. (1992). Measuring personality disorder: The use of self-report questionnaires. *Journal of Personality Disorders*, *6*, 125-133.

Hurt, S. W., Clarkin, J. F., Koenigsberg, H. W., Frances, A., & Nurnberg, H. G. (1986). Diagnostic Interview for Borderlines: Psychometric properties and validity. *Journal of Consulting and Clinical Psychology*, *54*, 256-260.

Hurt, S. W., Friedman, R. C., Clarkin, J., Corn, R., & Aronoff, M. S. (1982). Rating the severity of depressive symptoms in adolescents and young adults. *Comprehensive Psychiatry*, *23*, 263-270.

Hurt, S. W., Ilyler, S. E., Frances, A., Clarkin, J. F., & Brent, R. (1984). Assessing borderline personality disorder with self-report, clinical interview, or semistructured interview. *American Journal of Psychiatry*, *141*, 1228-1231.

Huxley, P., Korer, J., & Tolley, S. (1987). The psychiatric "caseness" of clients referred to an urban social services department. *British Journal of Sociology*, *17*, 507-520.

Hwu, H. G., Yeh, E. K., & Chang, L. Y. (1986). Chinese Diagnostic Interview Schedule: Agreement with psychiatrist's diagnosis. *Acta Psychiatrica Scandinavica*, *73*, 225-233.

Hwu, H. G., Yeh, E. K., & Chang, L. Y. (1988). Alcoholism by Chinese Diagnostic Interview Schedule: A prevalence and validity study. *Acta Psychiatrica Scandinavica*, *77*, 7-13.

Hwu, H. G., Yeh, E. K., & Chang, L. Y. (1989). Prevalence of psychiatric disorders in Taiwan defined by the Chinese Diagnostic Interview Schedule. *Acta Psychiatrica Scandinavica*, *79*, 136-147.

Hwu, H. G., Yeh, E. K., Chang, L. Y., & Yeh, Y. L. (1986). Chinese Diagnostic Interview Schedule: A validity study on estimation of lifetime prevalence. *Acta Psychiatrica Scandinavica*, *73*, 348-357.

Hwu, H. G., Yeh, E. K., Chen, C. T., Chen, C. C., & Chen, T. Y. (1983). An applicability study of the Chinese modification of Diagnostic Interview Schedule. *Bulletin of the Chinese Society of Neurology and Psychiatry, 9,* 30-39.

Hyler, S. E., & Rieder, R. O. (1987). PDQ-R: Personality Diagnostic Questionnaire–Revised. New York: New York State Psychiatric Institute.

Hyler, S. E., Skodol, A. E., Kellman, H. D., Oldham, J. M., & Rosnick, L. (1990). Validity of the Personality Diagnostic Questionnaire–Revised: Comparison with two structured interviews. *American Journal of Psychiatry, 147,* 1043-1048.

Hyler, S. E., Skodol, A. E., Oldham, J. M., Kellman, D., & Doidge, N. (1992). Validity of the Personality Diagnostic Questionnaire–Revised: A replication in an outpatient sample. *Comprehensive Psychiatry, 33,* 73-77.

Isaacs, B., & Walkey, F. A. (1963). The assessment of the mental state of elderly hospital patients using a simple questionnaire. *American Journal of Psychiatry, 120,* 173-174.

Ivens, C., & Rehm, L. P. (1988). Assessment of childhood depression: Correspondence between reports by child, mother, and father. *Journal of the American Academy of Child and Adolescent Psychiatry, 27,* 738-741.

Jackson, D. N., & Paunonen, S. V. (1980). Personality structure and assessment. *Annual Review of Psychology, 31,* 503-551.

Jackson, H. J., Grazis, J., Rudd, R. P., & Edwards, J. (1991). Concordance between two personality disorder instruments. *Comprehensive Psychiatry, 32,* 252-260.

Jackson, H. J., Whiteside, H. L., Bates, G. W., Bell, R., Rudd, R. P., & Edwards, J. (1991). Diagnosing personality disorders in psychiatric inpatients. *Acta Psychiatrica Scandinavica, 83,* 206-213.

Jackson, J. E., & Ramsdell, J. W. (1988). Use of the Mini-Mental State Examination (MMSE) to screen for dementia in elderly outpatients. *Journal of the American Geriatrics Society, 36,* 662.

Jacobs, J. W., Bernhard, M. R., Delgado, A., & Strain, J. J. (1977). Screening for organic mental syndromes in the medically ill. *Annals of Internal Medicine, 107,* 481-485.

Jastak, J., Bijou, S., & Jastak, S. (1978). *Wide Range Achievement Test.* Wilmington, DE: Jastak Assessment Systems.

Jeste, D. V., Harris, J., & Zweifach, M. (1988). Late-onset schizophrenia. In R. Michels, J. O. Cavenar, A. M. Cooper, S. B. Guze, L. L. Judd, G. L. Klerman, & A. J. Solnit (Eds.), *Psychiatry* (Vol. 1, Chap. 56). Philadephia: J. B. Lippincott.

Johnson, M. H., Margo, P. A., & Stern, S. L. (1986). Use of the SADS-C as a diagnostic and symptom severity measure. *Journal of Consulting and Clinical Psychology, 54,* 546-551.

Johnson, J., Williams, T., Klingler, D., & Gianetti, R. (1988). Interventional relevance and retrofit programming: Concepts for the improvement of clinical acceptance of computer-generated assessment reports. *Behavioral Research Methods and Instrumentation, 9,* 123-132.

Johnson, T. D. (1990). *Partial helplessness conditioning as a possible etiological factor in psychopathy.* Unpublished doctoral dissertation, University of Alabama, Birmingham.

Jones, L. R., Badger, L. W., Ficken, R. P., Leeper, J. D., & Anderson, R. L. (1988). Mental health training of primary care physicians: An outcome study. *International Journal of Psychiatry in Medicine, 18,* 107-121.

Kahn, R. L., Goldfarb, A. I., Pollack, M., & Peck, A. (1960). Brief objective measures for the determination of mental status in the aged. *American Journal of Psychiatry, 117,* 326-328.

Kaplan, E., Goodglass, H., & Weintraub, S. (1976). *The Boston Naming Test.* Unpublished test, Veterans Administration, Boston.

Kaplan, H. I., & Sadock, B. J. (1988). *Synopsis of psychiatry, behavioral sciences, clinical psychiatry* (5th ed.). Baltimore: William & Wilkins.

Kaplan, L. M., & Reich, W. (1991). *Manual for Diagnostic Interview for Children and Adolescents—Revised (DICA-R).* St. Louis, MO: Washington University.

Karno, M., Burnam, A., Escobar, J. L., Hough, R. L., & Eaton, W. W. (1983). Development of the Spanish-language version of the National Institute of Mental Health Diagnostic Interview Schedule. *Archives of General Psychiatry, 40,* 1183-1188.

Karpman, B. (1961). The structure of neurosis: With special differentials between neurosis, psychosis, homosexuality, alcoholism, psychopathy, and criminality. *Archives of Criminal Psychodynamics, 4,* 599-646.

Kashini, J. H., Beck, N. C., & Burk, J. P. (1987). Predictors of psychopathology in children of patients with major affective disorders. *Canadian Journal of Psychiatry, 32,* 287-290.

Kashini, J. H., Konig, P., Shepperd, J. A., Wilfley, D., & Morris, D. A. (1988). Psychopathology and self-concept in asthmatic children. *Journal of Pediatric Psychology, 13,* 509-520.

Kashini, J. H., Sherman, A. D., Parker, D. P., & Reid, J. C. (1990). Utility of the Beck Depression Inventory with clinic-referred adolescents. *Journal of the American Academy of Child and Adolescent Psychiatry, 29,* 278-282.

Kashini, J. H., Strober, M., Rosenberg, T. K., & Reid, J. C. (1988). Correlates of psychopathology in adolescents. *Psychiatry Research, 26,* 141-148.

Katon, W., Lin, E., Von Korff, M., Russo, J., Lipscomb, P., & Bush, T. (1991). Somatization: A spectrum of severity. *American Journal of Psychiatry, 148,* 34-40.

Katz, M. M., Marsella, A., Dube, K. C., Olatawura, M., Takahashi, R., Nakane, Y., Wynne, L. C., Gift, T., Brennan, J., Sartorius, N., & Jablensky, A. (1988). On the expression of psychosis in different cultures: Schizophrenia in an Indian and in a Nigerian community. *Culture, Medicine, and Psychiatry, 12,* 331-355.

Katzman, R., Brown, T., Fuld, P., Peck, A., Schechter, R., & Schimmel, H. (1983). Validation of a short orientation-memory-concentration test of cognitive impairment. *American Journal of Psychiatry, 140,* 734-739.

Kaufman, D. M., Weinberger, M., Strain, J. J., & Jacobs, J. W. (1979). Detection of cognitive deficits by a brief mental status examination. *General Hospital Psychiatry, 1,* 247-255.

Kavoussi, R. J., Coccaro, E. F., Klar, H. M., Berstein, D., & Siever, L. J. (1990). Structured interviews for borderline personality disorder. *American Journal of Psychiatry*, *147*, 1522-1525.

Keisler, D. J. (1983). The 1982 interpersonal personal circle: A taxonomy for complementarity of human transactions. *Psychological Review*, *90*, 185-214.

Keller, M. B., Lavori, P. W., McDonald-Scott, P., Scheftner, W. A., Andreason, W. C., Shapiro, R. W., & Croughan, J. (1981). Reliability of lifetime diagnoses and symptoms in patients with a current psychiatric disorder. *Journal of Psychiatric Research*, *16*, 229-240.

Keller, M. B., & Manschreck, T. C. (1981). The bedside mental status examination—reliability and validity. *Comprehensive Psychiatry*, *22*, 500-511.

Keller, M. B., Nielsen, E., Herzog, D. B., & Stasior, J. K. (undated). *Schedule of Eating Disorders, Affective Disorders and Schizophrenia-L (EAT-SADS-L)*. Unpublished test, Massachusetts General Hospital, Boston.

Kelly, T., Soloff, P. H., Cornelius, J., George, A., Lis, J. A., & Ulrich, R. (1992). Can we study (treat) borderline patients? Attrition from research and open treatment. *Journal of Personality Disorders*, *6*, 417-433.

Kendell, R. E. (1985). Schizophrenia: Clinical features. In R. Michels, J. O. Cavenar, A. M. Cooper, S. B. Guze, L. L. Judd, G. L. Klerman, & A. J. Solnit (Eds.), *Psychiatry* (Vol. 1, Chap. 53). Philadelphia: J. B. Lippincott.

Kendell, R. E., Everitt, B., Cooper, J. E., Sartorius, N., & David, M. E. (1968). Reliability of the Present State Examination. *Social Psychiatry*, *3*, 123-129.

Kendler, K. S., Gruenberg, A. M., & Kinney, D. K. (1994). Independent diagnoses of adoptees and relatives as defined by DSM-III in the provincial and national samples of the Danish adoption study of schizophrenia. Archives of General Psychiatry, 51, 456-468.

Kendler, S. L. (1990). Toward a scientific psychiatric nosology: Strengths and limitations. *Archives of General Psychiatry*, *47*, 969-973.

Kent, G. H. (1946). *E-G-Y scales*. Baltimore: Williams & Wilkins.

Kernberg, O. F. (1967). Borderline personality organization. *Journal of the American Psychoanalytic Association*, *15*, 641-685.

Kernberg, O. F. (1975). *Borderline conditions and pathological narcissism*. New York: Jason Aronson.

Kernberg, O. F. (1979). Two reviews of the literature on borderlines: An assessment. *Schizophrenia Bulletin*, *5*, 53-58.

Kernberg, O. F. (1981). Structural interviewing. *Psychiatric Clinics of North America*, *4*, 169-195.

Kessler, L. G., Cleary, P. D., & Burke, Jr., J. D. (1985). Psychiatric disorders in primary care: Results of a follow-up study. *Archives of General Psychiatry*, *42*, 583-587.

Kessler, R. C., McGonagle, K. A., Zhao, S., Nelson, C. B., Hughes, M., Eshleman, S., Wittchen, H. U., & Kendler, K. S. (1994). Lifetime and 12-month prevalence of DSM-III-R psychiatric disorders in the United States. *Archives of General Psychiatry*, *51*, 8-19.

Kewman, D. G., Vaishampayan, N., Zald, D., & Han, B. (1991). Cognitive impairment in musculoskeletal pain patients. *International Journal of Psychiatry in Medicine, 21,* 253-262.

Kiernan, R. J., Mueller, J., Langston, J. W., & Van Dyke, C. (1987). The neuro-behavioral cognitive screening examination: A brief but quantitative approach to cognitive assessment. *Annals of Internal Medicine, 107,* 481-485.

Kiesler, D. J. (1983). The 1982 interpersonal circle: A taxonomy for complementarity in human transactions. *Psychological Review, 90,* 185-214.

Kiesler, D. J. (1986). Interpersonal methods of diagnosis and treatment. In E. Michels, J. O. Cavenar, & A. M. Cooper (Eds.), *Psychiatry* (Vol. 1, Chap. 4). Philadelphia: J. B. Lippincott.

Kight-Law, A., Mathisen, K. S., Calandra, F., Evans, F. J., & Salierno, C. A. (1989). Computerized collection of mental health information from emotionally disturbed adolescents. *Computers in Human Services, 5,* 171-181.

Klerman, G. L., Endicott, J., Spitzer, R. L., & Hirschfeld, R. M. A. (1979). Neurotic depressions: A systematic analysis of multiple criteria and meanings. *American Journal of Psychiatry, 136,* 57-61.

Knight, R. (1953). Borderline states. *Bulletin of the Menninger Clinic, 17,* 1-12.

Knopman, D. S., Kitto, J., Deinar, S., & Heiring, J. (1988). Longitudinal study of death and institutionalization in patients with primary degenerative dementia. *Journal of the American Geriatrics Society, 36,* 108-112.

Kocsis, J. H., & Mann, J. J. (1985). Drug treatment in personality disorders and neuroses. In R. Michels, J. O. Cavenar, A. M. Cooper, S. B. Guze, L. L. Judd, G. L. Klerman, & A. J. Solnit (Eds.) *Psychiatry* (Vol. 1, Chap. 10). Philadelphia: J. B. Lippincott.

Koenigsberg, H. W., Kernberg, O. F., & Schomer, J. (1983). Diagnosing borderline conditions in an outpatient setting. *Archives of General Psychiatry, 40,* 49-53.

Kolb, J. E., & Gunderson, J. G. (1980). Diagnosing borderline patients with a semi-structured interview. *Archives of General Psychiatry, 37,* 37-41.

Korenblum, M., Marton, P., Golombek, H., & Stein, B. (1990). Personality status: Changes through adolescence. *Psychiatric Clinics of North America, 13,* 389-399.

Kosson, D. S., Smith, S. S., & Newman, J. P. (1990). Evaluating the construct validity of psychopathy on black and white male inmates: Three preliminary studies. *Journal of Abnormal Psychology, 99,* 250-259.

Kosten, T. R., Rounsaville, B. J., & Kleber, H. D. (1986). A 2.5-year follow-up of depression, life crises, and treatment effects on abstinence among opioid addicts. *Archives of General Psychiatry, 43,* 733-738.

Kovacs, M. (1978). *Children's Depression Inventory (CDI).* Pittsburgh, PA: University of Pittsburgh.

Kovacs, M. (1983). *Interview Schedule for Children (ISC): Form C and follow-up form.* Unpublished manuscript, University of Pittsburgh, PA.

Kovacs, M., Akiskal, H. S., Gatsonis, C., & Parrone, P. L. (1994). Childhood-onset dysthymic disorder. *Archives of General Psychiatry, 41,* 365-374.

Kovacs, M., Feinberg, T. L., Crouse-Novak, M., Paulauskas, S. L., & Finkelstein, R. (1984). Depressive disorders in childhood: I. A longitudinal prospective study of characteristics and recovery. *Archives of General Psychiatry*, *41*, 229-237.

Kovacs, M., Feinberg, T. L., Crouse-Novak, M., Paulauskas, S. L., Pollock, M., & Finkelstein, R. (1984). Depressive disorders in childhood: II. A longitudinal study of the risk for subsequent major depression. *Archives of General Psychiatry*, *41*, 643-649.

Kovess, V., & Fournier, L. (1990). The DISSA: An abridged self-administered version of the DIS. *Social Psychiatry and Psychiatric Epidemiology*, *25*, 179-186.

Kroger, R. O., & Turnbull, W. (1975). Invalidity of validity scales: The case of the MMPI. *Journal of Consulting and Clinical Psychology*, *43*, 48-55.

Kroll, J., Pyle, R., & Zander, J. (1981). Borderline personality disorder: Interrater reliability of the Gunderson Diagnostic Interview for Borderlines (DIB). *Schizophrenia Bulletin*, *7*, 269-272.

Kroll, J., Pyle, R., Zander, J., Martin, K., Lari, S., & Sines, L. (1981). Borderline personality disorder: Interrater reliability of the Diagnostic Interview for Borderlines (DIB). *Schizophrenia Bulletin*, *7*, 269-272.

Kroll, J., Sines, L., Martin, K., Lari, S., Pyle, R., & Zander, J. (1981). Borderline personality disorder: Construct validity of the concept. *Archives of General Psychiatry*, *38*, 1021-1026.

Kropp, P. R. (1992). *Antisocial personality disorder and malingering*. Unpublished doctoral dissertation, Simon Fraser University, Burnaby, Canada.

Kruedelbach, N., McCormick, R. A., Schulz, S. C., & Grueneich, R. (1993). Impulsivity, coping styles, and triggers for craving in substance abusers with borderline personality disorders. *Journal of Personality Disorders*, *7*, 214-222.

Kullgren, G., & Armelius, B. A. (1990). The concept of personality organization: A long-term comparative follow-up study with special reference to borderline personality organization. *Journal of Personality Disorders*, *4*, 203-212.

Kurtz, R., & Meyer, R. G. (1994, March). *Vulnerability of the MMPI-2, M Test, and SIRS to different strategies of malingering psychosis*. Paper presented at the American Psychology-Law Society, Santa Fe, NM.

Kutcher, S. P., Yanchyshyn, G., & Cohen, C. (1985). Diagnosing affective disorder in adolescents: The use of the Schedule for Affective Disorders and Schizophrenia. *Canadian Journal of Psychiatry*, *30*, 605-608.

Laboratory of Community Psychiatry. (1973). *Competency to stand trial and mental illness*. Rockville, MD: Department of Health, Education, and Welfare.

Lachar, D., & Gdowski, C. L. (1979). *Actuarial assessment of child and adolescent personality: An interpretive guide for the Personality Inventory for Children profile*. Los Angeles: Western Psychological Services.

LaForge, R., & Suczek, R. (1955). The interpersonal dimension of personality: III. Interpersonal checklist. *Journal of Personality*, *24*, 94-112.

Lahey, B. B., Loeber, R., Stouthamer-Loeber, M., Christ, M. A. G., Green, S., Russo, M. R., Frick, P. J., & Duncan, M. (1990). Comparison of DSM-III and DSM-III-R diagnoses for prepubertal children: Changes in prevalence and validity. *Journal of the American Academy of Child and Adolescent Psychiatry, 29,* 620-626.

Lahey, B. B., Piacentini, J. C., McBurnett, K., Stone, P., Hartdagen, S., & Hynd, G. (1988). Psychopathology in the parents of children with conduct disorder and hyperactivity. *Journal of the American Academy of Child and Adolescent Psychiatry, 27,* 163-170.

Lancker, D. V. (1990). The neurology of proverbs. *Behavioral Neurology, 3,* 169-187.

Larkin, A. R. (1979). The form and content of schizophrenic hallucinations. *American Journal of Psychiatry, 136,* 940-943.

Larson, L. M., & Heppner, P. P. (1989). Problem-solving appraisal in an alcoholic population. *Journal of Counseling Psychology, 36,* 73-78.

LaRue, A., Spar, J., & Hill, C. D., (1986). Cognitive impairment in late-life depression: Clinical correlates and treatment implications. *Journal of Affective Disorders, 11,* 179-184.

Lasage, A. D., Cyr, M., & Toupin, J. (1991). Reliable use of the Present State Examination by psychiatric nurses for clinical studies of psychotic and non-psychotic patients. *Acta Psychiatrica Scandinavica, 83,* 121-124.

Last, C. G., Strauss, C. C., & Francis, G. (1987). Comorbidity among childhood anxiety disorders. *Journal of Nervous and Mental Disease, 175,* 726-730.

Lautenschlaeger, E., Meier, H. M. R., & Donnelly, M. (1986). Folstein vs. Goldfarb mental status exams. *Clinical Gerontologist, 4,* 40-42.

Lavoro, S. A., Geddings, V. J., & Patrick, C. J. (1994, March). *Temperamental variables in the criminal psychopath.* Paper presented at the American Psychology-Law Society convention, Santa Fe, NM.

Lawson, J. S., Rodenburg, M., & Dykes, J. A. (1977). A dementia rating scale for use with psychogeriatric patients. *Journal of Gerontology, 32,* 153-159.

Leboyer, M., Maier, W., Teherani, M., Lichtermann, D., D'Amato, T., Franke, P., Lepine, J. P., Minges, J., & McGuffin, P. (1991). The reliability of the SADS-LA in a family study setting. *European Archives of Psychiatry and Clinical Neuroscience, 241,* 165-169.

Leckman, J. F., Sholomsaks, D., Thompson, W. D., Belanger, A., & Weissman, M. M. (1982). Best estimates of lifetime psychiatric diagnoses. *Archives of General Psychiatry, 39,* 879-883.

Le Couteur, A., Rutter, M., Lord, C., Rios, P., Robertson, S., Holdgrafer, M., & McLennan, F. (1989). Autism diagnostic interview: A standardized investigator-based instrument. *Journal of Autism and Developmental Disorders, 19,* 363-387.

Lees-Haley, P. R., English, L. T., & Glenn, W. J. (1991). A fake bad scale on the MMPI-2 for personal injury claimants. *Psychological Reports, 68,* 203-210.

Lehtinen, V., Lindholm, T., Veijola, J., & Vaisanen, E. (1990). The prevalence of PSE-CATEGO disorders in a Finnish adult population cohort. *Social Psychiatry and Psychiatric Epidemiology, 25,* 187-192.

Lesher, E. L., & Whelihan, W. M. (1986). Reliability of mental status instruments administered to nursing home residents. *Journal of Consulting and Clinical Psychology, 54,* 726-727.

Lesser, I. M., Rubin, R. T., Pecknold, J. C., Rifkin, A., Swinson, R. P., Lydiard, B., Burrows, G. D., Noyes, R., & DuPont, R. L., Jr. (1988). Secondary depression in panic disorder and agoraphobia: II. Frequency, severity and response to treatment. *Archives of General Psychiatry, 45,* 437-443.

Lewis, M. (1986). Personality and personality disorder (borderline personality disorder). In R. Michels, J. O. Cavenar, A. M. Cooper, S. B. Guze, L. L. Judd, G. L. Klerman, & A. J. Solnit (Eds.), *Psychiatry* (Vol. 2, Chap. 42). Philadelphia: J. B. Lippincott.

Lezak, M. D. (1983). *Neuropsychological assessment.* New York: Oxford University Press.

Liberty, P. G., Jr., Lunneborg, C. E., & Atkinson, G. C. (1964). Perceptual defense, dissimulation, and response styles. *Journal of Consulting Psychology, 28,* 529-537.

Linblad, A. D. (1993). *Detection of malingered mental illness with a forensic population: An analogue study.* Unpublished doctoral dissertation, University of Saskatchewan, Saskatoon, Canada.

Links, P. S., Steiner, M., Boiago, I., & Irwin, D. (1990). Lithium therapy for borderline patients: Preliminary findings. *Journal of Personality Disorders, 4,* 173-181.

Liss, J. L., Welner, A., & Robins, E. (1972). Undiagnosed psychiatric patients: Part II. Follow-up study. *British Journal of Psychiatry, 121,* 647-651.

Livesley, W. J. (1985a). The classification of personality disorder: I. The choice of category concept. *Canadian Journal of Psychiatry, 30,* 353-358.

Livesley, W. J. (1985b). The classification of personality disorder: II. The problem of diagnostic criteria. *Canadian Journal of Psychiatry, 30,* 359-362.

Livesley, W. J. (1986). Trait and behavioral prototypes of personality disorder. *American Journal of Psychiatry, 143,* 728-732.

Livesley, W. J. (1991). Classifying personality disorders: Ideal types, prototypes, or dimensions? *Journal of Personality Disorders, 5,* 52-59.

Livesley, W. J., & Jackson, D. N. (1986). The internal consistency and factorial structure of behaviors judged to be associated with DSM-III personality disorders. *American Journal of Psychiatry, 143,* 1473-1474.

Livesley, W. J., Jackson, D. N., & Schroeder, M. L. (1992). Factorial structure of traits delineating personality disorders in clinical and general population samples. *Journal of Abnormal Psychology, 101,* 432-440.

Livesley, W. J., Reiffer, L. I., Sheldon, A. E. R., & West, M. (1987). Prototypicality ratings of DSM-III criteria for personality disorders. *Journal of Nervous and Mental Disease, 175,* 395-401.

Livingston, R. L., & Bracha, H. S. (1992). Psychotic symptoms and suicidal behavior in hospitalized children. *American Journal of Psychiatry, 149*, 1585-1586.

Livingston, R. L., Dykman, R. A., & Ackerman, P. T. (1990). The frequency and significance of additional self-reported psychiatric diagnoses in children with attention deficit disorder. *Journal of Abnormal Child Psychology, 18*, 465-478.

Livingston, R. L., Dykman, R. A., & Ackerman, P. T. (1992). Psychiatric comorbidity and response to two doses of methylphenidate in children with attention deficit disorder. *Journal of Child and Adolescent Psychopharmacology, 2*, 115-122.

Loebel, A. D., Lieberman, J. A., Alvir, J. M. J., Mayerhoff, D. I., Geisler, S. H., & Szymanski, S. R. (1992). Duration of psychosis and outcome in first-episode schizophrenia. *American Journal of Psychiatry, 149*, 1183-1188.

Loeber, R., Lahey, B. B., & Thomas, C. (1991). Diagnostic conundrum of oppositional defiant disorder and conduct disorder. *Journal of Abnormal Psychology, 100*, 379-390.

Longabaugh, R., Fowler, D. R., Stout, R. L., & Kriebel, G. W. (1982). Validation of a problem-focused nomenclature. *Archives of General Psychiatry, 40*, 453-461.

Longabaugh, R., Stout, R. L., Kriebel, G. W., McCullough, L., & Bishop, D. (1986). DSM-III and clinically identified problems as a guide to treatment. *Archives of General Psychiatry, 43*, 1097-1103.

Lopez, P. S., Llinas, A. J., & Vidal, C. (1990). Camdex: Una nueva entrevista psicogeriatrica [CAMDEX: A new psychogeriatric interview]. *Actas Luso Espanolas de Neurologia, Psiquiatria y Ciencias Afines, 18*, 290-295.

Loranger, A. W. (1988). *Personality Disorder Examination (PDE) manual.* Yonkers, NY: DV Communications.

Loranger, A. W. (1990). The impact of DSM-III on diagnostic practice in a university hospital. *Archives of General Psychiatry, 47*, 672-675.

Loranger, A. W. (1991). Diagnosis of personality disorders: General considerations. In R. Michels, J. O. Cavenar, A. M. Cooper, S. B. Guze, L. L. Judd, G. L. Klerman, & A. J. Solnit (Eds.), *Psychiatry* (Vol. 1, Chap. 15). Philadelphia: J. B. Lippincott.

Loranger, A. W. (1992). Are current self-report and interview measures adequate for epidemiological studies of personality disorders? *Journal of Personality Disorders, 6*, 313-325.

Loranger, A. W., Hirschfeld, R. M. A., Sartorius, N., & Regier, D. A. (1991). The WHO/ADAMHA international pilot study of personality disorders: Background and purpose. *Journal of Personality Disorders, 5*, 296-306.

Loranger, A. W., Lenzenweger, M. F., Gartner, A. F., Susman, V. L., Herzig, J., Zammit, G. K., Gartner, J. D., Abrams, R. C., & Young, R. C. (1991). Trait-state artifacts and the diagnosis of personality disorders. *Archives of General Psychiatry, 48*, 720-728.

Loranger, A. W., Oldham, J. M., Russakoff, L. M., & Susman, V. (1984). Structured interviews and borderline personality disorder. *Archives of General Psychiatry, 41*, 565-568.

Loranger, A. W., Sartorius, N., Andreoli, A., Berger, P., Buchheim, P., Channabasavanna, S. M., Coid, B., Dahl, A., Diekstra, R. F. W., Ferguson, B., Jacobsberg, L. B., Mombour, W., Pull, C., Ono, Y., & Regier, D. A. (in press). The International Personality Disorder Examination (IPDE): The WHO/ADAMHA international pilot study of personality disorders. *Archives of General Psychiatry*.

Loranger, A. W., Susman, V. L., Oldham, J. M., & Russakoff, L. M. (1985). *The Personality Disorder Examination (PDE): A structured interview for DSM-III-R personality disorders*. Unpublished manuscript, New York Hospital, Cornell Medical Center, White Plains, NY.

Loranger, A. W., Susman, V. L., Oldham, J. M., & Russakoff, L. M. (1987). The Personality Disorder Examination: A preliminary report. *Journal of Personality Disorders, 1*, 1-13.

Luria, R. E. (1979). The use of the visual analogue mood and alert scales in diagnosing hospitalized affective psychoses. *Psychological Medicine, 9*, 155-164.

Luria, R. E., & Guziec, R. J. (1981). Comparative description of the SADS and the PSE. *Schizophrenia Bulletin, 8*, 248-257.

Luria, R. E., & McHugh, P. R. (1974). Reliability and clinical utility of the "Wing" present state examination. *Archives of General Psychiatry, 30*, 866-871.

Lyketsos, C. G., Lyketsos, G. C., Richardson, S. C., & Beis, A. (1987). Dysthymic states and depressive syndromes in physical conditions of presumably psychogenic origin. A*cta Psychiatrica Scandinavica, 76*, 529-534.

MacKinnon, R. A., & Yudofsky, S. C. (1986). *The psychiatric evaluation in clinical practice*. Philadelphia: J. B. Lippincott.

Maier, W., Buller, R., Sonntag, A., & Heuser, I. (1986). Subtypes of panic attacks and ICD-9 classification. *European Archives of Psychiatry and Neurological Sciences, 235*, 361-366.

Maier, W., Lichertermann, D., Klingler, T., Heun, R., & Hallmayer, J. (1992). Prevalences of personality disorders (DSM-III-R) in the community. *Journal of Personality Disorders, 6*, 187-196.

Mann, A. H., Jenkins, R., & Belsey, E. (1981). The twelve-month outcome of patients with neurotic illness in general practice. *Psychological Medicine, 11*, 535-550.

Mann, A. H., Jenkins, R., Cutting, J. C., & Cowen, P. J. (1981). The development and use of a standardized assessment of abnormal personality. *Psychological Medicine, 11*, 839-847.

Mann, A. H., & Pilgrim, J. A. (1992). *Standardized Assessment of Personality: ICD-10 version*. London: University of London, Institute of Psychiatry.

Manuzza, S., Fyer, A. J., Klein, D. F., & Endicott, J. (1986). Schedule of Affective Disorders and Schizophrenia—Lifetime version modified for the study of anxiety disorders (SADS-LA): Rationale and conceptual development. *Journal of Psychiatric Research, 20*, 317-325.

Manuzza, S., Fyer, A. J., Martin, L. Y., Gallops, M. S., Endicott, J., Gorman, J., Liebowitz, M. R., & Klein, D. F. (1989). Reliability of anxiety assessment: I. Diagnostic agreement. *Archives of General Psychiatry, 46*, 1093-1101.

Marcus, M. D., Smith, D., Santelli, R., & Kaye, W. (1992). Characterization of eating disordered behavior in obese binge eaters. *International Journal of Eating Disorders, 12,* 249-255.

Marcus, S., Robins, L. N., & Bucholz, K. (1991). *The Quick Diagnostic Interview Schedule III-R, Version 1.0.* St. Louis, MO: Washington University School of Medicine.

Margaziner, J., Bassett, S. S., & Hebel, J. R. (1987). Predicting performance on the Mini-Mental State Examination. *Journal of the American Geriatrics Society, 35,* 996-1000.

Marin, D. B., Kocsis, J. H., Frances, A. J., & Klerman, G. L. (1993). Personality disorders in dysthymia. *Journal of Personality Disorders, 7,* 223-231.

Marks, I. M., & Mathews, A. M. (1978). Brief standard self-rating for phobic patients. *Behavioral Research and Therapy, 17,* 263-267.

Marlatt, A. G., & Miller, W. R. (1984). *Comprehensive Drinker Profile.* Odessa, FL: Psychological Assessment Resources.

Marton, P., Churchard, M., Kutcher, S., & Korenblum, M. (1991). Diagnostic utility of the Beck Depression Inventory with adolescent psychiatric outpatients and inpatients. *Canadian Journal of Psychiatry, 36,* 428-431.

Maser, J. D., Kaelber, C., & Weise, R. E. (1991). International use and attitudes toward DSM-III and DSM-III-R: Growing consensus in psychiatric classification. *Journal of Abnormal Psychology, 100,* 271-279.

Matarazzo, J. D. (1983). The reliability of psychiatric and psychological diagnosis. *Clinical Psychology Review, 3,* 103-145.

Mathisen, K. S., Evans, F. J., & Meyers, K. (1987). Evaluation of a computerized version of the Diagnostic Interview Schedule. *Hospital and Community Psychiatry, 38,* 1311-1315.

Mattis, S. (1976). Mental status examination for organic mental syndrome in the elderly patient. In L. Bellack & T. B. Karasu (Eds.), *Geriatric psychiatry* (pp. 77-121). New York: Grune & Stratton.

Maurer, K., Biehl, H., Kuhner, C., & Loffler, W. (1989). On the way to expert systems: Comparing DSM-III computer diagnosis with CATEGO (ICD) diagnoses in depressive and schizophrenic patients. *European Archives of Psychiatry and Neurological Sciences, 239,* 127-132.

Mauri, M., Sarno, N., Rossi, V. M., Armani, A., Zambotto, S., Cassano, G. B., & Akiskal, H. S. (1992). Personality disorders associated with generalized anxiety, panic, and recurrent depressive disorders. *Journal of Personality Disorders, 6,* 162-167.

Mavreas, V. G., Beis, A., Mouyias, S., Rigoni, F., & Lysketsos, G. C. (1986). Prevalence of psychiatric disorders in Athens. *Social Psychiatry, 21,* 172-181.

Maxwell, A. E. (1977). Coefficients of agreement between observers and their interpretation. *British Journal of Psychiatry, 130,* 79-83.

Mayeux, R., Stern, Y., Rosen, J., & Leventhal, J. (1981). Depression, intellectual impairment, and Parkinson's disease. *Neurology, 31,* 645-650.

Mayou, R., Peveler, R., Davies, B., Mann, J., & Fairburn, C. (1991). Psychiatric morbidity in young adults with insulin-dependent diabetes mellitus. *Psychological Medicine, 21,* 639-645.

Maziade, M., Roy, A. A., Fournier, J. P. Cliche, D., Merette, C. Caron, C., Garneau, Y., Montgrain, N., Shriqui, C., Dion, C., Nicole, L., Potvin, A., Lavallee, J. C., Pires, A., & Raymond, V. (1992). Reliability of best-estimate diagnosis in genetic linkage studies of major psychoses. *American Journal of Psychiatry, 149,* 1674-1686.

Mazure, C., & Gershon, E. S. (1979). Blindness and reliability in lifetime psychiatric diagnosis. *Archives of General Psychiatry, 36,* 521-525.

McBride-Houtz, P. (1993). *Detecting cognitive impairment in older adults: A validation study of selected screening instruments.* Unpublished doctoral dissertation, University of North Texas, Denton.

McBroom, P. (1980). *Behavioral genetics.* Rockville, MD: National Institute of Mental Health.

McCann, U. D., Rossiter, E. M., King, R. J., & Agras, W. S. (1991). Nonpurging bulimia: A distinct subtype of bulimia nervosa. *International Journal of Eating Disorders, 10,* 679-687.

McCord, W. M., & McCord, J. (1964). *The psychopath: An essay on the criminal mind.* Princeton, NJ: Van Nostrand Reinhold.

McDonald-Scott, P., & Endicott, J. (1984). Informed versus blind: The reliability of cross-sectional ratings of psychopathology. *Psychiatry Research, 12,* 207-217.

McGee, R., Anderson, J., Williams, S., & Silva, P. A. (1986). Cognitive correlates of depressive symptoms in 11-year-old children. *Journal of Abnormal Child Psychology, 14,* 517-524.

McGee, R., & Stanton, W. (1990). Parent reports of disability among 13-year-olds with DSM-III disorders. *Journal of Child Psychology and Psychiatry, 31,* 793-801.

McGorry, P., Kaplan, I., Dossetor, C., Copolov, D., & Singh, B. (1988). *The Royal Park Multidiagnostic Instrument for Psychosis: A comprehensive assessment procedure for the acute psychotic episode (RPMIP).* Melbourne, Australia: Department of Psychological Medicine, Monash University.

McHugh, P. R., & Folstein, M. F. (1988). Organic mental disorders. In R. Michels, J. O. Cavenar, A. M. Cooper, S. B. Guze, L. L. Judd, G. L. Klerman, & A. J. Solnit (Eds.), *Psychiatry* (Vol. 1, Chap. 73). Philadelphia: J. B. Lippincott.

McKeon, J., Roa, B., & Mann, A. (1984). Life events and personality traits in obsessive-compulsive neurosis. *British Journal of Psychiatry, 144,* 185-189.

McManus, M., Lerner, H., Robbins, D., & Barbour, C. (1984). Assessment of borderline symptomatology in hospitalized adolescents. *Journal of the American Academy of Child Psychiatry, 23,* 685-694.

Medin, D. L., Altom, M. W., Edelson, S. M., & Freko, D. (1982). Correlated symptoms and simulated medical classification. *Journal of Experimental Psychology: Learning, Memory, and Cognition, 8,* 37-50.

Meehl, P. E. (1990). Toward an integrated theory of schizotaxia, schizotypy, and schizophrenia. *Journal of Personality Disorders, 4,* 1-99.

Meek, P. S., Clark, H. W., & Solana, B. L. (1989). Neurocognitive impairment: The unrecognized component of dual diagnosis in substance abuse treatment. *Journal of Psychoactive Drugs, 21,* 153-160.

Mellman, T. A., Leverich, G. S., Hauser, P., Kramlinger, K., Post, R. M., & Uhde, T. W. (1992). Axis II pathology in panic and affective disorders: Relationship to diagnosis, course of illness, and treatment response. *Journal of Personality Disorders, 6,* 53-63.

Melzack, R. (1975). The McGill Pain Questionnaire: Major properties and scoring methods. *Pain, 1,* 277-299.

Merikangus, K. R. (1981). *The reliability of assortative mating to social adjustment and course of illness in primary affective disorder.* Unpublished doctoral dissertation, University of Pittsburgh, PA.

Merskey, H., Ball, M. J., Blume, W. T., Fox, A. J., Fox, H., Hersch, E. L., Kral, V. A., & Palmer, R. B. (1980). Relationships between psychological measurements and cerebral organic changes in Alzheimer's disease. *Canadian Journal of Neurological Sciences, 7,* 45-49.

Meyer, R. G. (1993). *The clinician's handbook: Integrated diagnostics, assessment, and intervention in adult and adolescent psychopathology* (3rd ed.). Boston: Allyn & Bacon.

Meyers, J. S., Rogers, R. L., McClintic, K., Mortel, K. F., & Lofti, J. (1989). Randomized clinical trial of daily aspirin therapy in multi-infarct dementia: A pilot study. *Journal of the American Geriatrics Society, 37,* 549-555.

Mignolli, G., Faccinicani, C., Turit, L., Gavioli, I., & Micciolo, R. (1988). Interrater reliability of the PSE-9 (full version): An Italian study. *Social Psychiatry and Psychiatric Epidemiology, 23,* 30-35.

Miller, G. A. (1985). *The Substance Abuse Subtle Screening Inventory manual.* Bloomington, IN: SASSI Institute.

Miller, M. W., Geddings, V. J., Levenston, G. K., & Patrick, C. J. (1994, March). *The personality characteristics of psychopathic and nonpsychopathic sex offenders.* Paper presented at the American Psychology and Law Society Biannual Conference, Sante Fe, NM.

Miller, W. R. (1978). Behavior treatment of problem drinkers: A comparative outcome study of three controlled drinking therapies. *Journal of Consulting and Clinical Psychology, 46,* 74-86.

Miller, W. R., Benefield, G., & Tonigan, J. S. (1992). *Enhancing motivation for change in problem drinking: A controlled comparison of two therapist styles.* Manuscript submitted for publication.

Miller, W. R., Crawford, V. L., & Taylor, C. A. (1979). Significant others as corroborative sources for problem drinkers. *Addictive Behaviors, 4,* 67-70.

Miller, W. R., & Dougher, M. J. (1989). Covert sensitization: Alternative treatment procedures for alcoholism. *Behavioral Psychotherapy, 17,* 203-220.

Miller, W. R., Gribskow, C. J., & Mortell, R. L. (1981). Effectiveness of a self-control manual for problem drinkers with and without therapist contact. *International Journal of the Addictions, 16,* 1247-1254.

Miller, W. R., Hedrick, K. E., & Taylor, C. A. (1983). Addictive behaviors and life problems before and after behavioral treatment of problem drinkers. *Addictive Behaviors, 8,* 403-412.

Miller, W. R., Leckman, A. L., Delaney, H. D., & Tinkcom, M. (1992). Long-term follow-up of behavioral self-control training. *Journal of Studies on Alcohol, 53,* 249-261.

Miller, W. R., & Marlatt, G. A. (1984). *Manual for the Comprehensive Drinker Profile.* Odessa, FL: Psychological Assessment Resources.

Miller, W. R., & Marlatt, G. A. (1987). *Comprehensive Drinker Profile: Manual supplement.* Odessa, FL: Psychological Assessment Resources.

Miller, W. R., Sovereign, R. G., & Krege, B. (1988). Motivational interviewing with problem drinkers: II. The drinker's check-up as a preventive intervention. *Behavioral Psychotherapy, 16,* 251-268.

Miller, W. R., & Taylor, C. A. (1980b). Relative effectiveness of bibliotherapy, individual and group self-control training in the treatment of problem drinkers. *Addictive Behaviors, 5,* 13-24.

Miller, W. R., Taylor, C. A., & West, J. C. (1980). Focused versus broad-spectrum behavior therapy for problem drinkers. *Journal of Consulting and Clinical Psychology, 48,* 590-601.

Millon, T. (1982). *Millon Clinical Multiaxial Inventory—II.* Minneapolis, MN: National Computer Systems.

Millon, T. (1991). Classification in psychopathology: Rationale, alternatives, and standards. *Journal of Abnormal Psychology, 100,* 245-261.

Millon, T., Green, C. J., & Meagher, R. B. (1972). *Millon Adolescent Personality Inventory manual.* Minneapolis, MN: Interpretive Scoring Systems.

Mirin, S. M., & Weiss, R. D. (1983). Substance abuse. In E. L. Bassuk, S. C. Schoonover, & A. J. Gelenberg (Eds.), *The practitioner's guide to psychoactive drugs* (pp. 221-291). New York: Plenum.

Morey, L. C. (1991a). Classification of mental disorder as a collection of hypothetical constructs. *Journal of Abnormal Psychology, 100,* 289-293.

Morey, L. C. (1991b). *Personality Assessment Inventory: Professional manual.* Odessa, FL: Psychological Assessment Resources.

Morey, L. C. (1992, August). *Personality disorder NOS: Specifying patterns of the otherwise unspecified.* Paper presented at the American Psychological Association convention, Washington, DC.

Morey, L. C., Waugh, M. H., & Blashfield, R. K. (1985). MMPI scores for the DSM-III personality disorders: Their derivation and correlates. *Journal of Personality Assessment, 49,* 245-251.

Morgan, H. G., & Hayward, A. E. (1988). Clinical assessment of anorexia nervosa. *British Journal of Psychiatry, 152,* 367-371.

Morgan, H. G., & Russell, G. R. M. (1975). Value of family background and clinical features as predictors of long term outcome in anorexia nervosa: Four year follow-up study of 41 patients. *Psychological Medicine, 5,* 355-371.

Mueller, J. (1988). A new test for dementia syndromes. *Diagnosis, 10*, 33-40.

Murphy, G. E., Woodruff, M., & Herjanic, M. (1974). Primary affective disorder: Selection efficiency of two sets of diagnostic criteria. *Archives of General Psychiatry, 31*, 182-184.

Murphy, G. E., Woodruff, M., Herjanic, M., & Fischer, J. R. (1974). Validity of clinical course of a primary affective disorder. *Archives of General Psychiatry, 30*, 757-761.

Murphy, G. L., & Medlin, D. L. (1985). The role of theories in conceptual coherence. *Psychological Review, 92*, 289-316.

Murphy, J. L. (1986). Cross-cultural psychiatry. In R. Michels, J. O. Cavenar, A. M. Cooper, S. B. Guze, L. L. Judd, G. L. Klerman, & A. J. Solnit (Eds.), *Psychiatry* (Vol. 3, Chap. 2). Philadelphia: J. B. Lippincott.

Murphy, J. M., & Helzer, J. E. (1985). Epidemiology of schizophrenia in adulthood. In R. Michels, J. O. Cavenar, A. M. Cooper, S. B. Guze, L. L. Judd, G. L. Klerman, & A. J. Solnit (Eds.), *Psychiatry* (Vol. 3, Chap. 15). Philadelphia: J. B. Lippincott.

Murray, R. M., Oon, M. C. H., Rodnight, R., Bireley, J. L. T., & Smith, A. (1979). Increased excretion of dimethyltryptamine and certain features of psychosis: A possible association. *Archives of General Psychiatry, 36*, 644-649.

Myers, J. K., & Weissman, M. M. (1980). Use of a self-report symptom scale to detect depression in a community sample. *American Journal of Psychiatry, 137*, 1081-1084.

Myers, J. K., Weissman, M. M., Tischler, G. L., Holzer, C. E., III, Leaf, P. J., Orvaschel, H., Anthony, J. C., Boyd, J. H., Burke, J. D., Kramer, M., & Stoltzman, R. (1984). Six-month prevalence of psychiatric disorders in three communities: 1980-1982. *Archives of General Psychiatry, 41*, 959-967.

Myers, W. C., Burket, R. C., Lyles, B., Stone, L., & Kemph, J. P. (1990). DSM-III diagnoses and offenses in committed female juvenile delinquents. *Bulletin of the American Academy of Psychiatry and Law, 18*, 47-54.

Myers, W. C., & Kemph, J. P. (1990). DSM-III-R classification of murderous youth: Help or hindrance? *Journal of Clinical Psychiatry, 51*, 239-242.

Nair, N. P. V., Bloom, D. M., Debonnel, G., Schwartz, G., & Mosticyan, S. (1984). Cholecystokinin-octapeptide in chronic schizophrenia: A double-blind placebo-controlled study. *Progress in Neuro-Psychopharmacology and Biological Psychiatry, 8*, 711-714.

Nathan, P. E. (1994). DSM-IV: Empirical, accessible, not yet ideal. *Journal of Clinical Psychology, 50*, 103-110.

National Institute of Mental Health (1991). *NIMH Diagnostic Interview for Children, Version 2.3*. Rockville, MD: Author.

Nelson, A., Fogel, B. S., & Faust, D. (1986). Bedside cognitive screening instruments: A critical assessment. *Journal of Nervous and Mental Disease, 174*, 73-83.

Nelson, H. F., Tennen, H., Tasman, A., Borton, M., Kubeck, M., & Stone, M. (1985). Comparison of three systems for diagnosing borderline personality disorder. *American Journal of Psychiatry, 142*, 855-858.

Nelson-Gray, R. O. (1991). DSM-IV: Empirical guidelines from psychometrics. *Journal of Abnormal Psychology, 100,* 308-315.

Nicholson, R. A., & Kugler, K. E. (1991). Competent and incompetent criminal defendants: A quantitative review of comparative research. *Psychological Bulletin, 109,* 357-370.

Ni Nuallain, M., O'Hare, A., & Walsh, D. (1990). The prevalence of schizophrenia in three counties in Ireland. *Acta Psychiatrica Scandinavica, 82,* 136-140.

Noyes, R., Reich, J., Christiansen, J., Suelzer, M., Pfohl, B., & Coryell, W. A. (1990). Outcome of panic disorder: Relationship of diagnostic subtypes and comorbidity. *Archives of General Psychiatry, 47,* 809-818.

Nussbaum, D. N., & Rogers, R. (1992). Screening psychiatric patients for axis II disorders. *Canadian Journal of Psychiatry, 37,* 658-660.

O'Boyle, M., & Self, D. (1990). A comparison of two interviews for DSM-III-R personality disorders. *Psychiatry Research, 32,* 85-92.

O'Conner, D. W. (1990). The contribution of CAMDEX to the diagnosis of mild dementia in community surveys. *Psychiatric Journal of the University of Ottawa, 15,* 216-220.

O'Conner, D. W., Pollitt, P. A., Hyde, J. B., Fellows, J. L., Miller, N. D., Brook, C. P. B., Reiss, B. B., & Roth, M. (1989). The prevalence of dementia as measured by the Cambridge Mental Disorders of the Elderly examination. *Acta Psychiatrica Scandinavica, 79,* 190-198.

Ogloff, J. R. P., Wong, S., & Greenwood, A. (1990). Treating criminal psychopaths in a therapeutic community program. *Behavioral Sciences and the Law, 8,* 181-190.

Ohta, R. J., Carlin, M. F., & Harmon, B. M. (1981). Auditory acuity and performance on the mental status questionnaire in the elderly. *Journal of the American Geriatrics Society, 29,* 476-478.

Okasha, A., & Ashour, A. (1981). Psycho-demographic study of anxiety in Egypt: The PSE in its Arabic version. *British Journal of Psychiatry, 139,* 70-73.

Olin, J. T., & Zelinski, E. M. (1991). The 12-month reliability of the Mini-Mental State Examination. *Psychological Assessment: A Journal of Clinical and Consulting Psychology, 3,* 427-432.

Olson, D. H., Portner, J., & Lavee, (1985). *Family Adaptability and Cohesion Evaluation Scales III.* Unpublished manuscript, Department of Family Social Science, University of Minnesota, St. Paul.

Omer, H., Foldes, J., Toby, M., & Menczel, J. (1983). Screening for cognitive deficits in a sample of hospitalized geriatric patients. *Journal of the American Geriatrics Society, 31,* 266-268.

Orley, J. H., & Wing, J. K. (1979). Psychiatric disorders in two African villages. *Archives of General Psychiatry, 36,* 513-520.

Ormel, J., Koeter, M. W. J., Van Den Brink, W., & Giel, R. (1989). Concurrent validity of GHQ-28 and PSE as measures of change. *Psychological Medicine, 19,* 1007-1013.

Orvaschel, H. (1989). Structured and semistructured psychiatric interviews for children. In C. F. Last & M. Hersen (Eds.), *Handbook of child psychiatric diagnosis* (pp. 483-495). New York: Wiley.

Orvaschel, H. (1990). Early onset psychiatric disorder in high risk children and increased familial morbidity. *Journal of the American Academy of Child and Adolescent Psychiatry*, *29*, 184-188.

Orvaschel, H., Puigh-Antich, J., Chambers, W., Tabrizi, M. A., & Johnson, R. (1982). Retrospective assessment of child psychopathology with the Kiddie-SADS-E. *Journal of the American Academy of Child Psychiatry*, *21*, 392-397.

Osherson, D. N., & Smith, E. E. (1981). On the adequacy of prototype theory as a theory of concepts. *Cognition*, *9*, 35-58.

Othmer, E., & Othmer, S. C. (1989). *The clinical interview using DSM-III-R*. Washington, DC: American Psychiatric Press.

Othmer, E., Penick, E. C., & Powell, B. J. (1981). *The Psychiatric Diagnostic Interview*. Los Angeles: Western Psychological Services.

Overall, J. E., & Gorham, D. R. (1962). The Brief Psychiatric Rating Scale. *Psychological Reports*, *10*, 799-812.

Palmateer, L. M., & McCartney, J. R. (1985). Do nurses know when patients have cognitive deficits? *Journal of Gerontological Nursing*, *11*, 6-16.

Palmer, R. L., Christie, M., Cordle, C., Davis, D., & Kedrick, J. (1987). The Clinical Eating Disorders Rating Instrument (CEDRI): A preliminary description. *International Journal of Eating Disorders*, *6*, 9-14.

Panzetta, A. F. (1974). Toward a scientific psychiatric nosology: Conceptual and pragmatic issues. *Archives of General Psychiatry*, *30*, 154-161.

Paradis, C. M., Friedman, S., Lazar, R. M., Grubea, J., & Kesselman, M. (1992). Use of a structured interview to diagnose anxiety disorders in a minority population. *Hospital and Community Psychiatry*, *43*, 61-64.

Paris, J. (1993). Personality disorders: A biopsychosocial model. *Journal of Personality Disorders*, *7*, 255-264.

Parker, G., & Blignault, I. (1983). A comparative study of neurotic depression in symptomatic volunteers and psychiatric patients. *Australian and New Zealand Journal of Psychiatry*, *17*, 74-81.

Parnas, J., Cannon, T. D., Jacobsen, B., Schulsinger, H., Schulsinger, F., & Mednick, S. A. (1993). Lifetime DSM-III-R diagnostic outcomes in the offspring of schizophrenic mothers. *Archives of General Psychiatry*, *50*, 707-714.

Pecknold, J. C., Chang, H., Fleury, D., Koszychi, D., Quirion, R., Nair, N. P. V., & Suranyi-Cadotte, B. E. (1987). Platelet imipramine binding in patients with panic disorder and major familial depression. *Psychiatry Research*, *21*, 319-326.

Perry, J. C. (1990). Challenges in validating personality disorders: Beyond description. *Journal of Personality Disorders*, *4*, 273-289.

Perry, J. C., & Klerman, G. L. (1978). The borderline patient: A comparative analysis of four sets of diagnostic criteria. *Archives of General Psychiatry*, *35*, 141-150.

Perry, J. C., & Klerman, G. L. (1980). Clinical features of the borderline personality disorder. *American Journal of Psychiatry, 137*, 165-173.

Perry, J. C., Lavori, P. W., Cooper, S. H., Hoke, L., & O'Connell, M. E. (1987). The Diagnostic Interview Schedule and DSM-III antisocial personality disorder. *Journal of Personality Disorders, 1*, 121-131.

Peveler, R. C., & Fairburn, C. G. (1990). Measurement of neurotic symptoms by self-report questionnaire: Validity of the SCL-90-R. *Psychological Medicine, 20*, 873-879.

Pfeiffer, E. (1975). A Short Portable Mental Status Questionnaire for the assessment of organic brain deficit in elderly patients. *Journal of the American Geriatrics Society, 23*, 433-441.

Pfeiffer, R. I., Kurosaki, T. T., Harrah, C. H., Jr., Chance, J. M., & Filos, S. (1982). Measurement of functional activities in older adults in the community. *Journal of Gerontology, 22*, 191-195.

Pfohl, B. (1993). *Iowa Personality Disorder Screen*. Iowa City: University of Iowa.

Pfohl, B., Barrash, J., True, B., & Alexander, B. (1989). Failure of two Axis II measures to predict medication noncompliance among hypertensive outpatients. *Journal of Personality Disorders, 3*, 45-52.

Pfohl, B., Blum, N., Zimmerman, M., & Stangl, D. (1989). *The Structured Interview for DSM-III Personality: SIDP-R*. Iowa City: University of Iowa.

Pfohl, B., Coryell, W., Zimmerman, M., & Stangl, D. (1986). DSM-III personality disorders: Diagnostic overlap and internal consistency of individual DSM-III criteria. *Comprehensive Psychiatry, 27*, 21-34.

Pfohl, B., Coryell, W., Zimmerman, M., & Stangl, D. (1987). Prognostic validity of self-report and interview measures of personality disorder in depressed inpatients. *Journal of Clinical Psychiatry, 48*, 468-472.

Pfohl, B., Stangl, D., & Zimmerman, M. (1982). *The Structured Interview for DSM-III Personality Disorders (SIDP)*. Iowa City: University of Iowa.

Pfohl, B., Stangl, D., & Zimmerman, M. (1984). The implications of DSM-III personality disorders for patients with major depression. *Journal of Affective Disorders, 7*, 309-319.

Philipp, M., & Maier, W. (1986). The polydiagnostic interview: A structured interview for the polydiagnostic classification of psychiatric patients. *Psychopathology, 19*, 175-185.

Piacentini, J., Shaffer, D., Fisher, P., Schwab-Stone, M., Davies, M., & Giola, P. (1993). The Diagnostic Interview Schedule for Children—Revised version (DISC-R): III. Concurrent criterion validity. *Journal of the American Academy of Child and Adolescent Psychiatry, 32*, 658-665.

Pica, S., Edwards, J., Jackson, H. J., Bell, R. C., Bates, G. W., & Rudd, R. P. (1990). Personality disorders in recent-onset bipolar disorder. *Comprehensive Psychiatry, 31*, 499-510.

Pilgrim, J. A., & Mann, A. H. (1990). Use of the ICD-10 version of the Standardized Assessment of Personality to determine the prevalence of personality disorder in psychiatric inpatients. *Psychological Medicine, 20*, 985-992.

Pilgrim, J. A., Mellers, J. D., Boothby, H. A., & Mann, A. H. (1993). Interrater and temporal reliability of the Standardized Assessment of Personality and the influence of informant characteristics. *Psychological Medicine, 23*, 779-786.

Pilkonis, P. A., & Frank, E. (1988). Personality pathology in recurrent depression: Nature prevalence, and relationship to treatment response. *American Journal of Psychiatry, 145*, 435-441.

Pilkonis, P. A., Heape, C. L., Ruddy, J., & Serrao, P. (1991). Validity in the diagnosis of personality disorders: The use of the LEAD standard. *Psychological Assessment: A Journal of Consulting and Clinical Psychology, 3*, 46-54.

Pincus, A. L., & Wiggins, J. S. (1990). Interpersonal problems and conceptions of personality disorders. *Journal of Personality Disorders, 4*, 342-352.

Pitman, R. K., Altman, B., & Macklin, M. L. (1989). Prevalence of posttraumatic stress disorder in wounded Vietnam veterans. *American Journal of Psychiatry, 146*, 667-669.

Pope, H. G., Jr., Jonas, J. M., Hudson, J. I., Cohen, B. M., & Gunderson, J. G. (1983). The validity of DSM-III borderline personality disorder: A phenomenologic, family history, treatment response and long-term follow-up study. *Archives of General Psychiatry, 40*, 23-30.

Powell, K. E. (1991). *The malingering of schizophrenia*. Unpublished doctoral dissertation, University of South Carolina, Columbia.

Prange, M. E., Greenbaum, P. E., Silver, S. E., Friedman, R. M., Kutash, K., & Duchnowski, A. J. (1992). Family functioning and psychopathology among adolescents with severe emotional disturbances. *Journal of Abnormal Child Psychology, 20*, 83-102.

Prohovnik, I., Smith, G., Sackeim, H. A,. Mayeux, R., & Stern, Y. (1989). Gray-matter degeneration in presenile Alzheimer's disease. *Annals of Neurology, 25*, 117-124.

Puig-Antich, J., Blau, S., Marx, N,. Greenhill, L. L., & Chambers, W. (1978). Prepubertal major depressive disorders: A pilot study. *Journal of the American Academy of Child Psychiatry, 17*, 695-707.

Puig-Antich, J., & Chambers, W. J. (1978). *Schedule for Affective Disorders and Schizophrenia for School-Age Children: Kiddie SADS (K-SADS)*. New York: Department of Child and Adolescent Psychiatry, New York State Psychiatric Institute.

Pulver, A. E., & Carpenter, W. T. (1983). Lifetime psychotic symptoms assessed with the DIS. *Schizophrenic Bulletin, 9*, 377-382.

Raczek, S. W. (1992). Childhood abuse and personality disorders. *Journal of Personality Disorders, 6*, 109-116.

Radloff, L. S. (1977). The CES-D scale: A self-report depression scale for research in the general population. *Applied Psychological Measurement, 3*, 385-401.

Rapp, M. S. (1979). Re-examination of the Clinical Mental Status Examination. *Canadian Journal of Medicine, 24*, 773-775.

Rapp, S. R., Parisi, S. A., & Walsh, D. A. (1988). Psychological dysfunction and physical health among elderly medical inpatients. *Journal of Consulting and Clinical Psychology, 56*, 851-855.

Rapp, S. R., Parisi, S. A., Walsh, D. A., & Wallace, C. E. (1988). Detecting depression in elderly medical inpatients. *Journal of Consulting and Clinical Psychology*, *56*, 509-513.

Regier, D. A., Myers, J. K., Kramer, M., Robins, L. N., Blazer, D. G., Hough, R. L., Eaton, W. W., & Locke, B. Z. (1984). The NIMH epidemiologic catchment area program: Historical context, major objectives and study population characteristics. *Archives of General Psychiatry*, *41*, 934-941.

Reich, J. (1986). The relationship between early life events and DSM-III personality disorders. *Hillsdale Journal of Clinical Psychiatry*, *8*, 164-173.

Reich, J. (1987a). Prevalence of DSM-III-R self-defeating (masochistic) personality disorder in normal and outpatient populations. *Journal of Nervous and Mental Disease*, *175*, 52-54.

Reich, J. (1987b). Sex distribution of DSM-III personality disorders in psychiatric outpatients. *American Journal of Psychiatry*, *144*, 485-488.

Reich, J. (1988a). DSM-III personality disorders and the outcome of treated panic disorder. *American Journal of Psychiatry*, *145*, 1149-1152.

Reich, J. (1988b). A family history method for DSM-III anxiety and personality disorders. *Psychiatry Research*, *26*, 131-139.

Reich, J. (1990). The effect of personality on placebo response in panic patients. *Journal of Nervous and Mental Disease*, *178*, 699-702.

Reich, J., & Noyes, R. (1987). A comparison of DSM-III personality disorders in acutely ill panic and depressed patients. *Journal of Anxiety Disorders*, *1*, 123-131.

Reich, J., Noyes, R., Hirschfeld, R., Coryell, W., & O'Gorman, T. (1987). State and personality in depressed and panic patients. *American Journal of Psychiatry*, *144*, 181-187.

Reich, J., Noyes, R., & Troughton, E. (1987). Dependent personality disorder associated with phobic avoidance in patients with panic disorder. *American Journal of Psychiatry*, *144*, 323-326.

Reich, J., & Troughton, E. (1988a). Comparison of DSM-III personality disorders in recovered depressed and panic disorder patients. *Journal of Nervous and Mental Disease*, *176*, 300-304.

Reich, J., & Troughton, E. (1988b). Frequency of DSM-III personality disorders in patients with panic disorder: Comparison with psychiatric and normal control subjects. *Psychiatry Research*, *26*, 89-100.

Reich, J. H. (1981). Proverbs and the modern mental status exam. *Comprehensive Psychiatry*, *22*, 528-531.

Reich, W. (1992a). *DICA-R Pregnancy, Birth and Preschool Questionnaire*. St. Louis, MO: Washington University.

Reich, W. (1992b). Structured and semi-structured interviews. In L. K. G. Hsu & M. Hersen (Eds.), *Research in psychiatry: Issues, strategies, and methods* (pp. 175-193). New York: Plenum.

Reich, W., & Earls, F. (1984). *Home Environment Interview for Children (HEIC)*. St. Louis, MO: Washington University.

Reich, W., & Earls, F. (1987). Rules for making psychiatric diagnoses in children on the basis of multiple sources of information: Preliminary strategies. *Journal of Abnormal Child Psychology, 15*, 601-606.

Reich, W., & Earls, F. (1990). Interviewing adolescents by telephone: Is it a useful methodological strategy? *Comprehensive Psychiatry, 31*, 211-215.

Reich, W., Earls, F., Frankel, O., & Shayka, J. J. (1993). Psychopathology in children of alcoholics. *Journal of the American Academy of Child and Adolescent Psychiatry, 32*, 995-1002.

Reich, W., Earls, F., & Powell, J. (1988). A comparison of the home and social environments of children of alcoholic and non-alcoholic parents. *British Journal of Addiction, 83*, 831-839.

Reich, W., Herjanic, B., Welner, Z., & Gandhy, P. R. (1982). Development of a structured psychiatric interview for children: Agreement on diagnosis comparing child and parent interviews. *Journal of Abnormal Child Psychology, 10*, 325-336.

Reich, W., & Kaplan, L. (in press). The effects of psychiatric and psychosocial interviews on children. *Comprehensive Psychiatry*.

Reich, W., Shayka, J. J., & Taibleson, C. (1991a). *Diagnostic Interview for Children and Adolescents (DICA-R-A): Adolescent version*. St. Louis, MO: Washington University.

Reich, W., Shayka, J. J., & Taibleson, C. (1991b). *Diagnostic Interview for Children and Adolescents (DICA-R-C): Child version*. St. Louis, MO: Washington University.

Reich, W., Shayka, J. J., & Taibleson, C. (1991c). *Diagnostic Interview for Children and Adolescents (DICA-R-P): Parent version*. St. Louis, MO: Washington University.

Reid, D. W., Tierney, M. C., Zorzitto, M. S., Snow, W. G., & Fisher, R. H. (1991). On the clinical value of the London psychogeriatric rating scale. *Journal of the American Geriatrics Society, 39*, 368-371.

Reisberg, B., Ferris, S. H., De Leon, M. J., & Crook, T. (1982). The global deterioration scale for assessment of primary degenerative dementia. *American Journal of Psychiatry, 139*, 1136-1139.

Reisberg, B., Schneck, M. K., Ferris, S. H., Schwartz, G. D., & De Leon, M. J. (1983). The Brief Cognitive Rating Scale (BCRS): Findings in primary degenerative dementia (PDD). *Psychopharmacology Bulletin, 19*, 47-51.

Reitan, R. M., & Wolfson, D. (1988). *Traumatic brain injury: Vol. 2. Recovery and rehabilitation*. Tucson, AZ: Neuropsychology Press.

Remington, M., Tyrer, P. J., Newson-Smith, J., & Cicchetti, D. V. (1979). Comparative reliability of categorical and analogue rating scales in the assessment of psychiatric symptomatology. *Psychological Medicine, 9*, 765-770.

Renneberg, B., Chambless, D. L., Dowdall, D. J., Fauerbach, J. A., & Gracely, E. J. (1992). The Structured Clinical Interview for DSM-III-R, Axis II and the Millon Clinical Multiaxial Inventory: A concurrent validity study of personality disorders among anxious outpatients. *Journal of Personality Disorders, 6*, 117-124.

Rice, M. E., Harris, G. T., & Quinsey, V. L. (1990). *A follow-up of rapists assessed in a maximum security psychiatric facility*. Unpublished manuscript.

Riley, K. (1988). Measurement of dissociation. *Journal of Nervous and Mental Disease, 176,* 449-450.

Riskland, J. H., Beck, A. T., Berchick, R. J., Brown, G., & Steer, R. A. (1987). Reliability of DSM-III diagnoses for major depression and generalized anxiety disorder using the structured clinical interview for DSM-III. *Archives of General Psychiatry, 44,* 817-820.

Riso, L. P., Klein, D. N., Anderson, R. L., Ouimette, P. C., & Lizardi, H. (1994). Concordance between patients and informants on the Personality Disorder Examination. *American Journal of Psychiatry, 151,* 568-573.

Robins, E., & Guze, S. B. (1970). Establishment of diagnostic validity in psychiatric illness: Its application to schizophrenia. *American Journal of Psychiatry, 126,* 107-111.

Robins, L. N. (1966). *Deviant children grow up*. Baltimore: Williams & Wilkins.

Robins, L. N. (1985). Epidemiology: Reflections on testing the validity of psychiatric interviews. *Archives of General Psychiatry, 42,* 918-924.

Robins, L. N. (1987). The assessment of psychiatric diagnosis in epidemiological studies. In M. M. Weissman (Ed.), *Psychiatric epidemiology: APA annual review* (pp. 592-607). Washington, DC: American Psychiatric Press.

Robins, L. N. (1989). Diagnostic grammar and assessment: Translating criteria into questions. *Psychological Medicine, 19,* 57-68.

Robins, L. N., Cottler, L. B., & Keating, S. (1991). *NIMH Diagnostic Interview Schedule, Version III—Revised (DIS-III-R): Question-by-question specifications*. St. Louis, MO: Washington University School of Medicine.

Robins, L. N., & Helzer, J. E. (1991, December). *The half-life of a structured interview—The NIMH Diagnostic Interview Schedule (DIS)*. Paper presented at the Annual Meeting of the American Public Health Association, Atlanta, GA.

Robins, L. N., Helzer, J. E., Cottler, L. B., & Goldring, E. (1989). *NIMH Diagnostic Interview Schedule, Version III—Revised*. St. Louis, MO: Washington University School of Medicine.

Robins, L. N., Helzer, J. E., Cottler, L. B., Works, J., Goldring, E., McEvoy, L., & Stoltzman, R. (1985). *The DIS version III-A training manual*. St. Louis, MO: Washington University School of Medicine.

Robins, L. N., Helzer, J. E., Croughan, J., & Ratcliff, J. S. (1981). National Institute of Mental Health Diagnostic Interview Schedule. *Archives of General Psychiatry, 38,* 381-389.

Robins, L. N., Helzer, J. E., Orvaschel, H., Anthony, J. C., Blazer, D., Burnam, M. A., Burke, J. D., Jr., & Eaton, W. W. (1982). Validity of the Diagnostic Interview Schedule, Version II: DSM-III diagnoses. *Psychological Medicine, 12,* 855-870.

Robins, L. N., Helzer, J. E., Weissman, M. M., Orvaschel, H., Gruenberg, E., Burke, J. D., Jr., & Regier, D. A. (1984). Lifetime prevalence of specific psychiatric disorders in three sites. *Archives of General Psychiatry, 41,* 949-958.

Robins, L. N., & Marcus, S. C. (1987). The diagnostic screening procedure writer: A tool to develop individualized screening procedures. *Medical Care, 25* (Suppl.), 106-122.

Robins, L. N., Wing, J. K., Wittchen, H. U., Helzer, J. E., Babor, T. R., Burke, J., Farmer, A., Jablenski, A., Pickens, R., Regier, D. A., Sartorius, N., & Towle, L. H. (1988). The composite international diagnostic interview: An epidemiologic instrument suitable for use in conjunction with different diagnostic systems and in different cultures. *Archives of General Psychiatry, 45,* 1069-1077.

Robinson, R. G., Starr, L. B., & Price, T. R. (1984). Two year longitudinal study of mood disorders following stroke: Prevalence and duration at six months follow-up. *British Journal of Psychiatry, 144,* 256-262.

Rodenhauser, P., & Fornal, R. E. (1991). How important is the mental status examination? *Psychiatric Hospital, 22,* 21-24.

Rodgers, B., & Mann, S. A. (1986). The reliability and validity of PSE assessments by lay interviewers: A national population survey. *Psychological Medicine, 16,* 689-700.

Rogers, R. (1984). Towards an empirical model of malingering and deception. *Behavioral Sciences and the Law, 2,* 93-112.

Rogers, R. (1986). *Conducting insanity evaluations.* New York: Van Nostrand Reinhold.

Rogers, R. (1987). Assessment of malingering within a forensic context. In D. N. Weisstub (Ed.), *Law and mental health: International perspectives* (Vol. 3, pp. 209-237). New York: Pergamon Press.

Rogers, R. (1988). Structured interviews and dissimulation. In R. Rogers (Ed.), *Clinical assessment of malingering and deception* (pp. 250-268). New York: Guilford.

Rogers, R. (1990a). Development of a new classificatory model of malingering. *Bulletin of the American Academy of Psychiatry and Law, 18,* 323-333.

Rogers, R. (1990b). Models of feigned mental illness. *Professional Psychology: Research and Practice, 21,* 182-188.

Rogers, R. (1992). *Structured Interview of Reported Symptoms.* Odessa, FL: Psychological Assessment Resources.

Rogers, R., & Bagby, R. M. (in press). MMPI Pd scale with forensic and nonforensic samples. *International Journal of Offender Therapy and Comparative Criminology.*

Rogers, R., Bagby, R. M., & Dickens, S. E. (1992). *Structured Interview of Reported Symptoms (SIRS) professional manual.* Odessa, FL: Psychological Assessment Resources.

Rogers, R., Bagby, R. M., & Prendergast, P. (1993). *Vulnerability of the Structured Interview of DSM-III-R (SCID) to dissimulation and distortion.* Manuscript submitted for publication.

Rogers, R., Bagby, R. M., & Rector, N. (1989). Diagnostic legitimacy of factitious disorder with psychological symptoms. *American Journal of Psychiatry, 146,* 1312-1314.

Rogers, R., Bagby, R. M., & Vincent, A. (in press). Factitious disorder with predominantly psychological symptoms: A forensic quandry. *Journal of Psychiatry and Law*.

Rogers, R., & Cavanaugh, J. L., Jr. (1981). Application of the SADS diagnostic interview to forensic psychiatry. *Journal of Psychiatry and Law, 9*, 329-344.

Rogers, R., & Cavanaugh, J. L., Jr. (1983). "Nothing but the truth"...A re-examination of malingering. *Journal of Psychiatry and Law, 11*, 443-460.

Rogers, R., Cavanaugh, J. L., Jr., & Dolmetsch, R. (1981). Schedule of Affective Disorders and Schizophrenia, a diagnostic interview in evaluations of insanity: An exploratory study. *Psychological Reports, 49*, 135-138.

Rogers, R., & Cunnien, A. J. (1986). Multiple SADS evaluation in the assessment of criminal defendants. *Journal of Forensic Sciences, 30*, 222-230.

Rogers, R., & Dion, K. L. (1991). Rethinking the DSM-III-R diagnosis of antisocial personality disorder. *Bulletin of the American Academy of Psychiatry and Law, 19*, 21-31.

Rogers, R., Dion, K. L., & Lynett, E. (1992). Diagnostic validity of antisocial personality disorder: A prototypical analysis. *Law and Human Behavior, 16*, 677-689.

Rogers, R., Duncan, J. C., & Lynett, E., & Sewell, K. W. (in press). Prototypical analysis of antisocial personality disorder: DSM-IV and beyond. *Law and Human Behavior*.

Rogers, R., & Ewing, C. P. (1992). The measurement of insanity: Debating the merits of the R-CRAS and its alternatives. *International Journal of Law and Psychiatry, 15*, 113-123.

Rogers, R., Gillis, J. R., & Bagby, R. M. (1990). Cross validation of the SIRS with a correctional sample. *Behavioral Sciences and the Law, 8*, 85-92.

Rogers, R., Gillis, J. R., Bagby, R. M., & Monteiro, E. (1991).Detection of malingering on the SIRS: A study of coached and uncoached simulators. *Psychological Assessment: A Journal of Consulting and Clinical Psychology, 3*, 673-677.

Rogers, R., Gillis, J. R., Dickens, S. E., & Bagby, R. M. (1991). Standardized assessment of malingering: Validation of the SIRS. *Psychological Assessment: A Journal of Clinical and Consulting Psychology, 3*, 89-96.

Rogers, R., Gillis, J. R., Turner, R. E., & Smith, T. (1990). The clinical presentation of command hallucinations. *American Journal of Psychiatry, 147*, 1304-1307.

Rogers, R., Harrell, E. H., & Liff, C. D. (1993). Feigning neuropsychological impairment: A critical review of methodological and clinical considerations. *Clinical Psychology Review, 13*, 255-274.

Rogers, R., Harris, M., & Wasyliw, O. E. (1983). Observed and self-reported psychopathology in NGRI acquittees in court-mandated outpatient treatment. *International Journal of Offender Therapy and Comparative Criminology, 27*, 143-149.

Rogers, R., Kropp, R., & Bagby, R. M. (1993). Faking specific disorders: A study of the Structured Interview of Reported Symptoms. *Journal of Clinical Psychology, 48*, 643-647.

Rogers, R., & Lynett, E. (1991). Role of Canadian psychiatry in dangerous offender testimony. *Canadian Journal of Psychiatry, 36*, 79-84.

Rogers, R., & Mitchell, C. (1991). *Mental health experts and the criminal courts: A handbook for lawyers*. Toronto, Canada: Carswell Legal Publications.

Rogers, R., & Ornduff, S. R. (in press). The role of psychopathy in forensic evaluations and expert testimony. In S. J. Hart & R. D. Hare (Eds.), *Psychopathy and the criminal justice system*. Toronto, Canada: Butterworths.

Rogers, R. & Resnick, P. J. (1988). *Manual on malingering and deception*. New York: Guilford.

Rogers, R., Sewell, K. W., & Goldstein, A. (in press). Prototypical analysis of malingering. *Law and Human Behavior*.

Rogers, R., Sewell, K. S., & Salekin, R. (in press). Feigning on the MMPI-2: A meta-analysis. *Assessment*.

Rogers, R., Thatcher, A. A., & Cavanaugh, J. L., Jr. (1984). Use of the SADS diagnostic interview in evaluating legal insanity. *Journal of Clinical Psychology, 40*, 1538-1541.

Rogers, R., & Wettstein, R. E. (1985). Relapse in NGRI patients: An empirical study. *International Journal of Offender Therapy and Comparative Criminology, 29*, 227-236.

Rogers, R., & Zinbarg, R. (1987). Bad or mad? Antisocial backgrounds of defendants evaluated for insanity. *International Journal of Law and Psychiatry, 10*, 75-80.

Roman, D. D., Tuley, M. R., Villanueva, M. R., & Mitchell, W. E. (1990). Evaluating MMPI validity in a forensic psychiatric population: Distinguishing between malingering and genuine psychopathology. *Criminal Justice and Behavior, 17*, 186-198.

Romans-Clarkson, S. E., Walton, V. A., Herbison, G. P., & Mullen, P. E. (1990). Psychiatric morbidity among women in urban and rural New Zealand: Psychosocial correlates. *British Journal of Psychiatry, 156*, 84-91.

Rosch, E. (1973). On the internal structure of perceptual and semantic categories. In T. E. Moore (Ed.), *Cognitive development and the acquisition of language* (pp. 111-144). New York: Academic Press.

Rosch, E. (1978). Principles of categorization. In E. Rosch & B. B. Lloyd (Eds.), *Cognition and categorization* (pp. 27-48). Hillsdale, NJ: Erlbaum.

Rosen, A. M., & Fox, H. A. (1986). Tests of cognition and their relationship to psychiatric diagnosis and demographic variables. *Journal of Clinical Psychiatry, 47*, 495-498.

Rosen, J. C., Vara, L., Wendt, S., & Leitenberg, H. (1990). Validity studies of the Eating Disorder Examination. *International Journal of Eating Disorders, 9*, 519-528.

Rosen, W. G., Mohs, R. C., & Davis, K. L. (1984). A new rating scale for Alzheimer's disease. *American Journal of Psychiatry, 141*, 1356-1364.

Rosen, W. G., Mohs, R. C., Johns, C. A., Small, N. S., Kendler, K. S., Horvath, T. B., & Davis, K. L. (1984). Positive and negative symptoms in schizophrenia. *Psychiatry Research, 13,* 277-284.

Rosenbaum, J. F., Biederman, J., Gersten, M., Hirshfeld, D. R., Meminger, S. R., Herman, J. B., Kagan, J., Reznick, S., & Snidman, N. (1988). Behavioral inhibition in children of parents with panic disorder and agoraphobia: A controlled study. *Archives of General Psychiatry, 45,* 463-470.

Rosenthal, M. J. (1989). Towards selective and improved performance of the mental status examination. *Acta Psychiatrica Scandinavica, 80,* 207-215.

Ross, C. A., & Leichner, P. (1984). Residents training in the mental status examination. *Canadian Journal of Psychiatry, 29,* 315-318.

Ross, C. A., & Leichner, P. (1988). Residents performance on the mental status examination. *Canadian Journal of Psychiatry, 33,* 108-111.

Ross, H. E., Gavin, D. R., & Skinner, H. A. (1990). Diagnostic validity of the MAST and the alcohol dependence scale in the assessment of DSM-III alcohol disorders. *Journal of Studies on Alcohol, 51,* 506-513.

Roth, M., Tym, E., Montjoy, C. Q., Huppert, F. A., Hendrie, H., Verma, S., & Goddard, R. (1986). CAMDEX: A standardized instrument for the diagnosis of mental disorders in the elderly with special reference to the early detection of dementia. *British Journal of Psychiatry, 149,* 698-709.

Rounsaville, B. J., Cacciola, J., Weissman, M. M., & Kleber, H. D. (1981). Diagnostic concordance in a follow-up study of opiate addicts. *Journal of Psychiatric Research, 16,* 191-201.

Rovner, B. W., & Folstein, M. F. (1987). Mini-Mental State Exam in clinical practice. *Hospital Practice, 22,* 99-110.

Rubio-Stipec, M., Bird, H., Canino, G., Bravo, M., & Alegria, M. (1991). Children of alcoholic parents in the community. *Journal of Studies on Alcohol, 52,* 78-88.

Rubio-Stipec, M., Shrout, P. E., Bird, H., Canino, G., & Bravo, M. (1989). Symptom scales of the Diagnostic Interview Schedule: Factor results in Hispanic and Anglo samples. *Psychological Assessment: A Journal of Consulting and Clinical Psychology, 1,* 30-34.

Ruegg, R. G., Ekstrom, D. E., Dwight, L., & Golden, R. N. (1990). Introduction of a standardized report form improves the quality of mental status examination reports by psychiatric residents. *Academic Psychiatry, 14,* 157-163.

Rutter, M., & Graham, P. (1968). The reliability and validity of the psychiatric assessment of the child: I. Interview with the child. *British Journal of Psychiatry, 114,* 563-579.

Ryan, N. D., Puig-Antich, J., Ambrosini, P., Rabinovich, H., Robinson, D., Nelson, B., Iyengar, S., & Twomey, J. (1987). The clinical picture of major depression in children and adolescents. *Archives of General Psychiatry, 44,* 854-861.

Saghir, M. T. (1971). A comparison of some aspects of structured and unstructured psychiatric interviews. *American Journal of Psychiatry, 128,* 180-184.

Sanderson, W. C., DiNardo, P. A., Rapee, R. M., & Barlow, D. H. (1990). Syndrome comorbidity in patients diagnosed with a DSM-III-R anxiety disorder. *Journal of Abnormal Psychology*, *98*, 308-312.

Sansone, R. A., & Fine, M. A. (1992). Borderline personality as a predictor of outcome in women with eating disorders. *Journal of Personality Disorders*, *6*, 176-186.

Sartorius, N., Ustun, T. B., Siva, J. A. C., Goldberg, D., Lecrubier, Y., Ormel, J., Von Korff, M., & Wittchen, H. U. (1993). International study of psychological problems in primary care. *Archives of General Psychiatry*, *50*, 819-824.

Schmidt, N. B., & Telch, M. J. (1990). Prevalence of personality disorders among bulimics, nonbulimic binge eaters, and normal controls. *Journal of Psychopathology and Behavioral Assessment*, *12*, 169-185.

Schmidtt, F. A., Ranseen, J. D., & DeKosky, S. T. (1989). Cognitive mental status examinations. *Clinics of Geriatric Medicine*, *5*, 545-564.

Schooler, N. R., Keith, S. J., Severe, J. B., & Matthews, S. (1989). Acute treatment response and short term outcome in schizophrenia. *Psychopharmacology Bulletin*, *15*, 3-13.

Schramm, E., Hohagen, F., Grasshoff, U., Riemann, D., Hajak, G., Hans-Gunther, W., & Berger, M. (1993). Test-retest reliability and validity of the Structured Interview for Sleep Disorders according to DSM-III-R. *American Journal of Psychiatry*, *150*, 867-872.

Schretlen, D. J. (1988). The use of psychological tests to identify malingered symptoms of a mental disorder. *Clinical Psychological Review*, *8*, 451-476.

Schretlen, D. J., Brandt, J., Krafft, L. & Van Gorp, W. (1991). Some caveats in using the Rey 15-item memory test to detect malingered amnesia. *Psychological Assessment: A Journal of Consulting and Clinical Psychology*, *3*, 667-672.

Schroeder, M. L., Schroeder, K. G., & Hare, R. D. (1983). Generalizability of a checklist for the assessment of psychopathy. *Journal of Consulting and Clinical Psychology*, *51*, 511-516.

Schroeder, M. L., Wormworth, J. A., & Livesley, W. J. (1992). Dimensions of personality disorder and their relationships to the big five dimensions of personality. *Psychological Assessment*, *4*, 47-53.

Schuckit, M. A. (1985). Trait and state markers of a predisposition to psychopathology. In R. Michels, J. O. Cavenar, A. M. Cooper, S. B. Guze, L. L. Judd, G. L. Klerman, & A. J. Solnit (Eds.), *Psychiatry* (Vol. 3, Chap. 57). Philadelphia: J. B. Lippincott.

Schwab-Stone, M., Fisher, P., Piacentini, J., Shaffer, D., Davies, M., & Briggs, M. (1993). The Diagnostic Interview Schedule for Children—Revised version (DISC-R): II. Test-retest reliability. *Journal of the American Academy of Child and Adolescent Psychiatry*, *32*, 651-657.

Schwamm, L. H., VanDyke, C., Kiernan, R. J., Merrin, E. L., & Mueller, J. (1987). The Neurobehavioral Cognitive Status Examination: Comparison with Cognitive Capacity Screening Examination and the Mini-Mental State Examination in a neurosurgical population. *Annals of Internal Medicine*, *107*, 486-491.

Schwartz, J. M., Aylward, E., Barta, P., Tune, L. E., & Pearlson, G. D. (1992). Sylvian fissure size in schizophrenia measured with the magnetic resonance imaging rating protocol of the consortium to establish a registry for Alzheimer's disease. *American Journal of Psychiatry, 149*, 1195-1198.

Schwartz, M. A., & Wiggins, O. P. (1986). Logical empiricism and psychiatric classification. *Comprehensive Psychiatry, 27*, 101-114.

Secunda, S. K., Katz, M. M., Swann, A., Koslow, S. H., Maas, J. W., Chaung, S., & Croughan, J. (1985). Mania: Diagnosis, state measurement, and prediction of treatment response. *Journal of Affective Disorders, 8*, 113-121.

Segal, H. G., Westen, D., Lohr, N. E., Silk, K. R., & Cohen, R. (1992). Assessing object relations and social cognition in borderline personality disorders from stories told to the picture arrangement subtest of the WAIS-R. *Journal of Personality Disorders, 6*, 458-470.

Selzer, M. L. (1971). Michigan Alcoholism Screening Test: The quest for a new diagnostic instrument. *American Journal of Psychiatry, 127*, 1653-1658.

Selzer, M. L., Vinokur, A., & Van Rooijen, L. (1975). A self-administered short Michigan Alcoholism Screening Test (SMAST). *Journal of Studies on Alcohol, 36*, 117-126.

Semler, G., Wittchen, H. U., Joschke, K., Zaudig, M., Geiso, T. von, Kaiser, S., Cranach, M. von, & Pfister, H. (1987). Test-retest reliability of a standardized psychiatric interview (DIS/CIDI). *European Archives of Psychiatry and Neurological Sciences, 236*, 214-222.

Serin, R. C. (1991). Psychopathy and violence in criminals. *Journal of Interpersonal Violence, 6*, 423-431.

Serin, R. C., Peters, R. D., & Barabaree, H. E. (1990). Predictors of psychopathy and release outcome in a criminal population. *Psychological Assessment: A Journal of Consulting and Clinical Psychology, 2*, 419-422.

Serper, M. R., Bernstein, D. P., Maurer, G., Harvey, P. D., Horvath, T., Klar, H., Coccaro, E. F., & Siever, L. J. (1993). Psychological test profiles of patients with borderline and schizotypal personality disorders: Implications for DSM-IV. *Journal of Personality Disorders, 7*, 144-154.

Shaffer, D. (1994). Debate and argument: Structured interviews for assessing children. *Journal of Child Psychology and Psychiatry, 35*, 783-784.

Shaffer, D., Gould, M. S., Brasic, J., Ambrosini, P., Fisher, P., Bird, H., & Aluwahlia, S. (1983). A Children's Global Assessment Scale (C-GAS). *Archives of General Psychiatry, 40*, 1228-1231.

Shaffer, D., Schwab-Stone, M., Fisher, P., Cohen, P., Piacentini, J., Davies, M., Conners, C. K., & Regier, D. (1993). The Diagnostic Interview Schedule for Children–Revised version (DISC-R): I. Preparation, field testing, interrater reliability, and acceptability. *Journal of the American Academy of Child and Adolescent Psychiatry, 32*, 643-650.

Shaffer, D., Schwab-Stone, M., Fisher, P., Davies, M., Piacentini, J,. & Giola, P. (1988). *A revised version of the Diagnostic Interview Schedule for Children (DISC-R): Results of a field trial and proposals for a new instrument*. Rockville, MD: Epidemiology and Psychopathology Research Branch, National Institute of Mental Health.

Shapiro, M. B., Post, F., Lofving, B., & Inglis, J. (1956). "Memory function" in psychiatric patients over sixty; some methodological and diagnostic implications. *Journal of Mental Sciences, 102*, 233-246.

Shapiro, S. K., & Garfinkel, B. D. (1986). The occurrence of behavior disorders in children: The interdependence of attention deficit disorder and conduct disorder. *Journal of the American Academy of Child Psychiatry, 25*, 809-819.

Shea, M. T., Glass, D. R., Pilkonis, P. A., Watkins, J., & Docherty, J. P. (1987). Frequency and implications of personality disorders in a sample of depressed outpatients. *Journal of Personality Disorders, 1*, 27-42.

Shear, M. K., Kligfield, P., Harshfield, G., Devereux, R. B., Polan, J. J., Mann, J. J., Pickering, T., & Frances, A. J. (1987). Cardiac rate and rhythm in panic patients. *American Journal of Psychiatry, 144*, 633-637.

Shrout, P. E., Spitzer, R. L., & Fleiss, J. L. (1987). Quantification of agreement in psychiatric diagnosis revisited. *Archives of General Psychiatry, 44*, 172-177.

Siever, L. J., Keefe, R., Bernstein, D. P., Coccaro, E. F., Klar, H. M., Zemishlany, Z., Peterson, A. E., Davidson, M., Mahon, T., Horvath, T., & Mohs, R. (1990). Eye tracking impairment in clinically identified patients with schizotypal personality disorder. *American Journal of Psychiatry, 147*, 740-745.

Silk, K. R., Lohr, N. E., Ogata, S. N., & Westen, D. (1990). Borderline inpatients with affective disorder: Preliminary follow-up data. *Journal of Personality Disorders, 4*, 213-224.

Simon, R., Endicott, J., & Nie, J. (1987). Intake diagnoses: How representative? *Comprehensive Psychiatry, 28*, 389-396.

Simourd, D. J., Bonta, D. A., Andrews, D. A., & Hoge, R. D. (1990). *Criterion validity of assessments of psychopathy: A meta-analysis.* Unpublished manuscript, Carleton University, Ottawa, Canada.

Singer, M. T., & Larson, D. G. (1981). Borderline personality and the Rorschach test. *Archives of General Psychiatry, 38*, 693-698.

Skinner, H. A. (1982). The Drug Abuse Screening Test. *Addictive Behaviors, 7*, 363-371.

Skinner, H. A., & Blashfield, R. K. (1982). Increasing the impact of cluster analysis research: The case of psychiatric classification. *Journal of Consulting and Clinical Psychology, 50*, 727-735.

Skinner, H. A., & Horn, J. L. (1984). *Alcohol Dependence Scale (ADS): User's guide.* Toronto, Canada: Addiction Research Foundation.

Skodol, A. E., Rosnick, L., Kellman, D., Oldman, J. M., & Hyler, S. E. (1988). Validating structured DSM-III-R personality disorder assessments with longitudinal data. *American Journal of Psychiatry, 145*, 1297-1299.

Skodol, A. E., Rosnick, L., Kellman, D., Oldman, J. M., & Hyler, S. E. (1991). Development of a procedure for validating structured assessments for Axis II. In J. M. Oldham (Ed.), *Personality disorders: New perspectives on diagnostic validity* (pp. 41-70). Washington, DC: American Psychiatric Press.

Skre, I., Onstad, S., Torgersen, S., & Kringlen, E. (1991). High interrater reliability for the Structured Clinical Interview for DSM-III-R Axis I (SCID-I). *Acta Psychiatrica Scandinavica, 84*, 167-173.

Skurla, E., Rogers, J. C., & Sunderland, T. (1988). Direct assessment of activities of daily living in Alzheimer's disease: A controlled study. *Journal of the American Geriatrics Society, 36*, 97-103.

Sletten, I. W., Altman, H., Evenson, R. C., & Cho, D. W. (1973). Computer assignment of psychotropic drugs. *American Journal of Psychiatry, 130*, 595-598.

Sletten, I. W., Ernhart, C. B., & Ulett, G. A. (1970). The Missouri Automated Mental Status Examination: Development, use and reliability. *Comprehensive Psychiatry, 11*, 315-327.

Sletten, I. W., & Evenson, R. C. (1972). The Missouri Automated Standard System of Psychiatry (SSOP): An overview. *Computer Medicine, 2*, 1-4.

Sletten, I. W., Ulett, G. A., Altman, H., & Sundland, D. (1970). The Missouri Standard System of Psychiatry (SSOP) computer generated diagnosis. *Archives of General Psychiatry, 23*, 73-79.

Smith, A. (1967). The serial sevens subtraction test. *Archives of Neurology, 17*, 78-80.

Smith, D. E., Marcus, M. D., & Kaye, W. (1992). Cognitive-behavioral treatment of obese binge eaters. *International Journal of Eating Disorders, 12*, 257-262.

Smith, G. P. (1990). *Detection of malingering of schizophrenia in male prisoners.* Unpublished manuscript, University of Missouri at St. Louis.

Smith, J., Carr, V., Morris, H., & Gilliland, J. (1988). The dexamethasone suppression test in relation to symptomatology: Preliminary findings controlling for serum dexamethasone concentrations. *Psychiatry Research, 25*, 123-133.

Smith, S. S., & Newman, J. P. (1990). Alcohol and drug abuse/dependence disorders in psychopathic and nonpsychopathic criminal offenders. *Journal of Abnormal Psychology, 99*, 430-439.

Smyer, M., Hofland, B., & Jonas, E. (1979). Validity study of the Short Portable Mental Status Questionnaire for the elderly. *Journal of the American Geriatrics Society, 27*, 263-269.

Snaith, R. P., Baugh, S. J., Clayden, A. D., Husain, A., & Sipple, M. A. (1982). The Clinical Anxiety Scale: An instrument derived from the Hamilton anxiety scale. *British Journal of Psychiatry, 141*, 518-523.

Soldz, S., Budman, S., Demby, A., & Merry, J. (1993). Diagnostic agreement between the Personality Disorder Examination and the MCMI-II. *Journal of Personality Assessment, 60*, 486-499.

Soloff, P. H., George, A., Cornelius, J., Nathan, S., & Schulz, P. (1991). Pharmacotherapy and borderline subtypes. In J. M. Oldham (Ed.), *Personality disorders: New perspectives on diagnostic validity* (pp. 89-103). Washington, DC: American Psychiatric Press.

Soloff, P. H., & Ulrich, R. F. (1981). Diagnostic interview for borderline patients: A replication study. *Archives of General Psychiatry, 38*, 686-692.

Sokal, R. R. (1974). Classification: Purposes, principles, progress, prospects. *Science, 185*, 1115-1123.

Spengler, P. A., & Wittchen, H. U. (1988). Procedural validity of standardized symptom questions for the assessment of psychotic symptoms: A comparison of the DIS with two clinical methods. *Comprehensive Psychiatry, 29*, 309-322.

Spielberger, C. D. (1973). *Preliminary manual for the State-Trait Anxiety Inventory for Children*. Palo Alto, CA: Consulting Psychologists Press.

Spielberger, C. D., Gorsuch, R. L., & Lushene, R. E. (1970). *Manual for the State-Trait Anxiety Inventory*. Palo Alto, CA: Consulting Psychologists Press.

Spiker, D. G., & Ehler, J. G. (1984). Structured psychiatric interviews for adults. In G. Goldstein & M. Hersen (Eds.), *Handbook of psychological assessment* (pp. 291-304). New York: Pergamon.

Spitzer, R. L. (1983). Psychiatric diagnosis: Are clinicians still necessary? *Comprehensive Psychiatry, 24*, 399-411.

Spitzer, R. L. (1991). An outsider-insider's views about revising the DSMs. *Journal of Abnormal Psychology, 100*, 294-296.

Spitzer, R. L., & Endicott, J. (1968). DIAGNO: A computer program for psychiatric diagnosis utilizing the differential diagnostic procedure. *Archives of General Psychiatry, 18*, 746-756.

Spitzer, R. L., & Endicott, J. (1969). DIAGNO II: Further developments in a computer program for psychiatric diagnosis. *American Journal of Psychiatry, 125*, 12-21.

Spitzer, R. L., & Endicott, J. (1970). *The mental status evaluation record (MSER)*. New York: Biometrics Research.

Spitzer, R. L., & Endicott, J. (1971). An integrated group of forms for automated psychiatric case records: Progress report. *Archives of General Psychiatry, 24*, 448-453.

Spitzer, R. L., & Endicott, J. (1975a). Psychiatric rating forms in the evaluation of psychiatric treatment. In A. M. Freedman, H. I. Kaplan, & B. J. Sadock (Eds.) *Comprehensive textbook in psychiatry* (2nd ed.) (Vol. 2, pp. 2015-2031). Baltimore: Williams & Wilkins.

Spitzer, R. L., & Endicott, J. (1975b). *Schedule of Affective Disorders and Schizophrenia (SADS)* (2nd ed.). New York: Columbia University.

Spitzer, R. L., & Endicott, J. (1978a). *Schedule of Affective Disorders and Schizophrenia* (3rd ed.). New York: Biometrics Research.

Spitzer, R. L., Endicott, J. (1978b). *Schedule of Affective Disorders and Schizophrenia—Change Version*. New York: Biometrics Research.

Spitzer, R. L., Endicott, J., Cohen, J., & Fleiss, J. L. (1974). Constraints on the validity of computer diagnosis. *Archives of General Psychiatry, 31*, 197-203.

Spitzer, R. L., Endicott, J., Fleiss, J. L., & Cohen, J. (1970). The Psychiatric Status Schedule: A technique of evaluating psychopathology and impairment in social role functioning. *Archives of General Psychiatry, 23*, 41-55.

Spitzer, R. L., Endicott, J., & Gibbon, M. (1979). Crossing the border into borderline personality and borderline schizophrenia. *Archives of General Psychiatry, 36*, 17-24.

Spitzer, R. L., Endicott, J., & Robins, E. (1975a). Clinical criteria for psychiatric diagnosis and DSM-III. *American Journal of Psychiatry, 132*, 1187-1192.

Spitzer, R. L., Endicott, J., & Robins, E. (1975b). *Research Diagnostic Criteria*. New York: Biometrics Research.

Spitzer, R. L., Endicott, J., & Robbins, E. (1978). Research Diagnostic Criteria for the use in psychiatric research. *Archives of General Psychiatry, 35*, 773-782.

Spitzer, R. L., Feister, S., Gay, M., & Pfohl, B. (1991). Results of a survey of forensic psychiatrists on the validity of the sadistic personality disorder diagnosis. *American Journal of Psychiatry, 148*, 875-879.

Spitzer, R. L., & Fleiss, J. L. (1974). A re-analysis of the reliability of psychiatric diagnosis. *British Journal of Psychiatry, 125*, 341-347.

Spitzer, R. L., Fleiss, J. L., Burdock, E. I., & Hardesty, A. S. (1964). The Mental Status Schedule: Rationale, reliability and validity. *Comprehensive Psychiatry, 5*, 384-395.

Spitzer, R. L., Williams, J. B. W., & Gibbon, M. (1987a). *SCID personality questionnaire*. New York: Biometrics Research.

Spitzer, R. L., Williams, J. B. W., & Gibbon, M. (1987b). *Structured Clinical Interview for DSM-III-R (SCID)*. New York: Biometrics Research.

Spitzer, R. L., Williams, J. B. W., & Gibbon, M. (1987c). *Structured Clinical Interview for DSM-III-R personality disorders (SCID-II)*. New York: Biometrics Research.

Spitzer, R. L., Williams, J. B. W., Gibbon, M., & First, M. B. (1990a). *SCID-II Questionnaire*. Washington, DC: American Psychiatric Press.

Spitzer, R. L., Williams, J. B. W., Gibbon, M., & First, M. B. (1990b). *Structured Clinical Interview for DSM-III-R (SCID)*. Washington, DC: American Psychiatric Press.

Spitzer, R. L., Williams, J. B. W., Gibbon, M., & First, M. B. (1990c). *Structured Clinical Interview for DSM-III-R personality disorders (SCID-II)*. Washington, DC: American Psychiatric Press.

Spitzer, R. L., Williams, J. B. W., Gibbon, M., & First, M. B. (in press). The Structured Clinical Interview for DSM-III-R (SCID): I. History, rationale, and description. *Archives of General Psychiatry*.

Spitznagel, E. L., & Helzer, J. E. (1985). A proposed solution to the base rate problem in the kappa statistic. *Archives of General Psychiatry, 42*, 725-728.

Squires-Wheeler, E., Skodol, A. E., Bassett, A., & Erlenmeyer-Kimling, L. (1990). DSM-III-R schizotypal personality traits in offspring and schizophrenic disorder, affective disorder, and normal control patients. *Journal of Psychiatric Research, 23*, 229-239.

Standage, K., & Ladha, N. (1988). An examination of the reliability of the Personality Disorder Examination and a comparison with other methods of identifying personality disorders in a clinical sample. *Journal of Personality Disorders, 2*, 267-271.

Stangl, D., Pfohl, B., Zimmerman, M., Bowers, W., & Corenthal, C. (1985). A structured interview for DSM-III personality disorders: A preliminary report. *Archives of General Psychiatry, 42*, 591-596.

Stavrakaki, C., Williams, E. C., Walker, S., Rogers, N., & Kotsopoulos, S. (1991). Pilot study of anxiety and depression in prepubertal children. *Canadian Journal of Psychiatry, 36*, 332-338.

Stefannson, J. G., Lindal, E., Bjornsson, J. ⏎ prevalence of specific mental disord ⏎ *Acta Psychiatrica Scandinavica, 8*

Stein, S. J. (1987). Computer-assisted dia ⏎ *Psychology: An International Rev*

Steinberg, M. (1992). *Field trials of the* ⏎ *Dissociative Disorders.* Unpublis ⏎ Medicine, New Haven, CT.

Steinberg, M. (1993). *Interviewer's gu* ⏎ *DSM-IV Dissociative Disorde* ⏎ Psychiatric Press.

Steinberg, M. (in press-a). Psychologic ⏎ Michelson and W. J. Ray (Eds.), *H*

Steinberg, M. (in press-b). Systematizi ⏎ assessment. In D. Spiegel (Ed.), *D* ⏎ American Psychiatric Press.

Steinberg, M., Bancroft, J., & Buchanan, J. (1993). Multiple personality ⏎ criminal law. *Bulletin of the American Academy of Psychiatry and the Law,* *21,* 345-356.

Steinberg, M., Cicchetti, D., Buchanan, J., Hall, R., & Rounsaville, B. (1993). Clinical assessment of dissociative symptoms and disorders: The Structured Clinical Interview for DSM-IV Dissociative Disorders (SCID-D). *Dissociation, 6,* 3-15.

Steinberg, M., Rounsaville, B., & Cicchetti, D. V. (1990). The Structured Clinical Interview for DSM-III-R Dissociative Disorders: Preliminary report on a new diagnostic instrument. *American Journal of Psychiatry, 147,* 76-82.

Stephens, J. H., Astrup, C., & Carpenter, W. T. (1982). A comparison of nine systems to diagnose schizophrenia. *Psychiatry Research, 6,* 127-143.

Stephens, J. H., Astrup, C., & Mangrum, J. C. (1966). Prognostic factors in recovered and deteriorating schizophrenics. *American Journal of Psychiatry, 122,* 1116-1121.

Stone, M. H. (1985). Borderline personality disorder. In R. Michels, J. O. Cavenar, A. M. Cooper, S. B. Guze, L. L. Judd, G. L. Klerman, & A. J. Solnit (Eds.), *Psychiatry* (Vol. 1, Chap. 17). Philadelphia: J. B. Lippincott.

Stonier, P. D. (1974). Score changes following repeated administration of Mental Status Questionnaire. *Age and Aging, 3,* 91-96.

Stout, A. L., Steege, J. F., Blazer, D. G., & George, L. K. (1986). Comparison of lifetime psychiatric diagnoses in premenstrual syndrome clinic and community samples. *Journal of Nervous and Mental Disease, 174,* 517-522.

Strakowski, S. M., Thohen, M., Stoll, A. L., Faedda, G. L., Mayer, P. V., Kolbrener, M. L., & Goodwin, D. C. (1993). Comorbidity in psychosis at first hospitalization. *American Journal of Psychiatry, 150,* 752-757.

Strain, J. J., Fulop, G., Lebovits, A., Ginsberg, B., Robinson, M., Stern, A., Charap, P. & Gany, F. (1988). Screening devices for diminished cognitive capacity. *General Hospital Psychiatry, 10,* 16-23.

Strein, D. C., Ham, T., & Engeland, H. (1992). Dropout characteristics in a follow-up study of 90 eating-disordered patients. *International Journal of Eating Disorders, 12,* 341-343.

Strober, M., Green, J., & Carlson, G. (1981). Reliability of psychiatric diagnosis in hospitalized adolescents. *Archives of General Psychiatry, 38,* 141-145.

Strub, R. L., & Black, F. W. (1977). *The Mental Status Examination in neurology.* Philadelphia: F. A. Davis.

Stuckenberg, K. W., Dura, J. R., & Kiecolt-Glaser, J. K. (1990). Depression screening scale validation in an elderly, community-dwelling population. *Psychological Assessment: A Journal of Clinical and Consulting Psychology, 2,* 134-138.

Sturt, E. (1981). Hierarchical patterns in the distribution of psychiatric symptoms. *Psychological Medicine, 11,* 783-794.

Sturt, E., & Wykes, T. (1987). Assessment schedules for chronic psychiatric patients. *Psychological Medicine, 17,* 485-493.

Sullivan, E. V., Sagar, H. J., Gabrieli, J. D. E., Corkin, S., & Growdon, J. H. (1989). Different cognitive profiles on standard behavioral tests in Parkinson's disease and Alzheimer's disease. *Journal of Clinical and Experimental Neuropsychology, 11,* 799-820.

Swartz, L., Ben-Arie, O., & Teggin, A. F. (1985). Subcultural delusions and hallucinations: Comments on the Present State Examination in a multicultural context. *British Journal of Psychiatry, 146,* 391-394.

Swartz, M. S., Blazer, D. G., George, L. K., & Winfield, I. (1990). Estimating the prevalence of borderline personality disorder in the community. *Journal of Personality Disorders, 4,* 257-272.

Swartz, M. S., Blazer, D. G., George, L. K., Winfield, I., Zakris, J., & Dye, E. (1989). Identification of borderline personality disorder with the NIMH Diagnostic Interview Schedule. *American Journal of Psychiatry, 146,* 200-205.

Sylvester, C. E., Hyde, T. S., & Reichler, R. J. (1987). The Diagnostic Interview for Children and the Personality Inventory for Children in studies of children at risk for anxiety disorders or depression. *Journal of the American Academy of Child and Adolescent Psychiatry, 26,* 668-675.

Syrakic, D. M., Whitehead, C., Przybeck, T. R., & Cloninger, C. R. (1993). Differential diagnosis of personality disorders by the seven-factor model of temperament and character. *Archives of General Psychiatry, 50,* 991-999.

Tancredi, L. R. (1987). The mental status examination. *Generations, 11,* 24-31.

Taylor, M. A. (1981). *The Neuropsychiatric Mental Status Examination.* New York: Spectrum.

Taylor, M. A., Abrams, R., Raber, R., & Almy G. (1980). Cognitive tasks in the mental status examination. *Journal of Nervous and Mental Disease, 168,* 167-170.

Teng, E. L., & Chui, H. C. (1987). The Modified Mini-Mental State (3MS) Examination. *Journal of Clinical Psychiatry, 48,* 314-318.

Teplin, L. A. (Ed.). (1984). *Mental health and criminal justice.* Beverly Hills, CA: Sage.

Teplin, L. A. (1990). Detecting disorder: The treatment of mental illness among jail detainees. *Journal of Clinical and Consulting Psychology, 58,* 233-236.

Teplin, L. A., & Swartz, J. (1989). Screening for severe mental disorder in jails: The development of the Referral Decision Scale. *Law and Human Behavior*, *13*, 1-18.

Tesser, P. R., & Paulhus, D. (1983). The definition of self: Private and public self-evaluation management strategies. *Journal of Personality and Social Psychology*, *44*, 672-682.

Tetlock, P. E., & Manstead, A. S. R. (1985). Impression management versus intrapsychic explanations in social psychology: A useful dichotomy? *Psychological Review*, *92*, 59-77.

Thal, L. J., Salmon, D. P., Lasker, B., Bower, D., & Klauber, M. R. (1989). The safety and lack of efficacy of vinpocetine in Alzheimer's disease. *Journal of the American Geriatrics Society*, *37*, 515-520.

Tilley, D. H., & Hoffman, J. A. (1981). Mental status examination: Myth or method. *Comprehensive Psychiatry*, *22*, 562-564.

Torgersen, S. (1980). Hereditary-environmental differentiation of general neurotic/obsessive, and impulsive hysterical personality traits. *Acta Genetica Medicae Gemellologiae*, *29*, 193-207.

Torgersen, S., & Alnaes, R. (1989). Localizing DSM-III personality disorders in a three-dimensional structural space. *Journal of Personality Disorders*, *3*, 274-281.

Torgersen, S., & Alnaes, R. (1990). The relationship between the MCMI personality scales and DSM-III, Axis II. *Journal of Personality Assessment*, *55*, 698-707.

Torgersen, S., Skre, I., Onstad, S., Edvardsen, J., & Kringlen, E. (1993). The psychometric-genetic structure of DSM-III-R personality criteria. *Journal of Personality Disorders*, *7*, 196-213.

Trull, T. J. (1992). DSM-III-R personality disorders and the five-factor model of personality: An empirical comparison. *Journal of Abnormal Psychology*, *101*, 553-560.

Trull, T. J., Widiger, T. A., & Frances, A. (1987). Covariation of criteria sets for avoidant, schizoid, and dependent personality disorders. *American Journal of Psychiatry*, *144*, 767-771.

Tsai, L., & Tsuang, M. T. (1979). The Mini-Mental State Test and computerized tomography. *American Journal of Psychiatry*, *136*, 436-439.

Tsuang, M. T. (1974). *Iowa Structured Psychiatric Interview (ISPI)*. Iowa City: Department of Psychiatry, University of Iowa College of Medicine.

Tsuang, M. T., & Loyd, D. W. (1985). Other psychotic disorders. In R. Michels, J. O. Cavenar, A. M. Cooper, S. B. Guze, L. L. Judd, G. L. Klerman, & A. J. Solnit (Eds.), *Psychiatry* (Vol. 1, Chap. 70). Philadelphia: J. B. Lippincott.

Tucker, G. J., & Neppe, V. M. (1991). Neurological and neuropsychiatric assessment of brain injury. In H. O. Doerr & A. S. Carlin (Eds.), *Forensic neuropsychology: Legal and scientific bases* (pp. 70-85). New York: Guilford.

Turner, R. M. (1989). Case study evaluations of a bio-cognitive-behavioral approach for the treatment of borderline personality disorder. *Behavior Therapy*, *20*, 477-489.

Tyrer, P. J., & Alexander, J. (1979). Classification of personality disorder. *British Journal of Psychiatry*, *135*, 163-167.

Tyrer, P. J., Alexander, J., Cicchetti, D., Cohen, M., & Remington, M. (1979). Reliability of a schedule for rating personality disorders. *British Journal of Psychiatry, 135*, 168-174.

Tyrer, P. J., Strauss, J., & Cicchetti, D. (1983). Temporal reliability in psychiatric practice. *Psychological Medicine, 13*, 393-398.

Uhlmann, R. R., & Larson, E. B. (1991). Effect of education on the Mini-Mental State Examination as a screening test for dementia. *Journal of the American Geriatrics Society, 39*, 876-880.

Uhlmann, R. R., Larson, E. B., & Buchner, D. M. (1987). Correlations of the Mini-Mental State and modified dementia rating scale to measures of transitional health status in dementia. *Journal of Gerontology, 42*, 33-36.

Vaglum, P., Friis, S., Karterud, S., Mehlum, L., & Vaglum, S. (1993). Stability of the severe personality disorder diagnosis: A 2- and 5-year prospective study. *Journal of Personality Disorders, 7*, 348-353.

Valliant, G. E. (1964). Prospective prediction of schizophrenic remission. *Archives of General Psychiatry, 11*, 509-518.

van de Loo, K., Derksen, J., Dassel, Y., & Becking, J. (1987). A structural approach to anorexia nervosa. In J. Derksen (Ed.), *A structural approach in psychodiagnostics and psychopathology* (pp. 13-19). Leiden, Netherlands: Leiden University.

Vandiver, T., & Sheer, K. J. (1991). Temporal stability of the diagnostic interview schedule. *Psychological Assessment: A Journal of Consulting and Clinical Psychology, 3*, 277-281.

Vazquez-Barquero, J. L., Diez-Manrique, J. F., Pena, C., Aldama, J., Samaniego, R. C., Menendez, A. J., & Mirapeix, C. (1987). A community mental health survey in Cantabria: A general description of morbidity. *Psychological Medicine, 17*, 227-241.

Velez, C. N., Johnson, J., & Cohen, P. (1989). A longitudinal analysis of selected risk factors for childhood psychopathology. *Journal of the American Academy of Child and Adolescent Psychiatry, 28*, 861-864.

Verhulst, F. C., Althaus, M., & Berden, G. F. M. G. (1987). The Child Assessment Schedule: Parent-child agreement and validity measures. *Journal of Child Psychology and Psychiatry, 28*, 455-466.

Verhulst, F. C., Berden, G. F. M. G., & Sanders-Woudstra, J. A. R. (1985). Mental health in Dutch children: II. The prevalence of psychiatric disorder and relationship between measures. *Acta Psychiatrica Scandinavica, 72* (Suppl. 324), 1-44.

Verhulst, F. C., Bieman, H. V. D., Ende, J. V. D., Berden, G. R. M. G., & Sanders-Woudstra, J. A. R. (1990). Problem behavior in international adoptees: III. Diagnosis of child psychiatric disorders. *Journal of the American Academy of Child and Adolescent Psychiatry, 29*, 420-428.

Vernon, S. W., & Roberts, R. E. (1982). Use of the SADS-RDC in a tri-ethnic community survey. *Archives of General Psychiatry, 39*, 47-52.

Viatori, M. S. (1985). A review of the Psychiatric Diagnostic Interview. *Journal of Counseling and Development, 63*, 531.

Walters, G. D., Mann, M. F., Miller, M. P., Hemphill, L. L., & Chlumsky, M. L. (1988). Emotional disorders among offenders: Inter- and intra-setting comparisons. *Criminal Justice and Behavior, 15*, 433-453.

Ward, C. H., Beck, A. T., Mendelson, M., Mock, J. E., & Erbaugh, J. K. (1962). The psychiatric nomenclature. *Archives of General Psychiatry, 7*, 198-205.

Watson, D., Clark, L. A., & Carey, G. (1988). Positive and negative affectivity and their relation to anxiety and depressive disorders. *Journal of Abnormal Psychology, 97*, 346-353.

Watt, D. C., Katz, K., & Shepherd, M. (1983). The natural history of schizophrenia: A 5-year prospective follow-up of a representative sample of schizophrenics by means of a standardized clinical and social assessment. *Psychological Medicine, 13*, 663-670.

Webster, J. S., Scott, R. R., Nunn, B., McNeer, M. R., & Varnell, N. (1984). A brief neuropsychological screening procedure that assesses left and right hemispheric function. *Journal of Clinical Psychology, 40*, 237-240.

Wechsler, D. (1981). *Wechsler Adult Intelligence Scale—Revised.* New York: The Psychological Corporation.

Wechsler, D. (1987). *Wechsler Memory Scale—Revised.* New York: The Psychological Corporation.

Weddington, W. W., Segraves, K. B., & Simon, M. A. (1986). Current and lifetime incidence of psychiatric disorders among a group of extremity sarcoma survivors. *Journal of Psychosomatic Research, 30*, 121-125.

Weinstein, S. R., Noam, G. G., Grimes, K., Stone, K., & Schwab-Stone, M. (1990). Convergence of DSM-III diagnoses and self-reported symptoms in child and adolescent inpatients. *Journal of the American Academy of Child and Adolescent Psychiatry, 29*, 627-634.

Weinstein, S. R., Stone, K., Noam, G. G., Grimes, K., & Schwab-Stone, M. (1989). Comparison of the DISC and clinicians' DSM-III diagnoses in psychiatric patients. *Journal of the American Academy of Child and Adolescent Psychiatry, 28*, 53-60.

Weiss, R. D., Griffin, M. L., & Hufford, C. (1992). Severity of cocaine dependence as a predictor of relapse to cocaine use. *American Journal of Psychiatry, 149*, 1595-1596.

Weissman, M. M., & Myers, J. K. (1980). Psychiatric disorders in a U.S. community: The application of the Research Diagnostic Criteria to a resurveyed community sample. *Acta Psychiatrica Scandinavica, 62*, 99-111.

Weissman, M. M., Paykel, E. S., & Prusoff, B. A. (1972). *Social Adjustment Scale handbook.* New York: College of Physicians and Surgeons, Columbia University.

Weissman, M. M., Warner, V., & Frendich, M. (1990). Applying impairment criteria to children's psychiatric diagnosis. *Journal of the American Academy of Child and Adolescent Psychiatry, 29*, 789-795.

Weitzel, W. D., Morgan, D. W., Guyden, T. E., & Robinson, J. S. (1973). Toward a more efficient mental status examination: Free-form or operationally defined. *Archives of General Psychiatry, 28*, 215-218.

Weller, R. A., Penick, E. C., Powell, B. J., Othmer, E., Rice, A. S., & Kent, T. A. (1985). Agreement between two structured interviews: DIS and the PDI. *Comprehensive Psychiatry*, *26*, 157-163.

Wells, K. B., Burnam, A., Leake, B., & Robins, L. N. (1988). Agreement between face-to-face and telephone-administered versions of the depression section of the NIMH Diagnostic Interview Schedule. *Journal of Psychiatric Research*, *22*, 207-220.

Welner, A., Liss, J. L., & Robins, E. (1972). Undiagnosed psychiatric patients: Part I. Record study. *British Journal of Psychiatry*, *120*, 315-319.

Welner, A., Liss, J. L., & Robins, E. (1973). Undiagnosed psychiatric patients: Part III. The undiagnosable patient. *British Journal of Psychiatry*, *123*, 91-98.

Welner, Z., Reich, W., Herjanic, B., Jung, K. G., & Amado, H. (1987). Reliability, validity, and parent-child agreement studies of the Diagnostic Interview for Children and Adolescents (DICA). *Journal of the American Academy of Child and Adolescent Psychiatry*, *26*, 649-653.

Westen, D., Moses, M. J., Silk, K. R., Lohr, N. E., Cohen, R., & Segal, H. (1992). Quality of depressive experience in borderline personality disorder and major depression: When depression is not just depression. *Journal of Personality Disorders*, *6*, 382-393.

Westermeyer, J. (1987). Clinical considerations in cross-cultural diagnosis. *Hospital and Community Psychiatry*, *38*, 160-165.

Whelihan, W. M., Lesher, E. L., Kleban, M. H., & Granick, S. (1984). Mental status and memory assessment as predictors of dementia. *Journal of Gerontology*, *39*, 572-576.

Widiger, T. A. (1985). *Personality Interview Questions (PIQ)*. Unpublished manuscript, University of Kentucky, Lexington.

Widiger, T. A. (1987). *Personality Interview Questions-II (PIQ-II)*. Unpublished manuscript, University of Kentucky, Lexington.

Widiger, T. A. (1991). Personality disorder dimensional models proposed for DSM-IV. *Journal of Personality Disorders*, *5*, 386-398.

Widiger, T. A. (1992). Categorical versus dimensional classification: Implications from and for research. *Journal of Personality Disorders*, *6*, 287-300.

Widiger, T. A., & Corbitt, E. M. (1993). Antisocial personality disorder: Proposals for DSM-IV. *Journal of Personality Disorders*, *7*, 63-77.

Widiger, T. A., & Corbitt, E. M. (in press). Antisocial personality disorder in DSM-IV. In W. J. Livesley (Ed.), *DSM-IV personality disorders*. New York: Guilford.

Widiger, T. A., Corbitt, E. M., Ellis, C. G., & Thomas, G. V. (1992). *Personality Interview Questions-III (PIQ-III)*. Unpublished manuscript, University of Kentucky, Lexington.

Widiger, T. A., & Frances, A. (1985). The DSM-III personality disorders: Perspectives from psychology. *Archives of General Psychiatry*, *42*, 615-623.

Widiger, T. A., & Frances, A. (1987). Interviews and inventories for the measurement of personality disorders. *Clinical Psychology Review*, *7*, 49-75.

Widiger, T. A., Frances, A. J., Pincus, H. A., & Davis, W. W. (1990). DSM-IV literature reviews: Rationale, process and limitations. *Journal of Psychopathology and Behavioral Assessment, 12,* 189-202.

Widiger, T. A., Frances, A. J., Pincus, H. A., Davis, W. W., & First, M. B. (1991). Towards an empirical classification for the DSM-IV. *Journal of Abnormal Psychology, 100,* 280-288.

Widiger, T. A., Frances, A., Spitzer, R. L., & Williams, J. B. W. (1988). The DSM-III-R personality disorders: An overview. *American Journal of Psychiatry, 145,* 786-795.

Widiger, T. A., Frances, A., Warner, L., & Bluhm, C. (1986). Diagnostic criteria for the borderline and schizoptypal personality disorders. *Journal of Abnormal Psychology, 95,* 43-51.

Widiger, T. A., Freiman, K., & Bailey, B. (1990). Convergent and discriminant validity of personality disorder prototypic acts. *Psychological Assessment: A Journal of Clinical and Consulting Psychology, 3,* 418-423.

Widiger, T. A., & Hyler, S. E. (1987). Axis I/Axis II interactions. In R. Michels, J. O. Cavenar, A. M. Cooper, S. B. Guze, L. L. Judd, G. L. Klerman, & A. J. Solnit (Eds.), *Psychiatry* (Vol. 1, Chap. 29). Philadelphia: J. B. Lippincott.

Widiger, T. A., Mangine, S., Corbitt, E. M., Ellis, C. G., & Thomas, G. V. (1995). *Personality Disorder Interview—IV.* Odessa, FL: Psychological Assessment Resources.

Widiger, T. A., & Sanderson, C. (1987). The convergent and discriminant validity of the MCMI as a measure of DSM-III personality disorders. *Journal of Personality Assessment, 51,* 228-242.

Widiger, T. A., Trull, T. J., Hurt, S., Clarkin, J. F., & Frances, A. (1987). A multidimensional scaling of the DSM-III personality disorders. *Archives of General Psychiatry, 44,* 557-563.

Wicns, A. N. (1990). Structured clinical interviews for adults. In G. Goldstein & M. Hersen (Eds.), *Handbook of psychological assessment* (2nd cd.) (pp. 324-341). New York: Pergamon Press.

Wiggins, J. S. (1962). Strategic, method, and stylistic variance in the MMPI. *Psychological Bulletin, 59,* 224-242.

Wiggins, J. S., & Broughton, R. (1985). The interpersonal circle: A structural model for the integration of personality research. In R. Hogan & W. Jones (Eds.), *Perspectives in personality* (Vol. 1, pp. 1-47). Greenwich, CT: JAI Press.

Wildman, R., Batchelor, E., Thompson, L., Nelson, F., Moore, J., Patterson, & De Laosa, M. (1980). *The Georgia Court Competency Test: An attempt to develop a rapid, quantitative measure for fitness to stand trial.* Unpublished manuscript, Forensic Services Division, Central State Hospital, Milledgeville, GA.

Williams, J. B. W. (1985). The multiaxial system of DSM-III: Where did it come from and where should it go?: II. Empirical studies, innovations, and recommendations. *Archives of General Psychiatry, 42,* 181-186.

Williams, J. B. W., Gibbon, M., First, M. B., Spitzer, R. L., Davies, M., Borus, J., Howes, M. J., Kane, J., Pope, H. G., Jr., Rounsaville, B., & Wittchen, H. U. (in press). The Structured Clinical Interview for DSM-III-R (SCID): II. Multisite test-retest reliability. *Archives of General Psychiatry*.

Williams, J. B. W., Rabkin, J. G., Remien, R. H., Gorman, J. M., & Ehrhardt, A. A. (1990). Multidisciplinary baseline assessment of homosexual men with and without human immunodeficiency virus infection: II. Standardized clinical assessment of current and lifetime psychopathology. *Archives of General Psychiatry*, *48*, 124-130.

Williams, J. B. W., Spitzer, R. L., & Gibbon, M. (1992). International reliability of a diagnostic intake procedure for panic disorder. *American Journal of Psychiatry*, *149*, 560-562.

Williams, S., McGee, R., Anderson, J., & Silva, P. A. (1989). The structure and correlates of self-reported symptoms in 11-year-old children. *Journal of Abnormal Child Psychology*, *17*, 55-71.

Wilmink, F. W., Ormel, J., Giel, R., Krol, B., Lindeboom, E. G., Van der Meer, K., & Soeteman, J. H. (1989). General practitioners' characteristics and the assessment of psychiatric illness. *Journal of Psychiatric Research*, *23*, 135-149.

Wilmink, F. W., & Snijders, T. A. B. (1989). Polytomous logistic regression analysis of the General Health Questionnaire and the Present State Examination. *Psychological Medicine*, *19*, 755-764.

Wilson, G. T., & Eldredge, K. L. (1991). Frequency of binge eating in bulimic patients: Diagnostic validity. *International Journal of Eating Disorders*, *5*, 557-561.

Wilson, G. T., Nonas, C. A., & Rosenblum, G. D. (1993). Assessment of binge eating in obese patients. *International Journal of Eating Disorders*, *13*, 25-33.

Wilson, G. T., & Smith, D. (1989). Assessment of bulimia nervosa: An evaluation of the Eating Disorders Examination. *International Journal of Eating Disorders*, *4*, 71-78.

Wilson, L., Roy, S., & Bursill, A. (1973). *The reliability of the Mental Status Questionnaire in geriatrics*. Unpublished manuscript.

Wing, J. K. (1976). A technique for studying psychiatric morbidity in inpatient and outpatient series and in general population samples. *Psychological Medicine*, *6*, 665-671.

Wing, J. K. (1980). Standardizing clinical diagnostic judgments—The PSE-CATEGO system. *Australian and New Zealand Journal of Psychiatry*, *14*, 17-20.

Wing, J. K., Babor, T., Brugha, T., Burke, F., Cooper, J. E., Giel, R., Jablenski, F., Regier, D., & Sartorius, N. (1990). SCAN: Schedules for clinical assessment in neuropsychiatry. *Archives of General Psychiatry*, *47*, 589-593.

Wing, J. K., Birely, J. L. T., Cooper, J. E., Graham, P., & Isaacs, A. (1967). Reliability of a procedure for measuring and classifying present psychiatric state. *British Journal of Psychiatry*, *113*, 499-515.

Wing, J. K., Cooper, J. E., & Sartorius, N. (1974). *The measurement and classification of psychiatric symptoms*. Cambridge, England: Cambridge University Press.

Wing, J. K., Henderson, A. S., & Winckle, M. (1977). The rating of symptoms by a psychiatrist and a non-psychiatrist: A study of patients referred from general practice. *Psychological Medicine*, *7*, 713-715.

Wing, J. K., Mann, S. A., Leff, J. P., & Nixon, J. M. (1978). The concept of a "case" in psychiatric population surveys. *Psychological Medicine, 8,* 203-217.

Wing, J. K., Nixon, J. N., Mann, S. A., & Leff, J. P. (1977). Reliability of the PSE (9th ed.) used in a population survey. *Psychological Medicine, 7,* 505-516.

Withers, E., & Hinton, J. (1971). Three forms of the clinical tests of the sensorium and their reliability. *British Journal of Psychiatry, 119,* 1-8.

Wittchen, H. U., Burke, J. D., Semler, G., Pfister, H., Von Cranach, M., & Zaudig, M. (1989). Recall and dating of psychiatric symptoms: Rest-retest reliability of time-related symptom questions in a standardized psychiatric interview. *Archives of General Psychiatry, 46,* 437-443.

Wittchen, H. U., Zhao, S., Kessler, R. C., & Eaton, W. W. (1994). DSM-III-R generalized anxiety disorder in the national comorbidity study. *Archives of General Psychiatry, 51,* 355-364.

Wolber, G., Romaniuk, M., Eastman, E., & Robinson, C. (1984). Validity of the Short Portable Mental Status Questionnaire with elderly psychiatric patients. *Journal of Clinical and Consulting Psychology, 52,* 712-713.

Wong, S. (1984). *Criminal and institutional behaviors of psychopaths. Programs Branch Users Report.* Ottawa, Ontario: Ministry of the Solicitor-General of Canada.

Wong, S. (1988). Is Hare's Psychopathy Checklist reliable without the interview? *Psychological Reports, 62,* 931-934.

Wong, S., & Elek, D. (1989, August). *The treatment of psychopathy: A review.* Paper presented at the American Psychological Association convention, New Orleans, LA.

World Health Organization. (1979). *Schizophrenia: An international follow-up study.* New York: Wiley.

World Health Organization—Alcohol, Drug, and Mental Health Administration. (1987). *Composite International Diagnostic Interview (CIDI).* Geneva: Author.

Wykes, T., Sturt, E. (1986). The measurement of social behavior in psychiatric patients: An assessment of the reliability and validity of the SBS schedule. *British Journal of Psychiatry, 148,* 1-11.

Wyndrowe, J. (1987). The microcomputerized Diagnostic Interview Schedule: Clinical use in an outpatient setting. *Canadian Journal of Psychiatry, 32,* 93-99.

Yager, J. (1989). Specific components of bedside manner in general hospital psychiatric consultation: 12 concrete suggestions. *Psychosomatics, 30,* 209-212.

Yazdanfar, D. J. (1990). Assessing the mental status of the cognitively impaired elderly. *Journal of Gerontological Nursing, 16,* 32-36.

Yesage, J. A., Brink, T. L., Rose, T. L., Lum, O., Huang, V., Adey, M., & Leirer, O. (1983). Development and validation of a geriatric depression screening scale: A preliminary report. *Journal of Psychiatric Research, 17,* 37-49.

Zahner, G. E. P. (1991). The feasibility of conducting structured diagnostic interviews with preadolescents: A community field trial of the DISC. *Journal of the American Academy of Child and Adolescent Psychiatry, 30,* 659-668.

Zanarini, M. C., Frankenburg, F. R., Chauncey, D. L., & Gunderson, J. G. (1987). The Diagnostic Interview for Personality Disorders: Interrater and test-retest reliability. *Comprehensive Psychiatry, 28,* 467-480.

Zanarini, M. C., Gunderson, J. G., & Frankenburg, F. R. (1989). Axis I. Phenomenology of borderline personality disorder. *Comprehensive Psychiatry, 30,* 149-156.

Zanarini, M. C., Gunderson, J. G., Frankenburg, F. R., & Chauncey, D. L. (1989). The revised Diagnostic Interview for Borderlines: Discriminating BPD from other axis II disorders. *Journal of Personality Disorders, 3,* 10-18.

Zelinski, E. M., Gilewski, M. J., & Anthony-Berstone, C. R. (1990). Memory functioning questionnaire: Concurrent validity with memory performance and self-reported memory failures. *Psychology and Aging, 5,* 388-399.

Zimmerman, M. (1994). *Interview guide for evaluating DSM-IV psychiatric disorders and mental status examination.* Philadelphia: Psych Products.

Zimmerman, M., & Coryell, W. (1987). The Inventory to Diagnose Depression (IDD): A self-report scale to diagnose major depressive disorder. *Journal of Consulting and Clinical Psychology, 55,* 55-59.

Zimmerman, M., & Coryell, W. (1988). The validity of a self-report questionnaire for diagnosing major depressive disorder. *Archives of General Psychiatry, 45,* 738-740.

Zimmerman, M., & Coryell, W. (1989). DSM-III personality disorder diagnoses in a nonpatient sample: Demographic correlates and comorbidity. *Archives of General Psychiatry, 46,* 682-689.

Zimmerman, M., & Coryell, W. (1990). Diagnosing personality disorders in the community: A comparison of self-report and interview measures. *Archives of General Psychiatry, 47,* 527-531.

Zimmerman, M., Coryell, W., Pfohl, B., Corenthal, C., & Stangl, D. (1986). ECT response in depressed patients with and without a DSM-III personality disorder. *American Journal of Psychiatry, 143,* 1030-1032.

Zimmerman, M., Pfohl, B., Coryell, W., Stangl, D., & Corenthal, C. (1986). Assessment of DSM-III personality disorders: The importance of interviewing an informant. *Journal of Clinical Psychiatry, 47,* 261-263.

Zimmerman, M., Pfohl, B., Coryell, W., Stangl, D., & Corenthal, C. (1988). Diagnosing personality disorder in depressed patients. *Archives of General Psychiatry, 45,* 733-737.

Zubenko, G. S., Rosen, J., Sweet, R. A., Mulsant, B. H., & Rifai, A. H. (1992). Impact of psychiatric hospitalization of behavioral complications of Alzheimer's disease. *American Journal of Psychiatry, 149,* 1484-1491.

Zung, W. (1965). A self-rating depression scale. *Archives of General Psychiatry, 12,* 63-70.

Zwick, R. (1983). Assessing the psychometric properties of psychodiagnostic systems: How do the research diagnostic criteria measure up? *Journal of Consulting and Clinical Psychology, 51,* 117-131.

Appendices

Appendix A

Standard Abbreviations for Diagnostic Standards, Measures, and Disorders

Abbreviation	Complete name
AD*	Alzheimer's disease
ADD	attention deficit disorders
ADHD	attention deficit with hyperactivity disorder
ADI	Autism Diagnostic Interview
ADIS	Anxiety Disorders Interview Schedule
AMDP	Assessment and Documentation of Psychopathology
AMS	Adolescent Mood Scale
APD	antisocial personality disorder
BAC	blood alcohol concentrations
BCRS	Brief Cognitive Rating Scale
BDI	Beck Depression Inventory
BDS	Blessed Dementia Scale
BPD*	borderline personality disorder
BPRS	Brief Psychiatric Rating Scale
BSI	Brief Symptom Inventory
CAI	Competency to Stand Trial Assessment Instrument
CAMCOG	Cambridge Cognitive Examination
CAMDEX	Cambridge Mental Disorders for the Elderly
CAPA	Child and Adolescent Psychiatric Assessment Scale
CAPPS	Current and Past Psychopathology Scales
CAS	Child Assessment Schedule *or* Clinical Anxiety Scale
CASH	Comprehensive Assessment of Symptoms and History
CASQ	Cognitive and Somatic Anxiety Questionnaire
CBCL	Child Behavior Checklist
CCSE	Cognitive Capacity Screening Examination
CDI	Children's Depression Inventory

*These disorders are typically not abbreviated except in chapter sections that involve extensive discussions.

Abbreviation	Complete name
CDP	Comprehensive Drinker Profile
CEDRI	Clinical Eating Disorders Rating Instrument
CES-D	Center of Epidemiologic Studies Depression scale
CFA	Cortical Function Assessment
CIDI	Composite International Diagnostic Interview
CTRS	Conners' Teacher Rating Scale
DES	Dissociative Experiences Scale
DIB	Diagnostic Interview of Borderline Patients
DICA	Diagnostic Interview for Children and Adolescents
DIPD	Diagnostic Interview of Personality Disorders
DIS	Diagnostic Interview Schedule
DISC	Diagnostic Interview Schedule for Children
DIS-CM	Diagnostic Interview Schedule, Chinese Modification
DISSA	Diagnostic Interview Schedule, Self-Administered
DST	dexamethasone suppression test
EDE	Eating Disorder Examination
EDE-Q	Eating Disorder Examination–Questionnaire
FACES	Family Adaptability and Cohesion Evaluation Scale
FDPS	factitious disorders with predominantly psychological signs and symptoms
GAD	generalized anxiety disorder
GAF	Global Assessment Functioning Scale
GAS	Global Assessment Scale
GAS-C	Global Assessment Scale for Children
GCCT	Georgia Court Competency Test
GDS	Global Deterioration Scale
GHQ	General Health Questionnaire
HDRS	Hamilton Depression Rating Scale
HEIC	Home Environment Interview for Children
IAS	Interpersonal Adjective Scales
ICD	International Classification of Diseases
IDD	Inventory to Diagnose Depression
IFI	Interdisciplinary Fitness Interview
IMPS	Inpatient Multidimensional Psychiatric Scale
IPDE	International Personality Disorder Examination
ISC	Interview Schedule for Children (ISC)
ISPI	Iowa Structured Psychiatric Interview

*These disorders are typically not abbreviated except in chapter sections that involve extensive discussions.

Abbreviation	Complete name
K-SADS	Schedule of Affective Disorders and Schizophrenia for School-Age Children
K-SADS-E	Schedule of Affective Disorders and Schizophrenia for School-Age Children–Epidemiological Version
MAST	Michigan Alcoholism Screening Test
MCMI	Millon Clinical Multiaxial Inventory
MMS	Missouri Mental Status
MMSE	Mini-Mental Status Examination
MSE	Mental Status Examination
MSER	Mental Status Evaluation Record
MSQ	Mental Status Questionnaire
NC-MSE	North Carolina MSE
NCSE	Neurobehavioral Cognitive Status Examination
NEO-PI	NEO Personality Inventory
OCD*	obsessive-compulsive disorder
PAF	Personality Assessment Form
PAI	Personality Assessment Inventory
PAS	Problem Appraisal Scales *or* Personality Assessment Schedule
PCL	Psychopathy Checklist
PCL-SV	PCL-Screening Version
PD*	Parkinson's disease
PDE	Personality Disorder Examination
PDI	Psychiatric Diagnostic Interview
PDI-IV	Personality Disorder Interview-IV
PDQ	Personality Diagnostic Questionnaire
PDS	personality disorder scales of the MMPI
PIC	Personality Inventory for Children
PIQ	Personality Interview Questions
PODI	Polydiagnostic Interview
PSE	Present State Examination
PSS	Psychiatric Status Schedule
PSPI	Psychosocial Pain Inventory
PTSD*	post-traumatic stress disorder
QED	Questionnaire of Experiences of Dissociation
RDC	Research Diagnostic Criteria
RDI	Renard Diagnostic Interview

*These disorders are typically not abbreviated except in chapter sections that involve extensive discussions.

Abbreviation	Complete name
RPMIP	Royal Park Multidiagnostic Instrument for Psychosis
SADS	Schedule of Affective Disorders and Schizophrenia
SADS-C	Schedule of Affective Disorders and Schizophrenia–Change Version
SADS-L	Schedule of Affective Disorders and Schizophrenia–Lifetime Version
SADS-LA	Schedule of Affective Disorders and Schizophrenia–Lifetime Version, Anxiety Disorders
SANS	Scale for the Assessment of Negative Symptoms
SAP	Standardized Assessment of Personality
SAPS	Scale for the Assessment of Positive Symptoms
SASSI	Substance Abuse Subtle Screening Inventory
SBS	Stony Brook Child Psychiatric Checklist
SCID	Structured Clinical Interview for *DSM-III-R*
SCID-D	Structured Clinical Interview for *DSM-IV* Dissociative Disorders
SCID-NP	Structured Clinical Interview for *DSM-III-R*–Non-Patient Version
SCID-P	Structured Clinical Interview for *DSM-III-R*–Patient Version
SCID-II	Structured Clinical Interview for *DSM-III-R*–Axis II Disorders
SCID-II-Q	SCID-II Questionnaire
SCL-90	Symptom Checklist-90
SDI	Survey Diagnostic Instrument
SEC	Standard Ethanol Content
SI	Structural Interview (Kernberg)
SIAB	Structured Interview for Anorexia and Bulimia Nervosa
SIB	Schedule for Interviewing Borderlines
SIDP	Structured Interview for *DSM-III* Personality Disorders
SIRS	Structured Interview of Reported Symptoms
SIS-D	Structured Interview of Sleep Disorders
SMAST	Short Michigan Alcoholism Screening Test
SPD*	schizotypal personality disorder
SPMSQ	Short Portable Mental Status Questionnaire
SSIAMI	Structured and Scaled Interview to Assess Maladjustment
STAI	State-Trait Anxiety Inventory
STAIC	State-Trait Anxiety Inventory for Children
SUDDS	Substance Use Disorders Diagnostic Schedule
TRF	Teacher's Report Form
YBOCS	Yale-Brown Obsessive-Compulsive Scale
YSR	Youth Self-Report

*These disorders are typically not abbreviated except in chapter sections that involve extensive discussions.

Appendix B

Sources for Commonly Used Diagnostic and Structured Interviews

Cambridge Cognitive Examination (CAMCOG)

> Cambridge University Press
> Shartesbury Road
> Cambridge CB2 2RU England

Children's Assessment Schedule (CAS)

> Kay Hodges, Ph.D.
> Department of Psychology
> 537 Mark Jefferson
> Eastern Michigan University
> Ypsilanti, MI 48197

Comprehensive Assessment of Symptoms and History (CASH)

> MH-CRC Administrator
> Department of Psychiatry
> University of Iowa College of Medicine
> 500 Newton Road
> Iowa City, IA 52242

Comprehensive Drinker's Profile (CDP)

> Psychological Assessment Resources, Inc.
> P.O. Box 998
> Odessa, FL 33556

Current and Past Psychopathology Scales (CAPPS)

> Jean Endicott, Ph.D.
> Columbia University Department of Psychiatry
> 722 West 168 Street, MB #123
> New York, NY 10032

Diagnostic Interview of Children and Adolescents (DICA)

> Wendy Reich, Ph.D.
> Washington University School of Medicine
> Department of Psychiatry
> 4940 Children's Place
> St. Louis, MO 63110

Diagnostic Interview Schedule (DIS)— Most recent versions and training materials

Lee N. Robins, M.D.
Department of Psychiatry
Washington University School of Medicine
4940 Audubon Avenue
St. Louis, MO 63110

Diagnostic Interview Schedule (DIS-III) and Diagnostic Interview Schedule for Children (DISC)

Publications Officer
Center for Epidemiological Studies
National Institute of Mental Health
Rockville, MD 20857

Diagnostic Interview Schedule (DIS-III) and Diagnostic Interview Schedule for Children (DISC)–Spanish Versions (The duplication cost for both is $30.00.)

Zenaida Gonzalez, M.S.
Supervisor, Behavioral Science Research Institute
University of Puerto Rico, Medical Sciences Campus
P.O. Box 365067
San Juan, Puerto Rico 00936-5067

Eating Disorders Examination (EDE)

Zafra Cooper
Senior Research Associate
Department of Psychiatry
University of Cambridge
Addenbrooke's Hospital
Cambridge CB2 2QQ England

Personality Disorder Examination (PDE)

Armand W. Loranger, Ph.D.
New-York Hospital–Cornell Medical Center
21 Bloomingdale Road
White Plains, NY 10805

Personality Disorder Interview—IV (PDI-IV)

Psychological Assessment Resources, Inc.
P.O. Box 998
Odessa, FL 33556

Psychopathy Checklist—Revised (PCL-R)

Multi-Health Systems, Inc.
95 Thorncliffe Park Drive, Suite 100
Toronto, Ontario M4H IL7 Canada

Revised Diagnostic Interview for Borderlines (DIB-R)

> John Gunderson, M.D.
> McLean Hospital
> 115 Mill Street
> Belmont, MA 02178 (unpublished)

Schedule for Affective Disorders and Schizophrenia (SADS)

> Jean Endicott, Ph.D.
> Columbia University Department of Psychiatry
> 722 West 168 Street MB #123
> New York, NY 10032

Schedule for Affective Disorders and Schizophrenia for School Aged Children (Kiddie-SADS or K-SADS)—original version

> William J. Chambers, M.D.
> Dept. of Child Psychiatry
> New York State Psychiatric Institute
> 722 West 168th Street
> New York, NY 10032

Schedule for Affective Disorders and Schizophrenia for School Aged Children (Kiddie-SADS or K-SADS-III-R)—most recent version

> Paul J. Ambrosini, M.D.
> Director of Child Outpatient Services
> Medical College of Pennsylvania
> 3200 Henry Street
> Philadelphia, PA 19129

Standardized Assessment of Personality (SAP)

> John A. Pilgrim, M.B.
> Institute of Psychiatry
> De Crespigny Park
> Denmark Hill
> London SE5 8AF England

Structured Clinical Interview for *DSM-III-R* Diagnosis (SCID) *and*

Structured Clinical Interview for *DSM-III-R* Personality Disorders (SCID-II)

> American Psychiatric Press
> 1400 K Street, N. W.
> Washington, DC 20005

For research versions and/or collaboration, contact:

> Miriam Gibbon
> Biometrics Research
> New York State Psychiatric Institute
> 722 W. 168 Street
> New York, NY 10032

Structured Interview for *DSM-III-R* Personality Disorders—Revised (SIDP-R)

Nancee Blum, M.S.W.
Department of Psychiatry
University of Iowa
Iowa City, IA 52242

Structured Interview of Reported Symptoms (SIRS)

Psychological Assessment Resources, Inc.
P.O. Box 998
Odessa, FL 33556

Indices

Author Index

This index references names of first authors only.

Subject Index

About the Author

Richard Rogers, Ph.D., ABPP, is currently Director of Clinical Training and Professor of Psychology at the University of North Texas. Dr. Rogers is a prolific writer and has authored four books and more than 75 refereed articles. He was honored by the American Psychiatric Association with the Manfred S. Guttmacher Award, given for outstanding contribution to literature, for his earlier book, *Clinical Assessment of Malingering and Deception.* A major clinical research focus of Dr. Rogers' continues to be the validation and refinement of psychological assessment methods, including diagnostic and structured interviews. As a result, he has developed and validated the *Structured Interview of Reported Symptoms,* a highly regarded standardized interview.